Contributions to
SENSORY PHYSIOLOGY

Volume 8

Contributors to This Volume

Daniel Algom
Harvey Babkoff
Judy K. Brunso-Bechtold
Vivien A. Casagrande
William C. Hall
R. Bruce Masterton
Paul J. May
Randolph J. Nudo
Ilsa R. Schwartz
Douglas B. Webster
Molly Webster

Contributions to
SENSORY PHYSIOLOGY

Edited by
WILLIAM D. NEFF
CENTER FOR NEURAL SCIENCES
INDIANA UNIVERSITY
BLOOMINGTON, INDIANA

VOLUME 8

1984

ACADEMIC PRESS, INC.
(Harcourt Brace Jovanovich, Publishers)

Orlando   San Diego   San Francisco   New York   London
Toronto   Montreal   Sydney   Tokyo   São Paulo

COPYRIGHT © 1984, BY ACADEMIC PRESS, INC.
ALL RIGHTS RESERVED.
NO PART OF THIS PUBLICATION MAY BE REPRODUCED OR
TRANSMITTED IN ANY FORM OR BY ANY MEANS, ELECTRONIC
OR MECHANICAL, INCLUDING PHOTOCOPY, RECORDING, OR ANY
INFORMATION STORAGE AND RETRIEVAL SYSTEM, WITHOUT
PERMISSION IN WRITING FROM THE PUBLISHER.

ACADEMIC PRESS, INC.
Orlando, Florida 32887

United Kingdom Edition published by
ACADEMIC PRESS, INC. (LONDON) LTD.
24/28 Oval Road, London NW1 7DX

LIBRARY OF CONGRESS CATALOG CARD NUMBER: 64-8943
ISBN 0-12-151808-6

PRINTED IN THE UNITED STATES OF AMERICA

84 85 86 87   9 8 7 6 5 4 3 2 1

Contents

Contributors vii

Preface ix

Contents of Previous Volumes xi

The Anatomical Basis for Sensorimotor Transformations in the Superior Colliculus

William C. Hall and Paul J. May

I. Introduction	1
II. The Laminar Organization of the Superior Colliculus	3
III. Models of Superior Colliculus Organization	13
IV. Indirect Visual Pathways to the Deep Layers of the Superior Colliculus	21
V. Conclusions	30
References	34

Development of Layers in the Dorsal Lateral Geniculate Nucleus in the Tree Shrew

Judy K. Brunso-Bechtold and Vivien A. Casagrande

I. Introduction	41
II. Features of Lamination in the Mature LGN	43
III. Development of LGN Layers	49
IV. The Role of Retinogeniculate Fibers in the Development of Individual Features of Lamination	62
V. A Model of LGN Development	71
References	74

2-Deoxyglucose Studies of Stimulus Coding in the Brainstem Auditory System of the Cat

Randolph J. Nudo and R. Bruce Masterton

I. Introduction	79
II. Interpretation of 2-DG Autoradiographs	81
III. Effects of Variations in Sound Onset	85

IV. Effects of Variations in Frequency 89
V. Effects of Variations in Intensity... 93
VI. Summary... 95
References... 96

Axonal Organization in the Cat Medial Superior Olivary Nucleus
ILSA R. SCHWARTZ

I. History of Multiple Classes of Axons... 99
II. Classical Approaches to Identifying Axonal Populations....................... 100
III. Differential Amino Acid-Labeling Studies 119
References... 127

Auditory Temporal Integration at Threshold: Theories and Some Implications of Current Research
DANIEL ALGOM AND HARVEY BABKOFF

I. Introduction... 131
II. Major Empirical Findings 132
III. Theories of Auditory Temporal Summation 140
IV. Some Implications of Current Research 151
V. Conclusions... 156
References... 157

The Specialized Auditory System of Kangaroo Rats
DOUGLAS B. WEBSTER AND MOLLY WEBSTER

I. Introduction... 161
II. The Middle Ears... 165
III. The Cochlea 183
IV. The Central Auditory System 189
V. Summary... 192
References... 194

INDEX 197

Contributors

Numbers in parentheses indicate the pages on which the authors' contributions begin.

DANIEL ALGOM (131), Department of Psychology, Bar-Ilan University, Ramat Gan, Israel

HARVEY BABKOFF (131), Department of Psychology, Bar-Ilan University, Ramat Gan, Israel

JUDY K. BRUNSO-BECHTOLD (41), Department of Anatomy, Bowman Gray School of Medicine, Wake Forest University, Winston-Salem, North Carolina 27103

VIVIEN A. CASAGRANDE (41), Department of Anatomy, Vanderbilt School of Medicine, Nashville, Tennessee 37232

WILLIAM C. HALL (1), Department of Anatomy, Duke University, Durham, North Carolina 27710

R. BRUCE MASTERTON (79), Department of Psychology, Florida State University, Tallahassee, Florida 32306

PAUL J. MAY (1), Department of Anatomy, Duke University, Durham, North Carolina 27710

RANDOLPH J. NUDO (79), Department of Psychology, Florida State University, Tallahassee, Florida 32306

ILSA R. SCHWARTZ (99), Head and Neck Surgery, University of California, Los Angeles School of Medicine, Los Angeles, California 90024

DOUGLAS B. WEBSTER (161), Department of Otorhinolaryngology and Department of Anatomy, Kresge Hearing Research Laboratory of the South Louisiana State University Medical Center, New Orleans, Louisiana 70119

MOLLY WEBSTER (161), Department of Otorhinolaryngology, Kresge Hearing Research Laboratory of the South Louisiana State University Medical Center, New Orleans, Louisiana 70119

Preface

The publication of *Contributions to Sensory Physiology* was undertaken with two principal objectives in mind: (1) to bring together reports of current research on all of the sensory systems and (2) to provide an opportunity for the scientist studying a sensory system to give a detailed account of a series of experiments or to present, at some length, a theory about the physiological basis of sensation. It is not the intent of *Contributions* to present review articles. Authors have been asked to write about their own research findings and theoretical notions and to review the work of others only as it seems suitable for the interpretation of results and theoretical discussion.

Sensory physiology has been given a broad definition—it includes the range from microscopic anatomy to psychophysics. The anatomist has been urged to speculate about the functional significance of his discoveries regarding structure; the psychophysicist has also been encouraged to consider the physiological mechanisms that might explain the findings of his experiments.

It is the hope of the editor and publisher that this serial publication will provide better communication among those who study sensory systems and that it will also be a valuable source of information for scientists from other fields who occasionally seek a representative sample of research that is being done in this important area of physiology rather than just a summary.

WILLIAM D. NEFF

Contents of Previous Volumes

Volume 1

CELLULAR PATTERN, NERVE STRUCTURES, AND FLUID SPACES OF THE ORGAN OF CORTI
  Hans Engström, Harlow W. Ades, and Joseph E. Hawkins, Jr.

FUNCTIONAL ANATOMY OF THE VESTIBULAR AND LATERAL LINE ORGANS
  Jan Wersäll and Åke Flock

PSYCHOPHYSIOLOGICAL STUDIES OF VESTIBULAR FUNCTION
  Fred E. Guedry, Jr.

BEHAVIORAL AND ELECTROPHYSIOLOGICAL STUDIES OF PRIMATE VISION
  Russell L. De Valois

VISION IN INTERMITTENT LIGHT
  H. Piéron

AUTHOR INDEX—SUBJECT INDEX

Volume 2

THE EVOLUTION OF VERTEBRATE HEARING
  Willem A. van Bergeijk

THE SENSORY NEOCORTEX
  I. T. Diamond

ORGANIZATION OF SOMATIC CENTRAL PROJECTION
  D. Albe-Fessard

ELECTRICAL RESPONSES OF THE NERVOUS SYSTEM AND SUBJECTIVE SCALES OF INTENSITY
  Burton S. Rosner and William R. Goff

GUSTATORY RESPONSE AS A TEMPERATURE-DEPENDENT PROCESS
  Masayasu Sato

AUTHOR INDEX—SUBJECT INDEX

Volume 3

ELECTROPHYSIOLOGY OF VIBRATORY PERCEPTION
  Wolf D. Keidel

TEMPORAL FEATURES OF INPUT AS CRUCIAL FACTORS IN VISION
  S. Howard Bartley

THE MEASUREMENT OF PERCEIVED SIZE AND DISTANCE
  Walter C. Gogel

EXPERIMENTAL AND THEORETICAL APPROACHES TO NEURAL PROCESSING IN THE CENTRAL AUDITORY PATHWAY
  S. D. Erulkar, P. G. Nelson, and J. S. Bryan

SUSCEPTIBILITY TO AUDITORY FATIGUE
  W. Dixon Ward

AUTHOR INDEX—SUBJECT INDEX

Volume 4

VISION, AUDITION, AND BEYOND
  Frank A. Geldard

PSYCHOPHYSICAL STUDIES OF TEMPERATURE SENSITIVITY
  Dan R. Kenshalo

PATHOPHYSIOLOGY OF THE FLUID SYSTEMS OF THE INNER EAR
  Harold F. Schuknecht

ANATOMICAL ASPECTS OF THE COCHLEAR NUCLEUS AND SUPERIOR OLIVARY COMPLEX
  J. M. Harrison and M. L. Feldman

CAT SUPERIOR OLIVE S-SEGMENT CELL DISCHARGE TO TONAL STIMULATION
  James C. Boudreau and Chiyeko Tsuchitani

AUTHOR INDEX—SUBJECT INDEX

Volume 5

SIMPLE CELLS OF THE STRIATE CORTEX
  G. H. Henry and P. O. Bishop

RELATIONS AND POSSIBLE SIGNIFICANCE OF TASTE BUD CELLS
  Raymond G. Murray and Assia Murray

THE NATURE OF TASTE RECEPTOR SITES
  Lloyd M. Beidler and Guenter W. Gross

AUDITORY RECEPTOR ORGANS OF REPTILES, BIRDS, AND MAMMALS
  Catherine A. Smith and Tomonori Takasaka

OLD AND NEW DATA ON TONE PERCEPTION
  Reinier Plomp
AUTHOR INDEX—SUBJECT INDEX

Volume 6

CUTANEOUS COMMUNICATION
  Carl E. Sherrick
EFFECTS OF ENVIRONMENTS ON DEVELOPMENT IN SENSORY SYSTEMS
  Austin H. Riesen
THE ACROSS-FIBER PATTERN THEORY: AN ORGANIZING PRINCIPLE FOR MOLAR NEURAL FUNCTION
  Robert P. Erickson
ELECTROPHYSIOLOGICAL ANALYSIS OF THE ECHOLOCATION SYSTEM OF BATS
  Philip H.-S. Jen
CODING IN THE AUDITORY CORTEX
  I. C. Whitfield
THE PSYCHOPHYSICS AND PHYSIOLOGY OF THE LATERALIZATION OF TRANSIENT ACOUSTIC STIMULI
  Harvey Babkoff

INDEX

Volume 7

PARALLEL ASCENDING PATHWAYS FROM THE COCHLEAR NUCLEUS: NEUROANATOMICAL EVIDENCE OF FUNCTIONAL SPECIALIZATION
  W. Bruce Warr
THE OPTIC CHIASM OF THE VERTEBRATE BRAIN
  R. W. Guillery
STUDIES ON THE MORPHOLOGICAL BASIS OF ORIENTATION SELECTIVITY
  Paul D. Coleman and Dorothy G. Flood
VISUAL CONTROL OF MOVEMENT: THE CIRCUITS WHICH LINK VISUAL TO MOTOR AREAS OF THE BRAIN WITH SPECIAL REFERENCE TO THE VISUAL INPUT TO THE PONS AND CEREBELLUM
  Mitchell Glickstein and Jack G. May III
VISUAL FUNCTIONS IN MONKEYS AFTER TOTAL REMOVAL OF VISUAL CEREBRAL CORTEX
  Pedro Pasik and Tauba Pasik
THE SEGREGATION OF FUNCTION IN THE NERVOUS SYSTEM: WHY DO SENSORY SYSTEMS HAVE SO MANY SUBDIVISIONS?
  Jon H. Kaas

INDEX

Contributions to
SENSORY PHYSIOLOGY

Volume 8

The Anatomical Basis for Sensorimotor Transformations in the Superior Colliculus

WILLIAM C. HALL AND PAUL J. MAY

DEPARTMENT OF ANATOMY
DUKE UNIVERSITY
DURHAM, NORTH CAROLINA

I. Introduction 1
II. The Laminar Organization of the Superior Colliculus 3
    A. Cytoarchitecture 3
    B. Efferent Connections of the Superficial and Deep Layers 3
    C. Behavioral Studies of Tectal Organization 5
    D. Physiological Distinctions between the Superficial
       and Deep Layers 7
III. Models of Superior Colliculus Organization 13
    A. Retinal Influences on the Deep Tectal Layers 13
    B. Intracollicular Connections between the Superficial
       and Deep Layers 15
    C. Influences of the Occipital Lobe on the Deep Tectal Layers 17
    D. Projections from the Ventral Lateral Geniculate Nucleus to the
       Deep Tectal Layers 19
IV. Indirect Visual Pathways to the Deep Layers of the
    Superior Colliculus 21
    A. The Distribution of the Tectoreticular Cells 21
    B. Relationships between the Optic Tectum and the Basal Ganglia . . 22
    C. Sources of Cortical Input to the Deep Tectum 27
    D. Cerebellar Connections with the Superior Colliculus 29
V. Conclusions 30
    References 34

I. INTRODUCTION

The superior colliculus, or optic tectum, is concerned with the initiation of orienting responses to visual stimuli and, probably, to nonvisual stimuli as well (Chalupa and Rhoades, 1977; Dräger and Hubel, 1975; Gordon, 1973; Harris and Gammow, 1971; Jay and Sparks, 1982; Kass et al., 1978; Schneider, 1969; Sprague and Meikle, 1965; Stein and Gaither, 1981; Wickelgren, 1971). This function of the superior colliculus is the subject of considerable study, not only because orientation is a universal behavior but, even more importantly, because the constant relationships between stimulus location and stereotyped motor responses suggest that orienting behavior may provide a relatively simple model for studying the more general problem of how sensorimotor transformations are mediated by the brain.

The superior colliculus is a layered structure and the layers are almost certainly a key to understanding the neural basis of its sensorimotor transformations. Anatomical studies have indicated the importance of differences between the layers by demonstrating that projections from the retina terminate almost entirely in the superficial layers (Abplanalp, 1970; Behan, 1981; Graybiel, 1975; Hubel et al., 1975; Sterling, 1971), whereas the major descending pathways from the colliculus to the lower brainstem regions known to control head and eye movements arise in the deep layers (Altman and Carpenter, 1961; Harting et al., 1973; Holcombe and Hall, 1981a,b; Kawamura and Hashikawa, 1978). In physiological studies, the superficial layers are considered to be sensory because the neurons in these layers respond at fixed latencies to visual stimulation and have receptive fields arranged into a systematic representation of the visual field (Dräger and Hubel, 1975; Horn and Hill, 1966; Humphrey, 1968; Marchiafava and Pepeu, 1966; McIlwain and Buser, 1968; Michael, 1972). In contrast, the deeper layers have properties of motor systems. In particular, neurons in the deeper layers discharge prior to saccadic head or eye movements, which shift gaze to a particular locus in the visual field (Crommelinck et al., 1977; Mohler and Wurtz, 1976; Schiller and Koerner, 1971; Sparks et al., 1977; Sparks, 1978; Wurtz and Goldberg, 1971, 1972). An association between the deep layers and motor functions is also suggested by electrical stimulation studies, which indicate that the current levels necessary to produce saccadic eye movements are much lower in the deep layers than in the superficial layers (Schiller and Stryker, 1972; Sparks and Pollack, 1977). In addition, the direction and amplitude of saccades produced by collicular stimulation vary systematically with the site of stimulation (Harris, 1980; Robinson, 1972; Schiller and Stryker, 1972; Stryker and Schiller, 1975). This systematic map of saccades is in register with the map of the visual field that is represented in the superficial layers (Schiller and Stryker, 1972).

The correspondence between the sensory and motor maps suggests that the sensorimotor transformation achieved by the superior colliculus may involve interactions between the superficial and deep layers. Consequently, a primary concern of research in this field has been to identify and describe the patterns of interconnections between these layers. The purpose of this article is to discuss this research and to relate it to various hypotheses that account for the apparent interactions between the layers. The discussion will be presented in three main sections. In the first, we shall briefly describe the anatomical, physiological, and behavioral data that distinguish between the superficial and deep layers. In the second section, we shall discuss several models that have been proposed to account both for the distinctions between the layers and also for how the sensory responses in the superficial layers might initiate appropriate motor responses in the deep layers. In the final section we shall present some recent results that suggest that the solution to the problem of how sensorimotor transformations are accomplished in the superior colliculus lies in part outside of the colliculus itself, and that this solution might also contribute to our understanding of similar transformations in other structures, such as the motor cortex.

II. THE LAMINAR ORGANIZATION OF THE SUPERIOR COLLICULUS

A. Cytoarchitecture

The cytoarchitecture of the superior colliculus is illustrated in Fig. 1 for a species with an exceptionally well-developed tectum, the gray squirrel (*Sciurus carolinensis*). Both the Nissl-stained section and the section stained for myelin illustrate that the mammalian colliculus can be divided into a series of alternating cell and fiber layers. The outermost layer is a cell-free neuropil designated stratum zonale. Beneath stratum zonale is a broad layer, heavily populated with cells, named stratum griseum superficiale. Stratum griseum superficiale can in turn be divided into two sublaminae, an upper zone of small neurons and a lower, thinner band of larger cells. These superficial layers, strata zonale and superficiale, are separated from the deeper layers by a layer consisting primarily of fibers, stratum opticum. Immediately beneath stratum opticum is a cell layer, stratum griseum intermediale. In this layer, an inner sublamina densely populated with cells can be distinguished from an outer, more sparsely populated one. Stratum griseum intermediale is separated by a fiber lamina, stratum album intermediale, from the deepest two layers, strata griseum and album profundum. The deepest two layers merge without clear cytoarchitectonic distinctions into the underlying midbrain tegmentum.

B. Efferent Connections of the Superficial and Deep Layers

Although seven or more layers can be recognized on the basis of cytoarchitecture in most mammals, studies of the connections of these layers have suggested that a fundamental distinction can be made between the superficial cell layer,

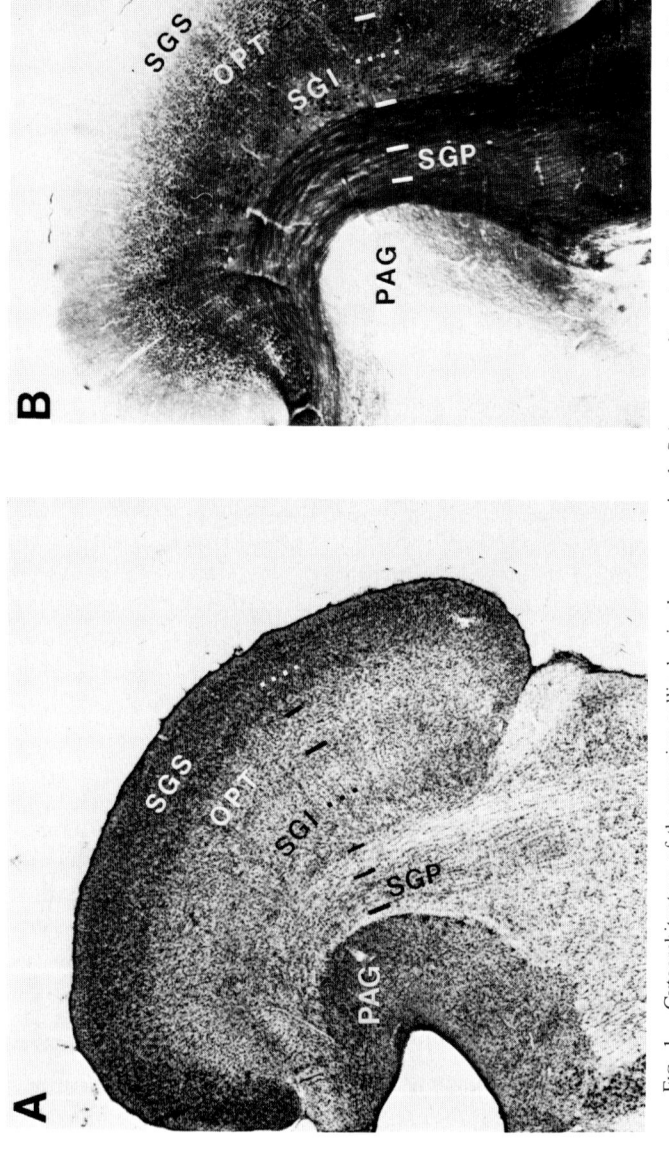

FIG. 1. Cytoarchitecture of the superior colliculus in the gray squirrel, *Sciurus carolinensis*. The photomicrographs in (A) and (B) are of frontal sections through the superior colliculus. Figure 1A is a Nissl-stained section and Fig. 1B was stained for myelin. The photomicrographs illustrate the large and distinctly laminated superior colliculus in this species. The borders between the layers are designated by a dash; those between the sublaminae, by dotted lines. OPT, Stratum opticum; PAG, periaqueductal gray; SGI, stratum griseum intermediale; SGP, stratum griseum profundum; SGS, stratum griseum superficiale.

stratum griseum superficiale, and the two cell layers lying beneath stratum opticum, strata griseum intermediale and profundum (Edwards, 1980; Glendenning *et al.*, 1975; Harting *et al.*, 1973; Holcombe and Hall, 1981a,b; Kawamura and Hashikawa, 1978; Kawamura and Kobayashi, 1975; Robson and Hall, 1977). To illustrate the anatomical basis for this distinction, Fig. 2 summarizes the results of an experiment that used the method of anterograde degeneration to compare the efferent projections of the superficial and deep layers in the tree shrew, *Tupaia glis*. Lesions were made in each superior colliculus, one restricted to the superficial and the other to the deep division (Harting *et al.*, 1973). This experiment shows that ascending pathways to visually related diencephalic structures, the pulvinar and the dorsal and ventral lateral geniculate nuclei, arise in the superficial layers. The only descending projections from these layers are to the parabigeminal nucleus and to the lateral pontine nuclei (not shown). The deeper layers, on the other hand, project to diencephalic structures not traditionally associated with the visual system, such as the intralaminar and suprageniculate nuclei, and also give rise to two major descending pathways to the brainstem reticular formation. One of these pathways crosses the midline of the brainstem as the predorsal bundle and descends to terminate in the paramedian reticular formation on the contralateral side (large arrow in Fig. 2A). A few fibers in the predorsal bundle descend to the cervical spinal cord as the tectospinal tract (Nudo and Masterton, 1983). The second main descending pathway travels along the lateral margin of the ipsilateral brainstem and terminates in the lateral brainstem reticular formation.

Further anatomical support for the distinction between superficial and deep divisions is provided by the projections to the superior colliculus from the visual system. Projections from the retina and from the occipital cortex terminate almost entirely in the layers above stratum opticum (Abplanalp, 1970; Behan, 1983; Garey *et al.*, 1968; Graham *et al.*, 1979; Graybiel, 1975; Harting and Noback, 1971; Hubel *et al.*, 1975; Kawamura *et al.*, 1974; Lund, 1969, 1972a,b; Sterling, 1971). Therefore, the superficial layers appear to be involved in relaying visual information to the diencephalon and, also, to the cerebellum by way of the relay in the lateral pontine nuclei. The deep layers, on the other hand, apparently have less direct connections with the visual system and project to brainstem regions of the reticular formation known to play an important role in the control of head and eye movements.

C. Behavioral Studies of Tectal Organization

Behavioral studies also relate the superficial layers to sensory functions and the deep layers to motor functions. For example, the role of the input from the retina to the superficial layers in *guiding* the orienting response has been elegantly demonstrated by experiments in which the projections from the eye are

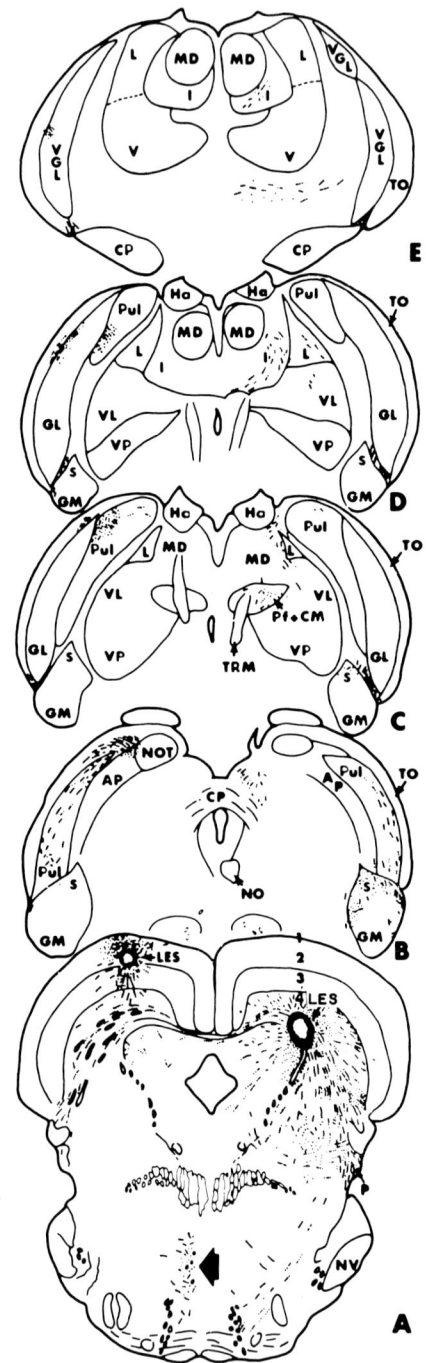

rerouted from the contralateral to the ipsilateral superior colliculus in neonatal hamsters (Schneider, 1973). As adults, these animals continue to make orienting responses, but orient away from rather than toward a visual stimulus. On the other hand, the importance of the deep layers for the *initiation* of the orienting response was indicated by experiments in which the predorsal bundles of tree shrews were sectioned as they cross the midline beneath the colliculus (Raczkowski *et al.*, 1976). These animals were unable to orient toward visual stimuli, even though tests demonstrated they could still detect and discriminate visual patterns. These studies suggest that both the superficial and deep layers contribute to the orienting response, but that their contributions are different and can be distinguished by behavioral tests.

D. Physiological Distinctions between the Superficial and Deep Layers

The anatomical and behavioral results correlate well with differences in the response characteristics of neurons in the superficial and deep layers. Figure 3, which is adapted from a paper by Wurtz and Albano (1980), illustrates some of these characteristics for the rhesus monkey. In these experiments, the responses of collicular cells were recorded while awake monkeys made saccades to targets appearing on a screen. In the superficial retinal recipient layers, the responses of neurons D and E are sensory. That is, their responses follow, with a fixed latency, the presentation of a visual target in a particular part of the visual field. In contrast, the responses of cells G and H, which lie beneath stratum opticum, precede saccadic eye movements by a fixed time period. Although some of these same neurons may also respond to the onset of a visual stimulus, as do the most superficial of the deep-layer cells in Fig. 3, the eye movement-related response is apparently not dependent on the occurrence of this sensory response, for these cells occasionally exhibit only the saccade-related response. A property of the deep layers, which is not illustrated in Fig. 3, is the presence of input from other

---

FIG. 2. A series of frontal sections through the brain of a tree shrew, *Tupaia glis*, with a lesion on the left restricted to stratum griseum superficiale and a lesion on the right to the layers below stratum opticum. Degenerating axons are indicated by rows of dots and terminal degeneration by small dots not aligned in rows. In Section A, the predorsal bundle is indicated by a large black arrow. Ascending pathways to visual nuclei of the diencephalon can be traced only from the superficial lesion, whereas the major descending pathways, including the predorsal bundle, can be traced only from the lesion in the deep layers (from Harting *et al.*, 1973). AP, Pretectal area; CM, central median nucleus; CP, cerebral peduncle; GL, dorsal lateral geniculate nucleus; GM, medial geniculate nucleus; Ha, habenula; I, intralaminar group; L, lateral nuclear group; MD, medial dorsal nucleus; NO, oculomotor nucleus; NOT, nucleus of the optic tract; NV, trigeminal nerve; Pf, parafascicular nucleus; Pul, pulvinar; S, suprageniculate nucleus; TO, optic tract; TRM, tractus retroflexus of Meynert; V, ventral nuclear group; VGL, ventral lateral geniculate nucleus; VL, ventral lateral nucleus; VP, ventral posterior nucleus.

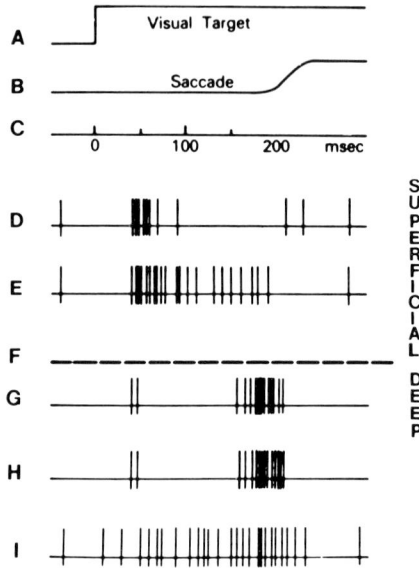

FIG. 3. Comparisons of responses of single neurons in the superior colliculus of monkey during saccadic eye movements. A shows the time of onset of the visual target for a saccade, while B indicates the onset of the saccade. C gives the time scale. D and E illustrate the responses of two neurons in the superficial layers. Both neurons respond shortly after the onset of the visual target, but neither gives a response that is temporally linked to the saccade. F indicates stratum opticum, the boundary between the superficial and deep layers. Deep-layer neurons G and H both have weak responses to the visual stimulus but—in contrast to neurons D and E— both also exhibit a vigorous burst of activity preceding the onset of the saccade. In this experiment, G responds only before saccades to a visual target. H also responds before spontaneous saccades in the dark. Neuron I, which is found in the deepest stratum, begins to discharge before the onset of the visual target in trials in which the monkey can anticipate the occurrence and location of the target. The saccade-related bursts in G and H are not dependent on the occurrence of a preceding sensory response. (Adapted from Wurtz and Albano, 1980.)

sensory modalities. Some of these deep-layer cells exhibit both sensory and motor responses to nonvisual stimuli. For example, more deeply located cells may give a sound-evoked response and then respond before a saccade toward the source of the auditory stimulus (Jay and Sparks, 1982).

In spite of the differences in their response characteristics, the superficial and deep collicular layers are in register spatially (Schiller and Stryker, 1972; Sparks and Mays, 1981). That is, the spatial map of the movement fields of neurons in the deep layers is congruent with the retinotopic map of the visual field in the overlying superficial layers. This is illustrated in Fig. 4, which shows the correspondence between visual receptive fields and the vectors of saccades elicited by electrical stimulation at the same site (Schiller and Stryker, 1972). Moreover, the duration and frequency of discharge by the eye movement-related cells does not vary with the direction or amplitude of the subsequent saccade. This suggests that spatial position is the important variable in the mechanisms underlying the functioning of the colliculus. If this is the case, a relatively simple spatial interaction could underlie the transition from visual sensory activity in the superficial layers to eye movement-related responses in the deep layers. Because auditory and somatosensory space also appear to be represented as spatiotopic maps in the colliculus, a similar transformation could initiate shifts of gaze

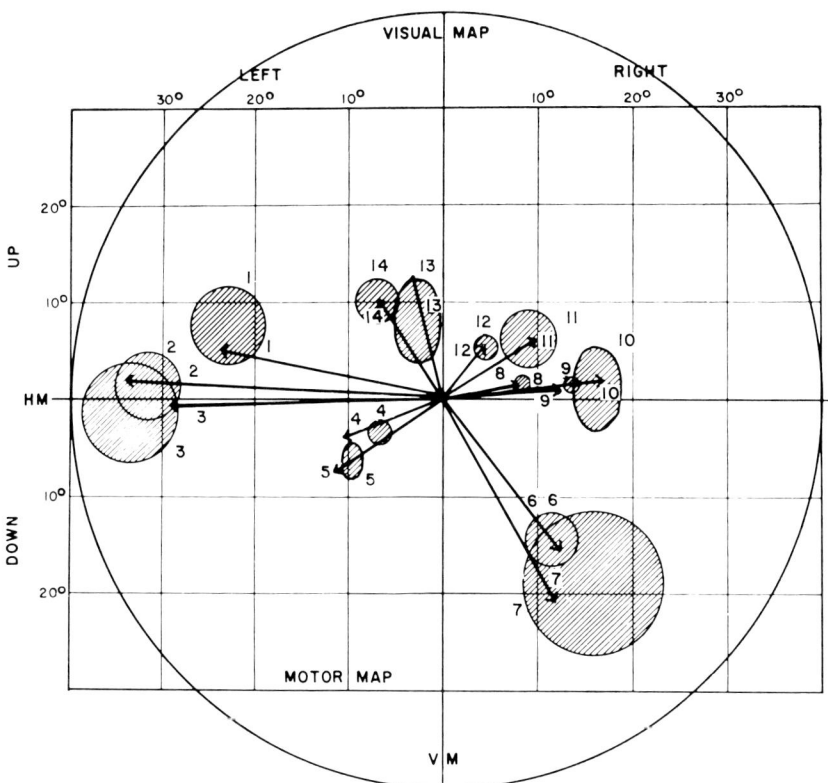

FIG. 4. Effects of recording and stimulating in the superficial layers of the superior colliculus in the monkey. The experimenters determined the location of the receptive field for each of 14 single neurons and then electrically stimulated at the same site. The figure illustrates the correspondence between visual receptive fields (shaded areas) and the direction and amplitude of the saccades elicited by electrical stimulation (arrows). In each case, the saccade terminates in or near the receptive field. In the deeper layers, the motor fields obtained by stimulating or by recording the saccade-related responses were in the same region as the overlying receptive fields. VM, Vertical meridian; HM, horizontal meridian. (From Schiller and Stryker, 1972.)

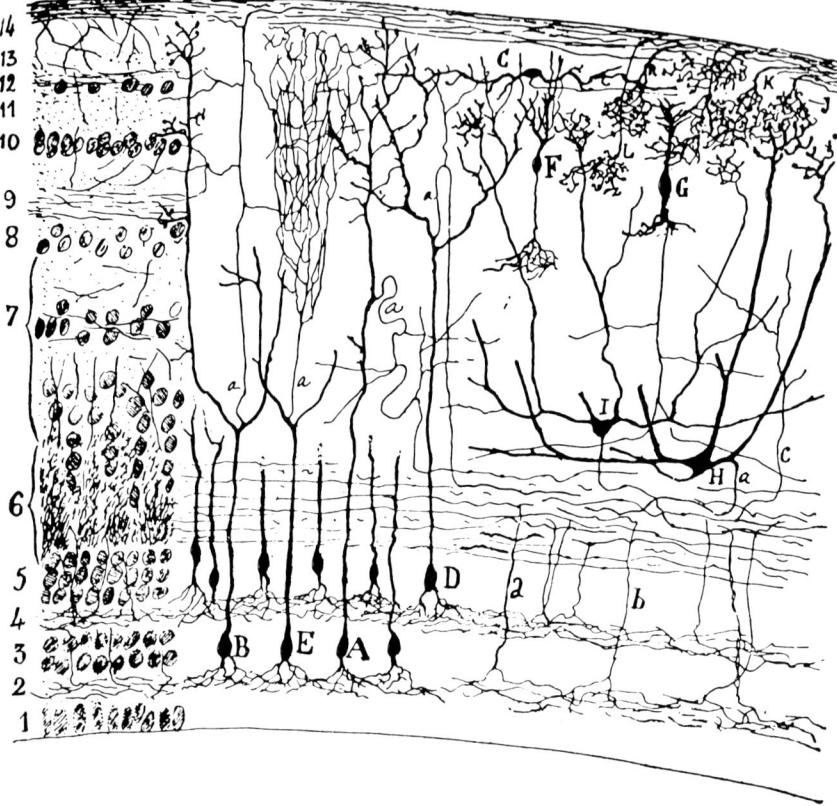

FIG. 5. Composite drawing by Ramón y Cajal (1911) of cell types in the optic tectum of the lizard. Cells A, B, D, H, and I are in deep tectal output layers and have apical dendrites extending into the retinal recipient layers 8–14 (Butler and Northcutt, 1971).

toward stimuli in these modalities as well (Dräger and Hubel, 1975; Finlay *et al.*, 1978; Jay and Sparks, 1982; Wickelgren, 1971). In the next section we will discuss several models that have been proposed as the anatomical substrate for these sensorimotor transformations. We will be concerned primarily with the responses to visual stimuli in this discussion, but similar arguments apply to other sensory modalities as well.

FIG. 6. Drawing (A) and photomicrograph (B) of tectal neurons in the frog, retrogradely filled by an injection of horseradish peroxidase in the predorsal bundle. The cell bodies of the neurons are located in layer 6 but the apical dendrites extend into the superficial retinal recipient layers (Hughes, Ingle, and Hall, unpublished experiments).

TRANSFORMATIONS IN THE SUPERIOR COLLICULUS   11

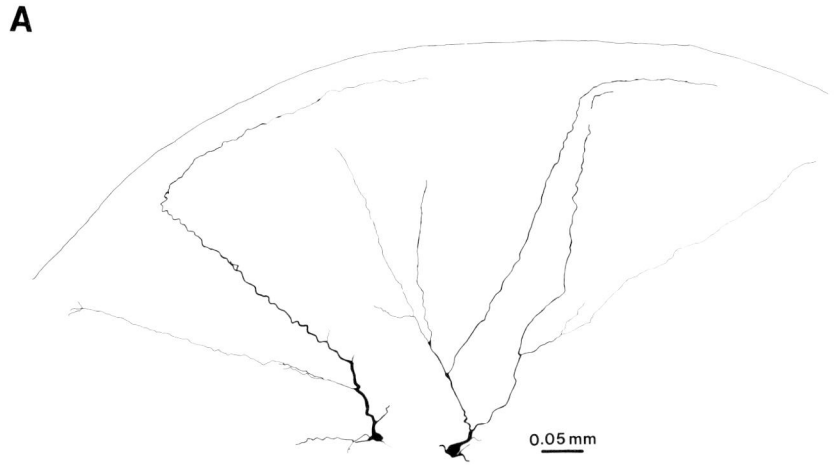

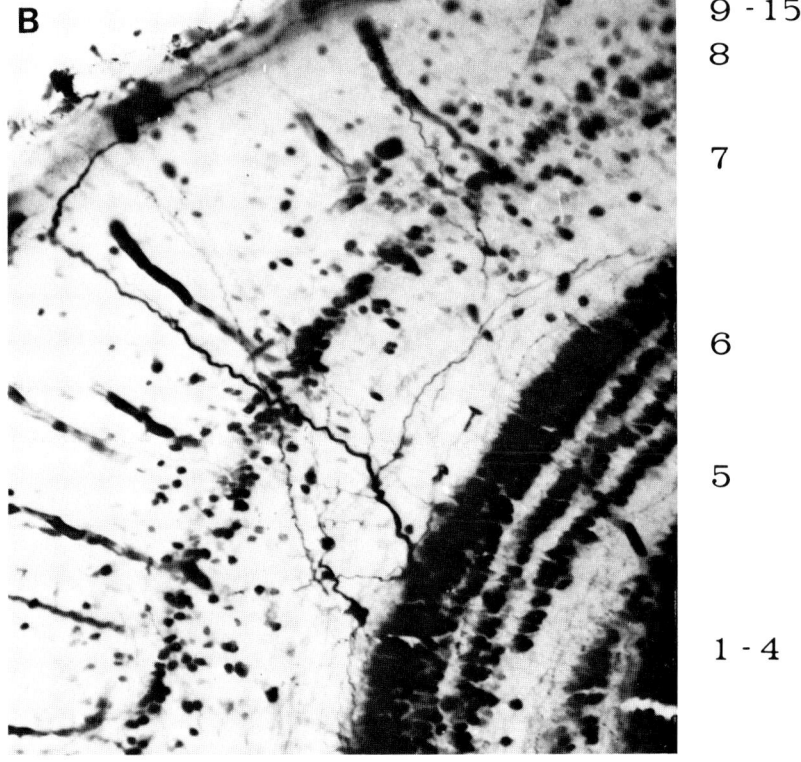

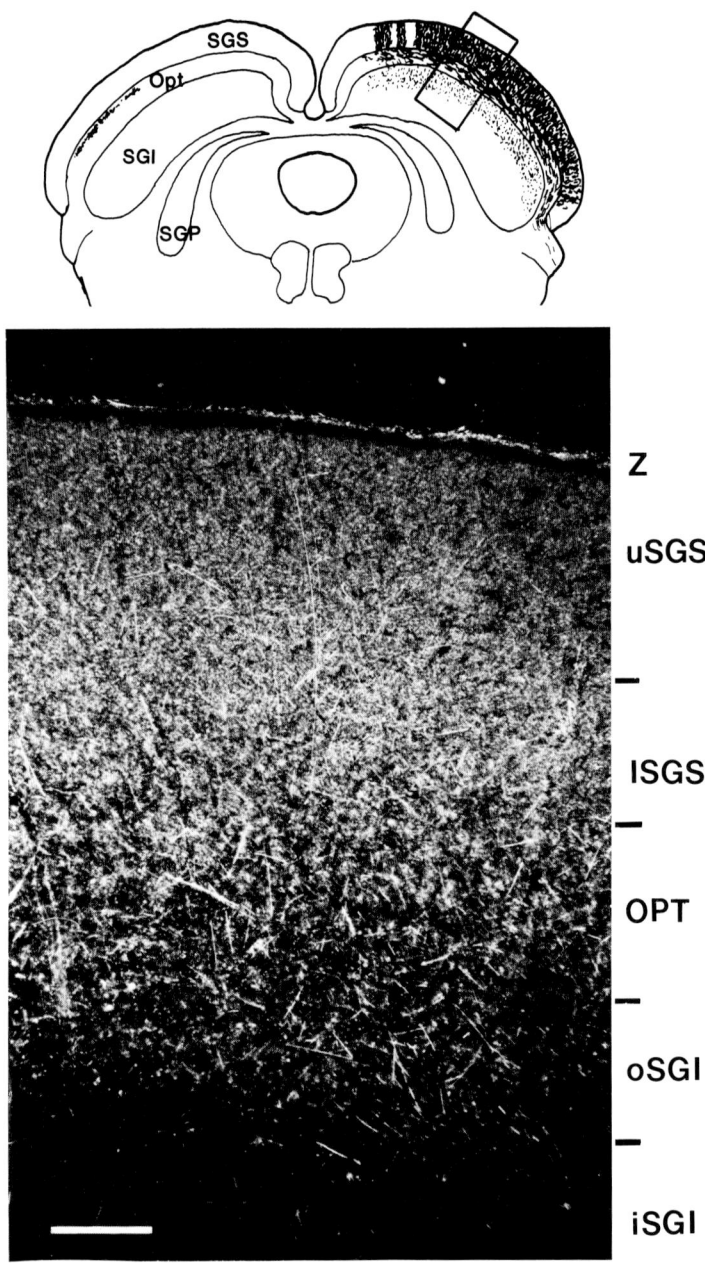

FIG. 7. Distribution of retinotectal projections in the gray squirrel. Retinal axons anterogradely labeled with horseradish peroxidase enter the superior colliculus in stratum opticum. The vast

III. MODELS OF SUPERIOR COLLICULUS ORGANIZATION

A. Retinal Influences on the Deep Tectal Layers

The most direct route through which the visual system could influence the motor cells of the deep tectal layers would be a monosynaptic input to these cells from the retina. The evidence for such a pathway is indirect and comes primarily from studies of the anatomy of the optic tectum in nonmammals. In general, the organization of the nonmammalian tectum resembles that of mammals (Foster and Hall, 1975; Stein and Gaither, 1981), for it consists of a superficial retinal recipient zone and deeper layers that contain the cells of origin of the major descending pathways to lower brainstem motor areas. The possibility of a direct retinal input to the output cells in nonmammals is suggested by Golgi studies, such as the one by Ramón y Cajal (1911) illustrated in Fig. 5. These studies indicate that many of the neurons in the deep tectal layers of nonmammals have apical dendrites that extend into the superficial layers and, consequently, are in a position to receive the retinal input (see also Butler and Northcutt, 1971; Székely, 1973; Székely *et al.*, 1973). Recent experiments by Ingle (Ingle and Quinn, 1982; Ingle, Hughes, and Hall, experiment in progress), in which the output neurons of the tectum in the frog were retrogradely filled with horseradish peroxidase, have demonstrated, as illustrated in Fig. 6, that many of the deep cells with apical dendrites extending to the superficial layers are indeed the cells of origin for descending pathways. Similar studies in the turtle suggest this may also be the case in reptiles (Sereno, 1982). Thus, although these experiments fall short of directly demonstrating a monosynaptic connection between optic tract axons and the output cells, the extensive overlap between their dendritic fields and the retinal terminal field is consistent with such a connection.

The overall similarities in tectal organization between mammals and nonmammals suggest that mammalian output cells might also receive direct retinal input. As Fig. 7 illustrates, very few retinal fibers terminate below stratum opticum in mammals (Behan, 1981; Frankfurter *et al.*, 1982; Graybiel, 1975; Hubel *et al.*, 1975; Lund, 1969, 1972a; May and Hall, 1982). Consequently, a major direct input would depend on the presence of output cells with apical dendrites that extend to the superficial layers, as in nonmammals. However, as Fig. 8 illustrates, Golgi studies of the superior colliculus in mammals indicate that the

---

majority of terminations are above stratum opticum. OPT, Stratum opticum; iSGI, inner stratum griseum intermediale; oSGI, outer stratum griseum intermediale; SGP, stratum griseum profundum; lSGS, lower stratum griseum superficiale; uSGS, upper stratum griseum superficiale; Z, zonale. Bar = 0.5 mm.

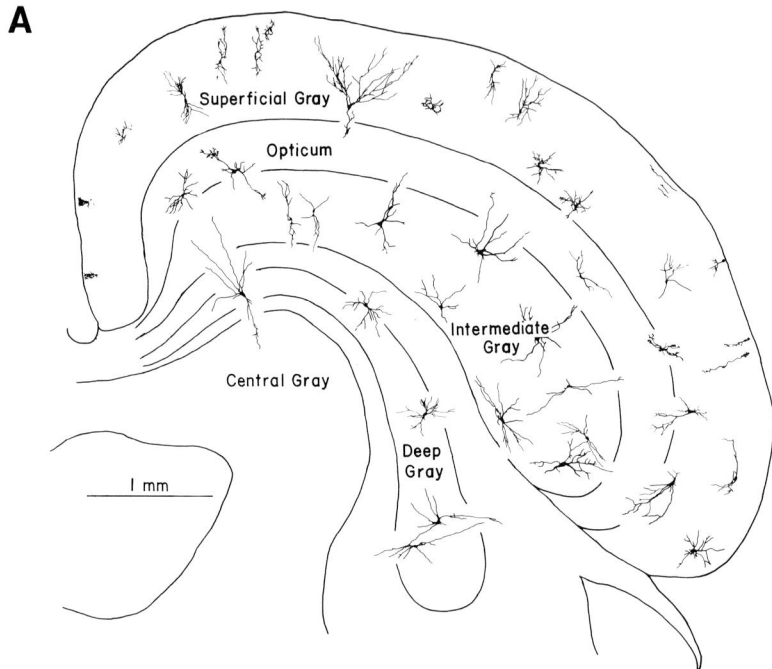

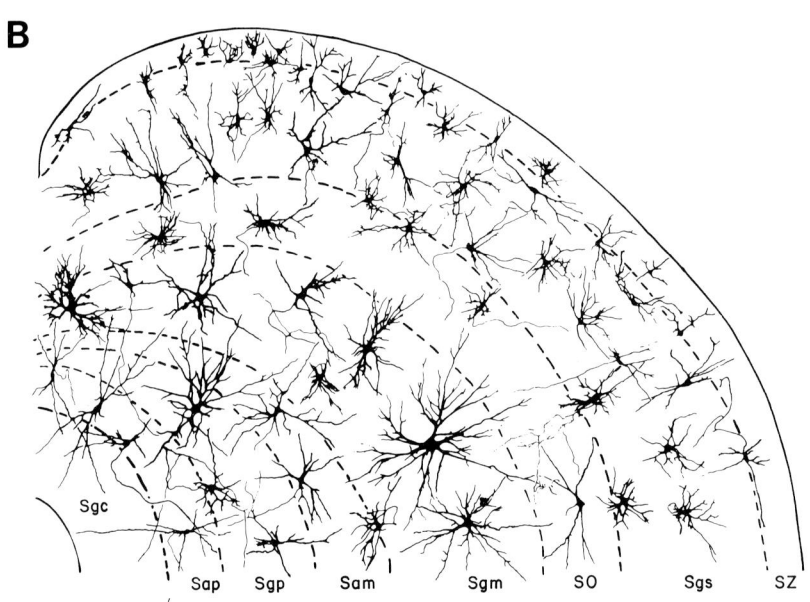

neurons below stratum opticum do not have apical dendrites that extend into the superficial layers. Instead, their dendritic fields are restricted almost entirely to the deep layers, although some extension into stratum opticum is present (Sprague, 1975). Similar dendritic fields are seen for deep-layer cells that are intracellularly filled with horseradish peroxidase (see Fig. 9, and Grantyn and Grantyn, 1982). Both of these methods indicate that the dendritic fields of the deep cells are, for the most part, confined to the lamina containing their somas. Because very few retinal axons can be traced to the deep layers, it seems unlikely that the retina of mammals is a major source of visual input to the cells of the deep layers. A similar conclusion is suggested by physiological studies, which indicate that only a very weak and labile monosynaptic retinal input is available to the cells of origin of the predorsal bundle (Berson and McIlwain, 1982).

B. Intracollicular Connections between the Superficial and Deep Layers

An alternative suggestion is that the visual system influences the deep tectal layers by means of projections from the overlying superficial layers (Sprague, 1975). Such intracollicular projections have been described in nonmammals (Dacey, 1982; Ramón y Cajal, 1911) and could potentially provide the basis for the topographic correspondence between the sensory and motor maps in mammals. However, the available evidence for a projection from the superficial to the deep layers in mammals is not convincing. For example, lesions or injections of tritiated amino acids restricted to the superficial layers have been made in several species, and in none of these have unequivocal projections been traced to the deep layers (Edwards, 1980; Glendenning *et al.*, 1975; Harting *et al.*, 1973; Robson and Hall, 1977). Thus, even though it is possible that newer, more sensitive techniques such as intraaxonal injections of horseradish peroxidase may eventually reveal intracollicular projections, the results obtained thus far suggest that they will not prove to be a major source of input to the deep layers.

The failure to find intracollicular projections in mammals is also consistent with the results of physiological experiments that suggest that the responses of neurons in the deep layers are not dependent on activity in the overlying superficial cells. For example, in the experiments illustrated in Fig. 10, monkeys were trained to make two consecutive saccades (Sparks *et al.*, 1977; Mays and Sparks,

---

FIG. 8. Composite drawings of Golgi-impregnated cells in the superior colliculus of the gray squirrel (A) and the cat (B). In mammals, the cells below stratum opticum do not send apical dendrites into the superficial, retinal recipient layers (Golgi drawing of the cat by Victorov, taken from Sprague, 1975). Sam, Stratum album intermediale; Sap, stratum album profundum; Sgc, periaqueductal gray, or stratum griseum centrale; Sgm, stratum griseum intermediale; Sgp, stratum griseum profundum; Sgs, stratum griseum superficiale; SO, stratum opticum; SZ, stratum zonale.

1980). The visual target of the second saccade was presented and extinguished before the onset of a saccade to the initial target. By recording from tectal cells while the animals performed this task, the experimenters demonstrated that in the deep layers the neuronal responses preceding the second saccade can occur in the absence of activity in the immediately overlying superficial cells. The same conclusion is suggested by experiments in the tree shrew, *Tupaia glis*, which show that an ablation that removes the superficial tectal layers but spares the deep layers disrupts pattern discrimination while leaving intact the ability to orient to visual stimuli (Casagrande and Diamond, 1974). As pointed out earlier,

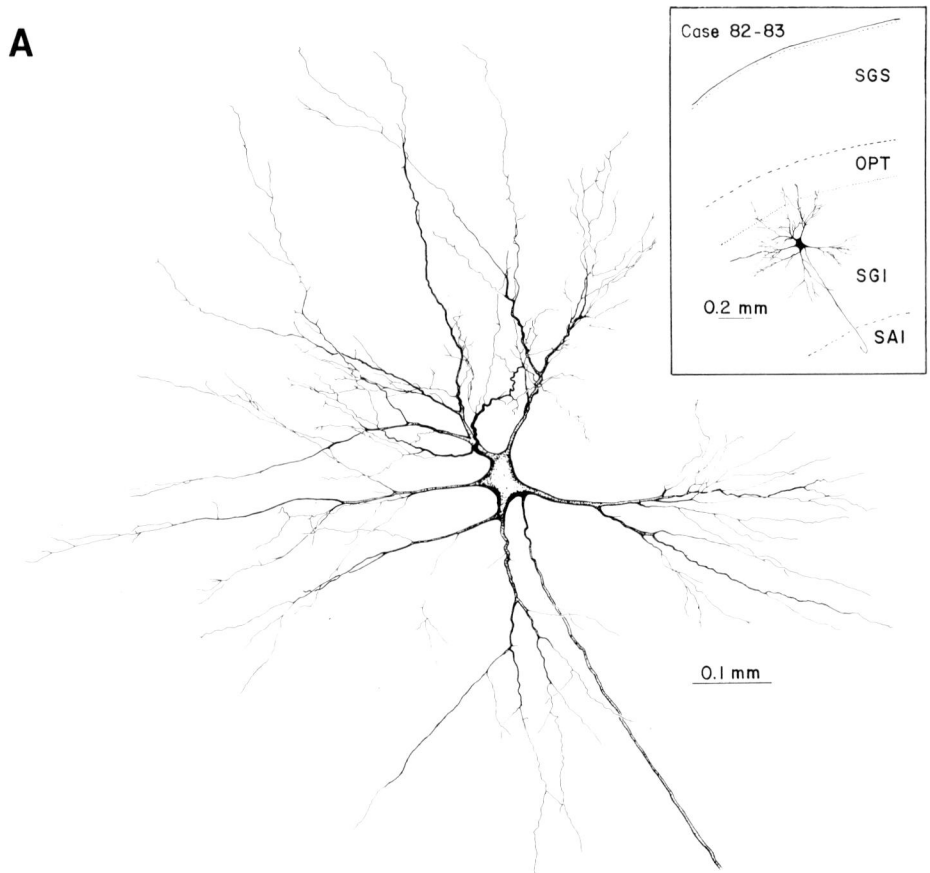

FIG. 9. Drawing (A) and photomicrograph (B) of a cell from the intermediate gray layer of the cat, intracellularly filled with horseradish peroxidase. The dendritic field, which is comparable in extent to those seen in Golgi preparations, is restricted to the intermediate gray layer and the lower

sectioning the predorsal bundle as it descends from the deep layers eliminates the orienting response in this species (Raczkowski et al., 1976). These studies suggest that the superficial layers are not necessary for the movement-related activity of the deep tectal layers.

Although much of the evidence is negative or indirect, taken together it is sufficient to raise strong doubts concerning the existence of major projections from the superficial to the deep layers. Consequently, these results have provided the stimulus for further efforts to identify alternate pathways linking the retina to the output of the deep layers.

C. Influences of the Occipital Lobe on the Deep Tectal Layers

In mammals, the output of the occipital lobe is functionally related to the deep tectal layers. For example, in primates saccades elicited by electrical stimulation

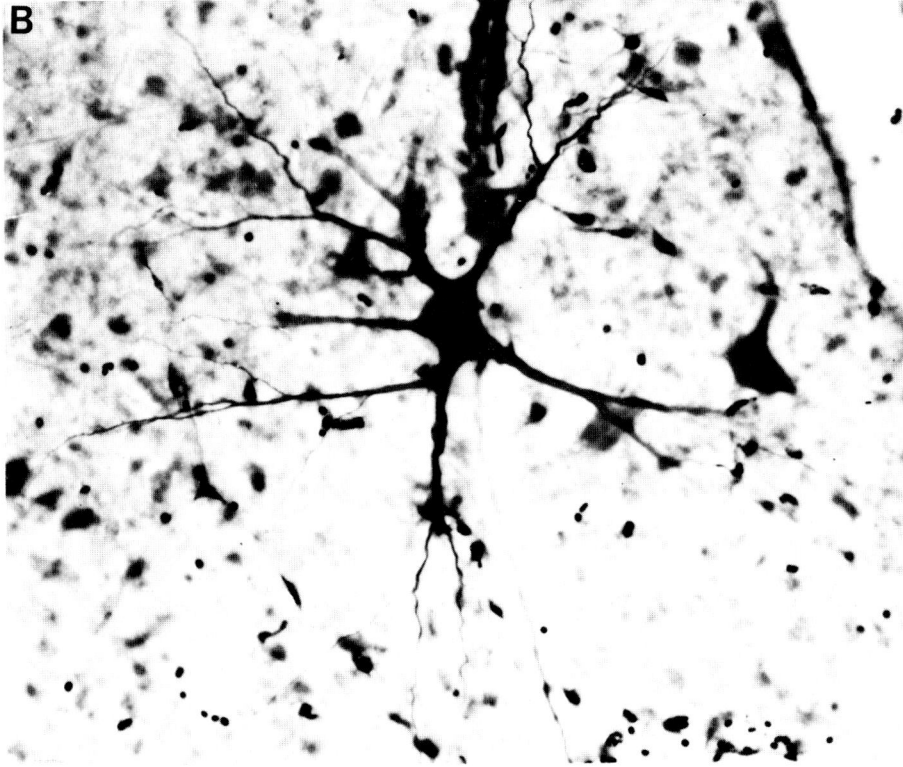

part of stratum opticum. There is little or no overlap with the distribution of retinal terminals (Lin, McIlwain, and Hall, unpublished experiments). OPT, Stratum opticum; SAI, stratum album intermediale; SGI, stratum griseum intermediale; SGS, stratum griseum superficiale.

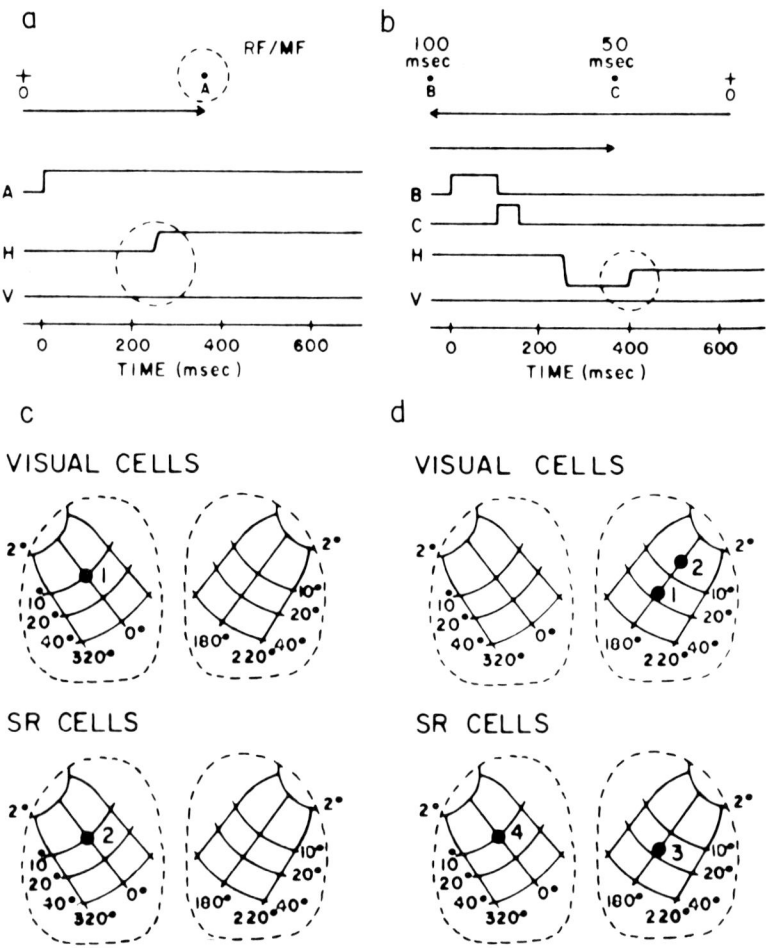

FIG. 10. Single and double saccade trials in the rhesus monkey. In part (a), the monkey makes a horizontal saccade from the fixation point (O) to target A, which is located in the right visual field. Line A indicates the onset of the target, whereas lines H and V indicate the horizontal and vertical components of the saccade, respectively. Part (c) of the figure indicates the location of the visual response to target A in the superficial layers in the left colliculus, and the location of the saccade-related cells (SR cells) in the underlying deep layers, which respond before a saccade to target A. In part (b), the monkey is required to make saccades to target B and, subsequently, from target B to target C. As can be seen from lines B, C, and H, both targets are extinguished before the onset of the initial saccade. In this trial, targets B and C are presented in the left half of the visual field and therefore represented by visual activity in the superficial layers of the right tectum [visual cells in part (d)]. Just before the initial saccade from the fixation point (O) to target B, a saccade-related burst occurs at site 3 in the deep layers of the right colliculus (SR cells). In contrast, the saccade-related burst preceding the saccade from target B to target C is located in the left tectum (point 4). This is the same area of the colliculus that was activated before the saccade from the fixation point (O) to target

of the striate cortex are eliminated by ablation of the ipsilateral superior colliculus (Schiller, 1977). Conversely, ablations of striate cortex eliminate the visual responses of cells in the deep layers (Schiller *et al.*, 1974). Moreover, stimulation of the occipital cortex in cats evokes short latency activity in the deeper tectal layers (Berson, 1982; Berson and McIlwain, 1983).

On the other hand, anatomical studies in the cat, gray squirrel (Fig. 11B), and monkey (Fig. 11A) suggest that the cortical influence may not be mediated by a direct pathway from the occipital lobe to the deep tectal layers (see also Behan, 1983; Garey *et al.*, 1968; Graham *et al.*, 1979). According to these experiments, the main terminal zone of the occipital–tectal pathway resides in the superficial rather than in the deep tectal layers. Thus, these data imply that the pathways from the occipital lobe, and adjacent cortical areas, which influence the deep layers, do not project directly, but instead involve additional relays in other structures. We will discuss the evidence for these indirect projections in a later section (IV,C).

D. Projections from the Ventral Lateral Geniculate Nucleus to the Deep Tectal Layers

One pathway to the deep tectal layers that has been documented arises in the ventral lateral geniculate nucleus of the ventral thalamus. This nucleus receives projections from several visual structures, including the retina (Giolli and Guthrie, 1962; Laties and Sprague, 1966; Mathers and Mascetti, 1975), the occipital lobe (Garey *et al.*, 1968; Graybiel, 1974; Holländer, 1970), and the superficial layers of the superior colliculus (Albano *et al.*, 1979; Altman and Carpenter, 1961; Benevento and Fallon, 1975; Harting *et al.*, 1973) and projects in turn to the deep tectal layers (Edwards *et al.*, 1974; Graybiel, 1974; Kawamura *et al.*, 1978; Swanson *et al.*, 1974). However, physiological and anatomical studies suggest that most of the cells in the ventral lateral geniculate nucleus have the properties of "W" cells (Albano *et al.*, 1979; Hoffman, 1973; Spear *et al.*, 1977), whereas the visual activity in the deep tectal layers is dominated by neurons classified as Y-like (Berson and McIlwain, 1982). Thus, it seems unlikely that the ventral lateral geniculate nucleus is a major source of the visual input to the deep layers. Moreover, the ventral lateral geniculate nucleus is small and poorly developed in many species, including most primates (Niimi *et al.*, 1963) and, for this reason as well, it seems unlikely to play a major role in initiating activity in the cells of the deep collicular layers.

A in part (a) of the figure. In the double saccade experiment, all visual stimuli were in the left half of the visual field and represented in the right tectum, but the saccade-related burst that preceded the movement from target B to target C is located in the deep layers of the left tectum (Mays and Sparks, 1980).

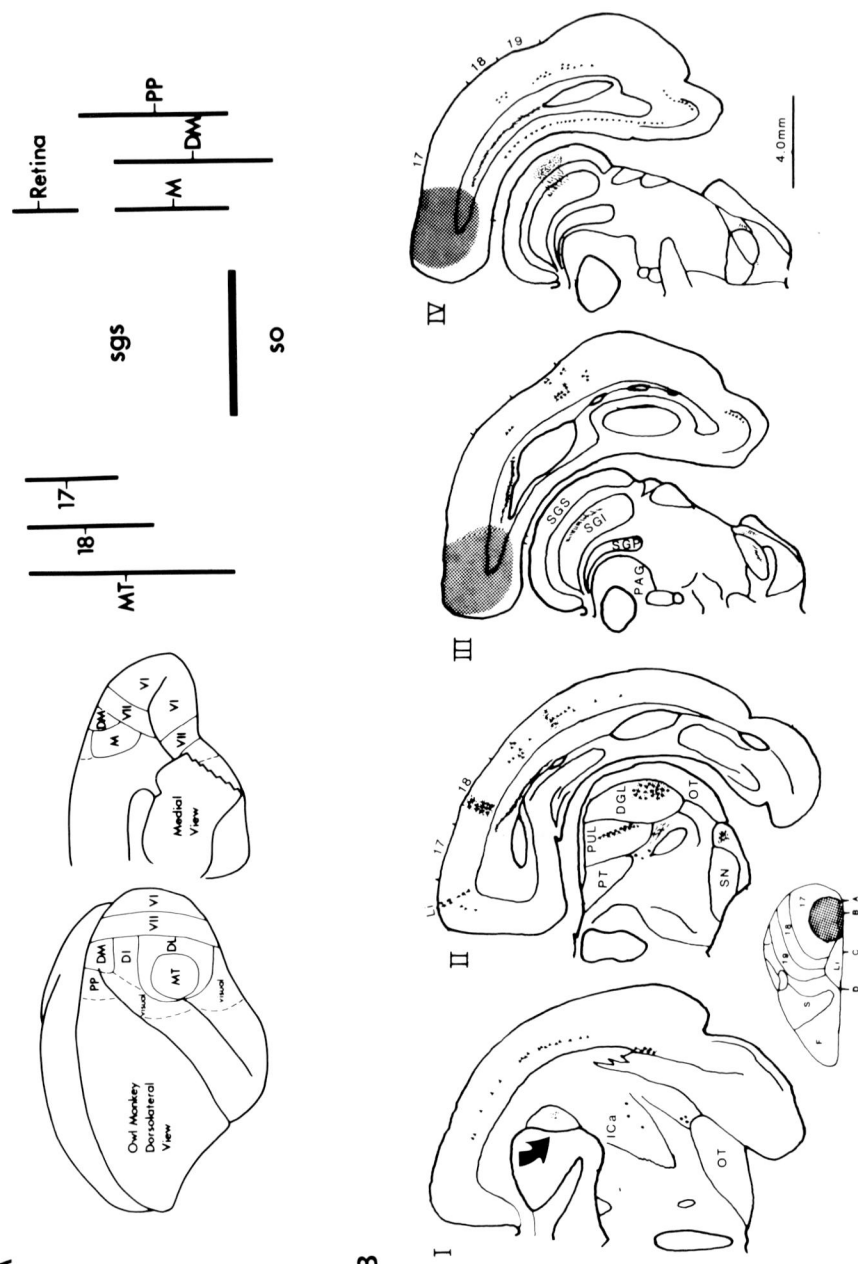

IV. INDIRECT VISUAL PATHWAYS TO THE DEEP LAYERS OF THE SUPERIOR COLLICULUS

In the previous sections we have discussed the evidence for and against various putative sources of influence on the movement-related cells of the deep tectal layers. The difficulty encountered in identifying pathways between visual structures and the deep tectal layers with anatomical methods is perhaps the most surprising conclusion of this research. There is very little evidence for either direct connections between the superficial and deep tectal layers of mammals, or direct input to the deep layers from other traditionally defined visual structures, such as the retina and the occipital lobe. This is in spite of the evidence for such connections in various nonmammalian vertebrates, and in spite of the close register between the sensory and motor maps represented in these layers in mammals. In the following sections we will present evidence that the links between the visual system and the deep colliculus are much more indirect than was hitherto suspected.

A. The Distribution of the Tectoreticular Cells

In our own research we have been studying the afferent connections of the deep tectal layers in the gray squirrel, *Sciurus carolinensis*. We chose the gray squirrel because its large and highly differentiated superior colliculus (see Fig. 1) offers an opportunity to determine precisely the relationships between its laminar organization and the distributions of various efferent and afferent pathways.

The first step in this work was to describe as precisely as possible the laminar distribution of the cells of origin of the major output pathway to lower brainstem gaze centers, the predorsal bundle. It has been possible to identify the laminar origin of the various efferent pathways by injecting horseradish peroxidase into

---

FIG. 11. Projections from visual cortex to the superior colliculus in the monkey and the squirrel. The surface view of the owl monkey brain at the top of the figure (A) summarizes the location of the cortical visual areas mapped in this species. The chart to the right indicates the tectal layers that receive projections from these areas. Visual areas in occipital, parietal, and temporal cortex project primarily to the superficial gray layer, with projections of several extending into the adjacent part of stratum opticum. These results are based on anterograde transport of tritiated amino acids following cortical injections (from Graham *et al.*, 1979). (B) Illustrates the pathways anterogradely labeled following an injection of horseradish peroxidase in area 17 of the gray squirrel. In the superior colliculus the projections are confined primarily to the lower part of stratum griseum superficiale. Pathways could also be traced to the pulvinar and dorsal lateral geniculate nucleus in the thalamus, and to the caudate (see arrow in Section I). DGL, Dorsal lateral geniculate nucleus; DL, dorsal lateral area; DM, dorsomedial area; F, frontal cortex; ICa, internal capsule; Li, limbic cortex; M, medial area; MT, medial temporal area; OT, optic tract; PAG, periaqueductal gray; PP, posterior parietal area; PT, pretectum; PUL, pulvinar; S, somatosensory cortex; SGI, stratum griseum intermediale; SGP, stratum griseum profundum; SGS, stratum griseum superficiale; SN, substantia nigra.

each potential target of the superior colliculus and locating the retrogradely labeled collicular neurons. These experiments have confirmed the finding that the major descending pathways arise from the deep layers and have further demonstrated that one particular deep layer, stratum griseum intermediale, is the main source of the efferent fibers of the predorsal bundle in the squirrel (Holcombe and Hall, 1981b).

More recently, by injecting horseradish peroxidase with a detergent such as saponin into an efferent pathway, it has been possible to increase the retrograde uptake to the extent that the dendritic fields, as well as the somas of neurons, are homogeneously filled with label (May and Hall, 1980). If this procedure is applied to label the cells that contribute to the predorsal bundle of the gray squirrel, a result such as that illustrated in Fig. 12 is obtained. In this case the retrogradely labeled neurons are not only restricted to stratum griseum intermediale, but also to the inner sublamina that lies along the ventral border of this layer (see also Fig. 1). Furthermore, the dendritic fields of the cells are restricted to the same inner sublamina. The extents of the dendritic fields of the cells filled by this method resemble those of cells described previously in Golgi-stained material (see Fig. 8) and also of intracellularly filled cells (see Fig. 9), which suggests that the entire field is included in our estimation.

The restriction of the dendritic fields of the neurons that give rise to the predorsal bundle to a clearly defined sublamina of stratum griseum intermediale in the squirrel provides an opportunity to establish more definite correlations between these cells and the distributions of various inputs to the deep layers.

B. Relationships between the Optic Tectum and the Basal Ganglia

Of the various inputs to the deep tectum that we have studied thus far, the terminal distribution of the nigrotectal pathway exhibits the most striking correlation with the location of the dendritic fields of the cells that contribute to the predorsal bundle (May and Hall, 1981). Figure 13 illustrates the distribution of labeled axon terminals in the superior colliculus following an injection of tritiated amino acid into the substantia nigra. The terminal field is dense and restricted to the same inner sublamina of the intermediate gray layer that contains the cells of origin of the predorsal bundle. A projection from substantia nigra pars reticulata to the superior colliculus also has been demonstrated in several species in addition to the gray squirrel, including the cat (Beckstead *et al.*, 1981; Graybiel, 1978; Rinvik *et al.*, 1976), the rhesus monkey (Beckstead and Frankfurter, 1982; Jayerman *et al.*, 1977), the rat (Bentivoglio *et al.*, 1979; Faull and Mehler, 1978), and the hamster (Rhoades *et al.*, 1982) and analogous pathways may even be present in nonmammalian vertebrates (Reiner *et al.*, 1980, 1982). Although none of these species exhibits the close correlation found in squirrel

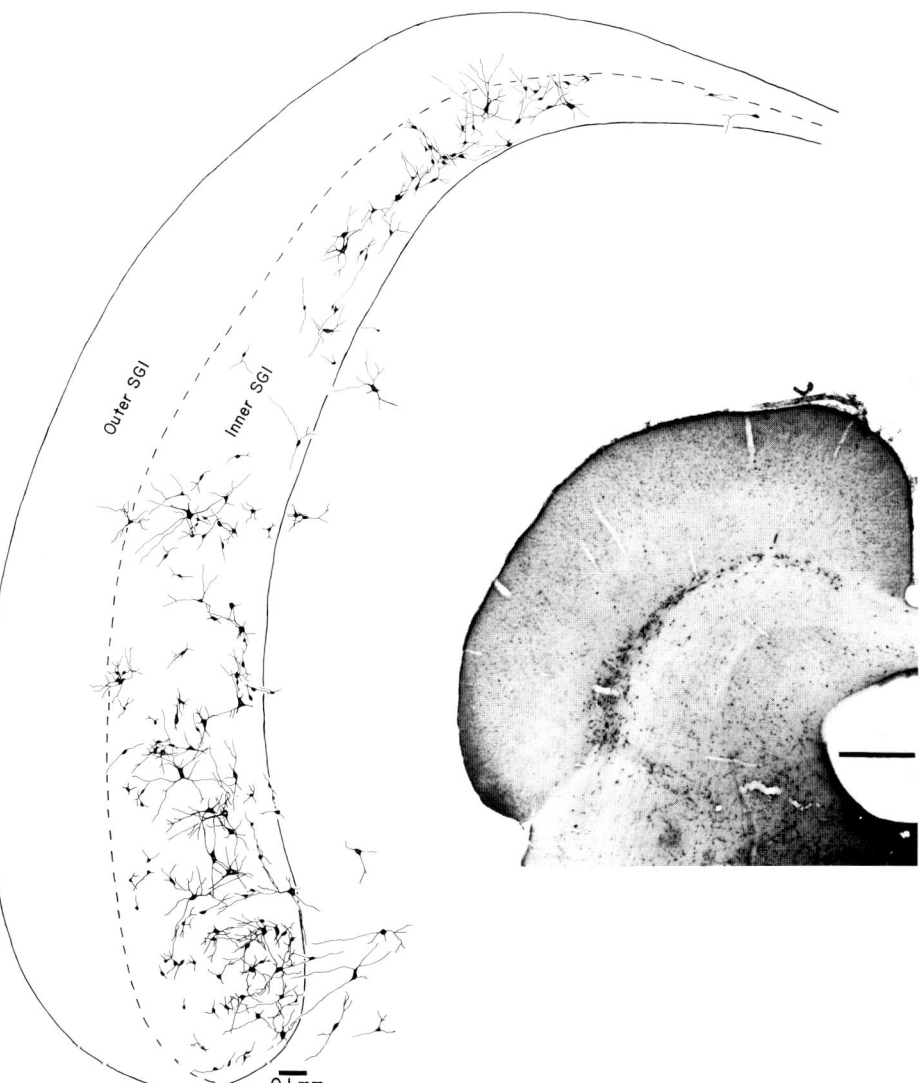

FIG. 12. Distribution and morphology of the cells of origin of the predorsal bundle. The injection site was in the predorsal bundle as its axons cross the midline beneath the oculomotor nucleus. The photomicrograph illustrates the distribution of cells retrogradely labeled with horseradish peroxidase. The cells are confined to the deep sublamina of stratum griseum intermediale. The drawing on the left shows that the dendritic fields as well as the cell bodies are, for the most part, restricted to this sublamina. SGI, Stratum griseum intermediale. Bar = 0.1 mm.

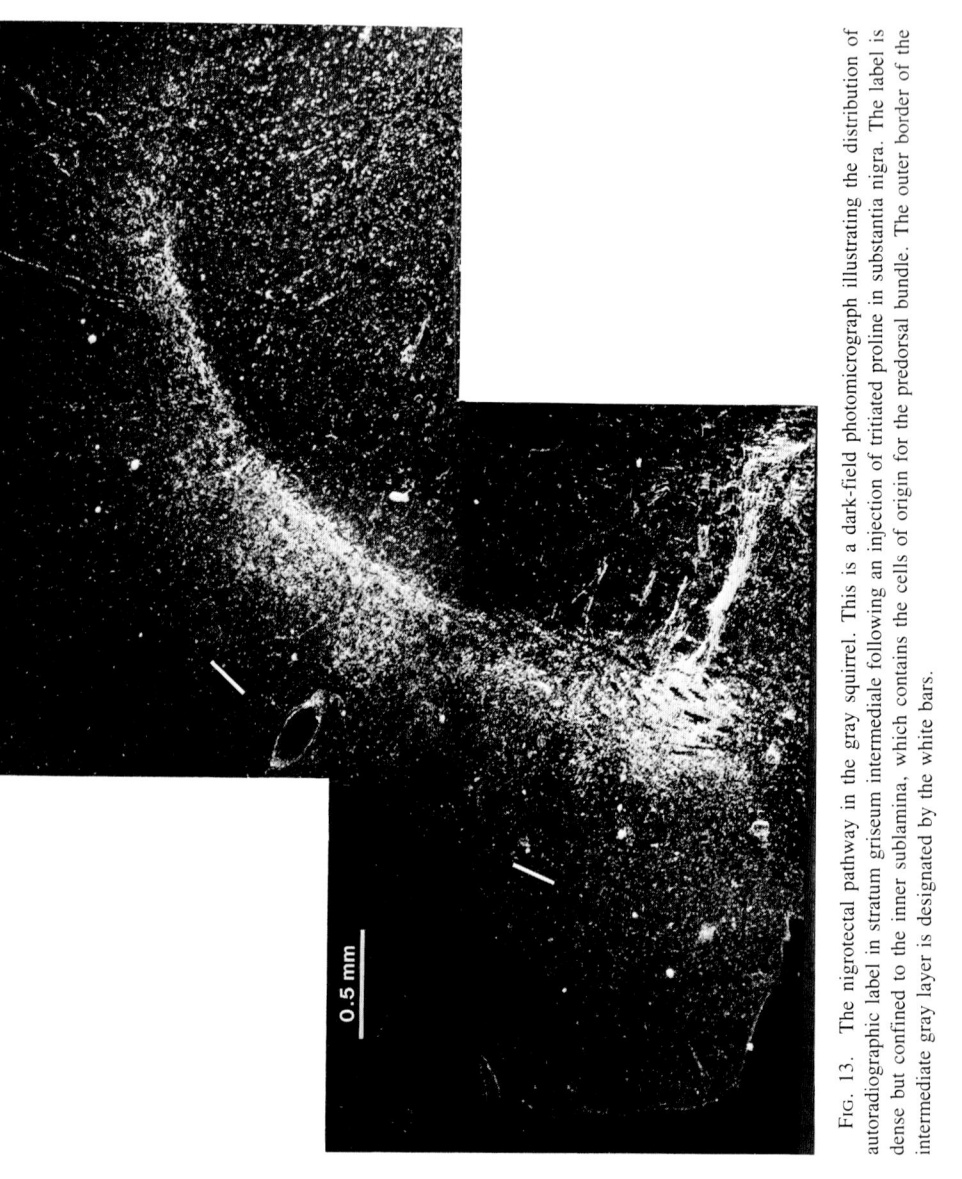

FIG. 13. The nigrotectal pathway in the gray squirrel. This is a dark-field photomicrograph illustrating the distribution of autoradiographic label in stratum griseum intermediale following an injection of tritiated proline in substantia nigra. The label is dense but confined to the inner sublamina, which contains the cells of origin for the predorsal bundle. The outer border of the intermediate gray layer is designated by the white bars.

between the nigrotectal terminal field and the cells of origin for the predorsal bundle, the projection is distributed to the deep tectal layers in every case, and therefore is potentially available to output cells in these species as well.

Although electron microscopic verification is necessary to establish a monosynaptic connection between the nigrotectal tract and the cells of origin of the predorsal bundle, the close correspondence between the distributions of axonal terminations and dendritic fields does imply that substantia nigra has a strong influence on these cells. Physiological investigations support this view and, further, suggest the nature of its influence. For example, electrical stimulation of substantia nigra pars reticulata in the rat results in inhibition of the activity of cells in the deep tectal layers (Deniau *et al.*, 1978; Chevalier *et al.*, 1981). The contribution this inhibition might make to the initiation of eye movement-related responses is suggested by the recent experiments of Hikosaka and Wurtz (1981a,b). By recording from cells in substantia nigra pars reticulata while monkeys made saccades to visual targets, they found that nigral neurons have a high level of spontaneous activity that decreases shortly before a saccade to a target within their receptive field. An example of the activity of such a neuron is presented in Fig. 14. Because the response pattern of these neurons is the inverse of that described for eye movement-related neurons in the colliculus (see Fig. 3), their results suggest that the tectal responses could be triggered by a release from nigral inhibition. It remains to be determined whether the release from tonic inhibition is, by itself, sufficient to account for the saccade-related bursts of the deep tectal cells (e.g., Hubbard *et al.*, 1969) or whether the nigral input serves to gate an unidentified excitatory input to the deep tectal cells.

In either case, the conclusion that substantia nigra pars reticulata is a major source of input to the cells of origin of the predorsal bundle still leaves the question of how, or by which pathways, the visual system influences the activity in the deep layers. Since the activity of nigral cells such as the one illustrated in Fig. 14 is a response to a target in a particular part of the visual field, it follows that the substantia nigra itself must be influenced by the visual system. There are reasons to believe that this link between the visual system and substantia nigra involves a relay in the corpus striatum. First of all, the corpus striatum is known to be the major source of projections to substantia nigra pars reticulata (Rhoades *et al.*, 1982; Nauta and Mehler, 1966). Because the pathway from the striatum to substantia nigra is predominantly inhibitory (Dray, 1979; Yoshida and Precht, 1971; Yoshida *et al.*, 1981), it may be responsible for the decrease in nigral activity that precedes saccadic eye movements to a visual target.

Visual projections to the corpus striatum are, in fact, known to arise from at least two structures: the visual cortex and the superficial layers of the superior colliculus. The visual cortex projects directly to the striatum (Graham *et al.*, 1979; Kemp and Powell, 1970; Rhoades *et al.*, 1982), whereas the projection

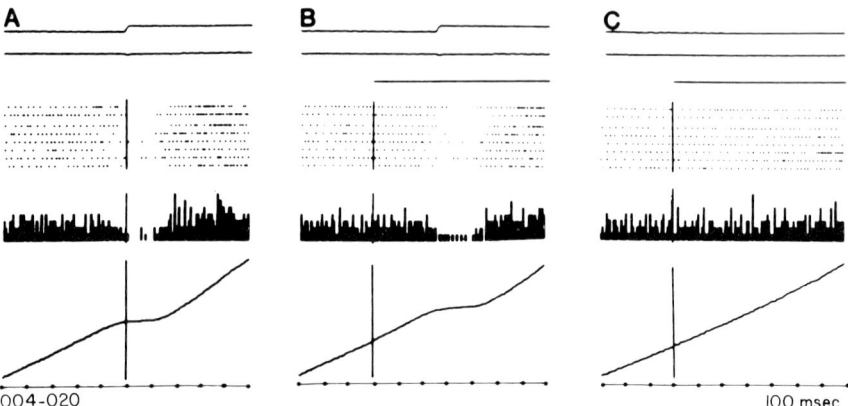

FIG. 14. Responses of a saccade-related cell in substantia nigra pars reticulata of the rhesus monkey. The upper two lines above the raster show the horizontal (upper line) and vertical (middle line) components of a saccadic eye movement. The lower line above the raster shows the onset of the visual stimulus. The vertical lines through all the recordings indicate the event used to align the traces. In the rasters, each dot indicates a single discharge of the cell. The histogram shows the sum of raster lines in 6-msec bins. The line below the histogram is a cumulative record of the number of discharges. The lower line with dots is the time base. The period between dots is 100 msec. In (A) the activity of the cell decreased 50 msec before the onset of a horizontal saccade. In (B) the response is aligned with the onset of the visual target. The variation in latencies suggests that the decrease in discharge rate of this cell is related to the onset of the saccade rather than to the onset of the target. In (C) no decrease occurred when the stimulus came on but the monkey did not make a saccade. (From Hikosaka and Wurtz, 1981a.)

from the superior colliculus involves an additional relay in the dorsal thalamus (Lin and Hall, 1982). Evidence for the latter pathway is based on studies that demonstrate that the band of neurons in the lower sublamina of stratum griseum superficiale (see Fig. 1) projects to the pulvinar, or lateral posterior nucleus, of the thalamus (Albano *et al.*, 1979; Graham and Berman, 1981; Graham and Casagrande, 1980; Kawamura *et al.*, 1980; Robson and Hall, 1977). Experiments such as the one illustrated in Fig. 15 demonstrate that the pulvinar in turn gives rise to a projection to the corpus striatum in addition to its well-known projections to the extrastriate and temporal cortex. As Fig. 11B illustrates, the region of the corpus striatum receiving the projections from the pulvinar also receives the previously discussed projections from visual cortex. Saccades to nonvisual targets may also be initiated by substantia nigra pars reticulata, because analogous pathways to the striatum from the cortex and thalamus can be traced for other sensory systems (Ebner, 1969; Jones *et al.*, 1977; Kemp and Powell, 1970; Nauta, 1979b; Reale and Imig, 1983; Wise and Jones, 1977).

C. Sources of Cortical Input to the Deep Tectum

The anatomical and physiological experiments just described support the idea that the nigrotectal pathway plays a critical role in the initiation of the eye movement-related responses of the deep-layer cells. On the other hand, the visual sensory responses exhibited by cells such as G and H in Fig. 3 occur prior to the movement-related responses and may depend on other pathways. In mammals, one of these visual pathways may involve the cortex.

Although, as mentioned earlier, the occipital lobe does not appear to give rise to a major direct projection to the deep tectal layers, occipital areas do project to other cortical areas, which in turn may give rise to direct pathways to the deep layers. For example, Berson and McIlwain (1983) have evoked short latency responses from cells in the deep-layer cells by electrically stimulating the posterior lateral suprasylvian gyrus in the cat. This result agrees with anatomical studies that indicate that cortical areas outside the occipital lobe project to tectal layers beneath stratum opticum (Garey et al., 1968; Holländer, 1974; Kawamura et al., 1974; Kuypers and Lawrence, 1967; Lund, 1966; Segal et al., 1982). The precise terminal distribution of these projections has not been determined, but these results indicate that nonoccipital visual areas may be a source of the visual sensory input to the deep layers.

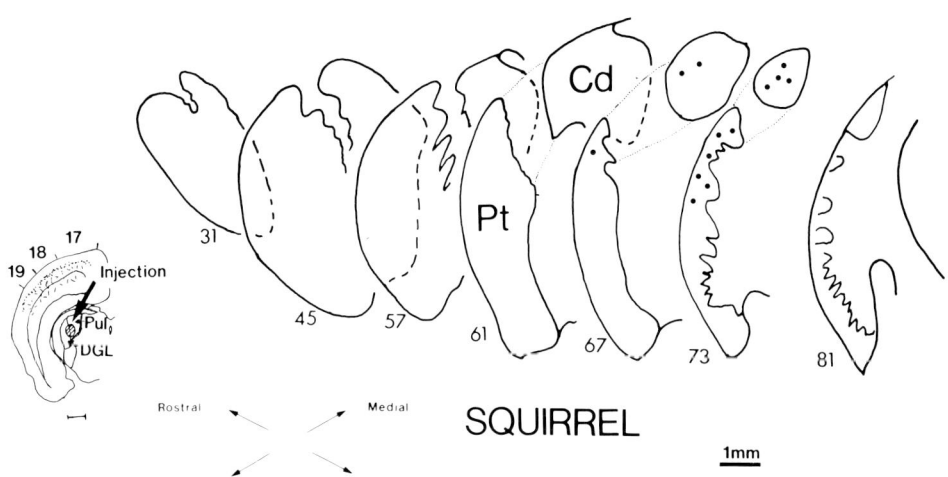

FIG. 15. Visual projections to the corpus striatum in the gray squirrel. The drawings show the distribution of terminations (large dots) present in the caudate and putamen following an injection of a tritiated amino acid in the pulvinar. Cd, Caudate; Pt, putamen; Pul, pulvinar; DGL, dorsal lateral geniculate nucleus.

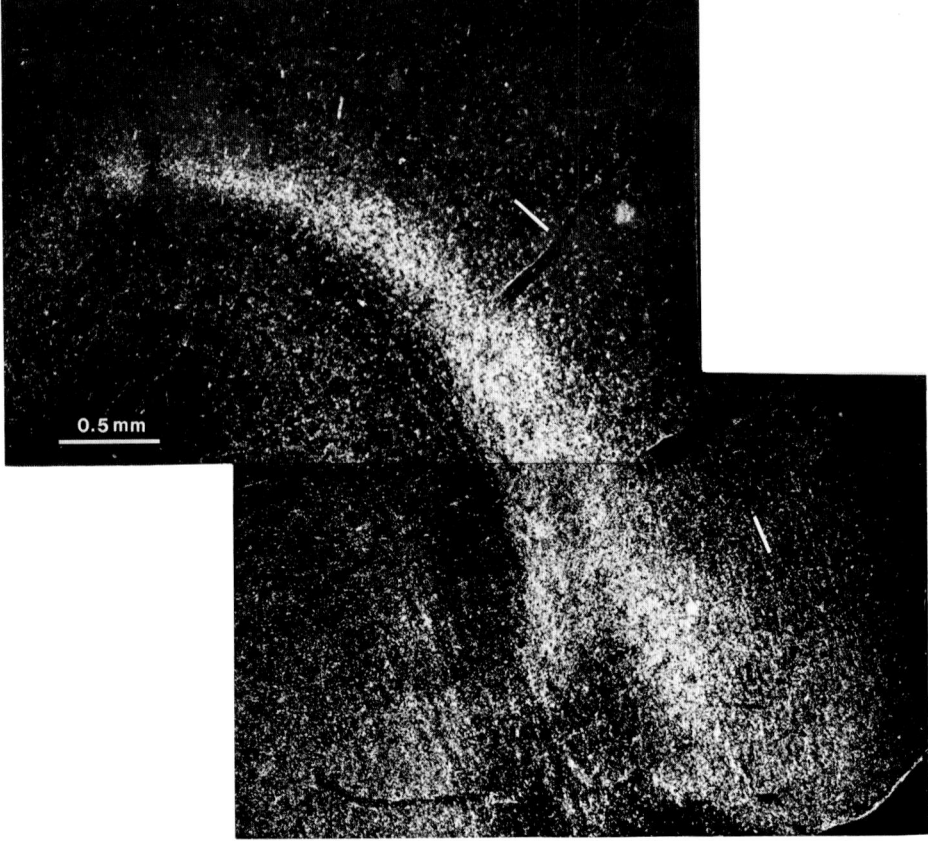

FIG. 16. The frontotectal pathway in the gray squirrel. A band of terminals labeled with horseradish peroxidase is present in the inner sublamina of the intermediate gray layer, following an injection centered in the medial bank of the frontal cortex. The outer border of the intermediate gray layer is designated by the white bars.

Prefrontal areas are another potential source of either sensory or motor influence on the deep layers. Our investigations of the gray squirrel have indicated that regions on the medial bank of the frontal lobe project to the same sublamina of stratum griseum intermediale that contains the cells of origin of the predorsal bundle (Fig. 16; May and Hall, 1983). Studies of primates have also demonstrated projections from the frontal lobe to the deep layers (Goldman and Nauta, 1976; Leichnetz et al., 1981; Leichnetz, 1980). However, in primates, ablation of the superior colliculus does not disrupt the saccades elicited by electrical stimulation of the frontal eye fields (Schiller, 1977). Consequently, it appears that the influence of these frontal areas on oculomotor mechanisms is at least partly independent of the superior colliculus. An independence is also suggested by the finding that the effects of combined lesions of the frontal eye fields and superior colliculus on the ability to make saccades are much more severe than the effects of removing either structure alone (Schiller *et al.*, 1980). Still, frontal areas do project to the layers below stratum opticum, and it remains to be determined what contribution these projections make to either the visual or the movement-related responses of the cells in these layers.

Taken together, the results just described indicate that the major sources of input to the deep layers of the superior colliculus in mammals involve projections from two regions of the forebrain, the cortex and the basal ganglia. In several ways, this pattern of connections is reminiscent of the projections to another area concerned with the initiation of movement, the motor cortex. For example, both the motor cortex and the deep collicular layers receive cortical projections that arise primarily outside of the primary sensory areas (Jones and Powell, 1970; Pandya and Seltzer, 1982). Both the motor cortex and the deep layers of the superior colliculus also receive major projections from the basal ganglia. The motor cortex receives input from the basal ganglia by way of relays through the globus pallidus and the ventral nuclei of the thalamus (Nauta, 1979a). The deep tectum receives similar projections from an apparent analog of the globus pallidus, substantia nigra pars reticulata (e.g., Nauta, 1979b). As we shall see in the next section, the similarities between the deep tectum and motor cortex also extend to the receipt of projections from a second extrapyramidal motor structure, the cerebellum.

D. Cerebellar Connections with the Superior Colliculus

Several studies have shown that the cerebellum projects to the deep layers of the superior colliculus (Angaut, 1969; Kawamura *et al.*, 1982; Roldan and Reinoso-Suárez, 1981; May and Hall, 1983). In the cat, the medial and intermediate deep cerebellar nuclei give rise to these projections (Angaut, 1969; Kawamura *et al.*, 1982; Roldan and Reinoso-Suárez, 1981). In the gray squirrel, the projections arise from the intermediate nucleus (May and Hall, 1983) and their terminations are concentrated in the inner sublamina of the intermediate gray layer. This suggests once again a close association between an extrapyramidal motor input and the cells of origin of the predorsal bundle (Fig. 17). The cerebellum receives visual information both from the cortex (Brodal, 1972a,b) and from the superficial layers of the superior colliculus (Holcombe and Hall, 1981a) by way of relays in the lateral pontine nuclei (Mower *et al.*, 1979). It also contains neurons whose responses are related in various ways to the production of eye movements (Hepp *et al.*, 1982). Although, like the substantia nigra pars reticulata, the cerebellum receives visual input and projects to the tectal sublamina containing the cells of origin of the predorsal bundle, recent work sug-

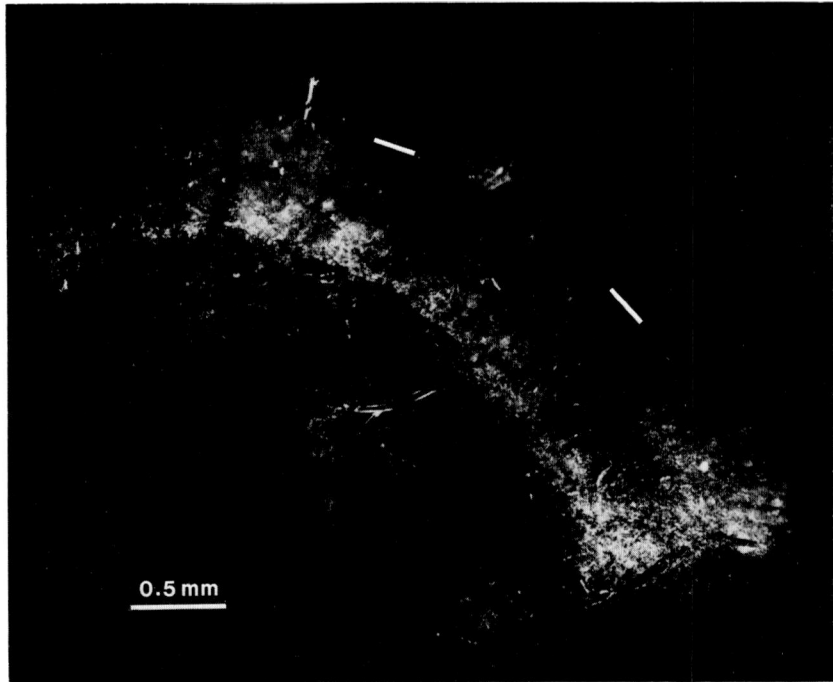

FIG. 17. The cerebellotectal pathway in the gray squirrel. A band of patches of terminals is present in the deepest part of striatum griseum intermediale following an injection into the intermediate deep cerebellar nucleus. The outer border of the intermediate gray layer is designated by the white bars.

gests its contributions may lie in the relatively long-term modulation of tectal activity to correct for saccadic errors, rather than in the initiation of the motor responses in these cells (Optican and Miles, 1979; Optican and Robinson, 1980). Whatever its contribution, it seems reasonable to suggest that the cerebellar–tectal pathway is analogous in function to the well-known pathway from the cerebellum to motor cortex that relays in the ventral nuclei of the thalamus.

V. CONCLUSIONS

A persistent problem in the study of the superior colliculus has been to identify the pathways through which sensory systems influence the eye movement-related responses of cells in the deep layers. In particular, it has been difficult to establish connectional relationships between the deep eye movement-related cells and neurons in the superficial, visual sensory layers of the colliculus. The research discussed above suggests that for understanding these relationships it is important to distinguish between two types of responses that can be recorded from the movement-related neurons of the deep layers. The saccade-related responses of these cells are probably primarily responsible for initiating the premotor activity of neurons in the brainstem gaze centers (Grantyn et al., 1979; Keller, 1979; Sparks et al., 1977; Sparks, 1978; Sparks and Pollack, 1977; Sparks and Mays, 1981). However, many of the cells with saccade-related responses also exhibit a sensory response that is temporally linked to the onset of the target of the eye movement. Sensory responses have been recorded not only to visual, but also to auditory, somatosensory, and even infrared stimuli (Dräger and Hubel, 1975; Finlay et al., 1978; Harris and Gammow, 1971). One implication of the studies discussed in this article is that the sensory and motor responses of the deep tectal cells depend on different types of pathways.

The pathway from substantia nigra pars reticulata may provide the input responsible for the initiation of the motor responses. A critical role for the nigrotectal pathway is indicated by the close similarities observed between the saccade-related response patterns of monkey nigrotectal and deep tectal cells. This conclusion is further supported by the close spatial correspondence between the terminal distribution of the nigrotectal pathway and the dendritic fields of the cells projecting to brainstem gaze centers via the predorsal bundle. Even in nonmammals, which may have monosynaptic connections between the retina and the tectal output cells, pathways from the basal ganglia to the deep tectum have been identified and probably play an important role in the initiation of motor responses in the tectal cells.

Other pathways, such as those from prefrontal cortex and the cerebellum, may also project preferentially to the cells of origin of the predorsal bundle. However, even though neurons that exhibit saccade-related responses are present in these areas (Goldberg and Bushnell, 1981; Hepp et al., 1982), the response patterns of these neurons do not correspond in a simple fashion to those of the deep tectum, and it seems unlikely that either structure plays a primary role in initiating the movement-related responses of deep tectal cells. Instead, there is considerable evidence that the cerebellum plays an important role in mediating adaptive corrections in the control of eye movements (Optican and Miles, 1978; Optican and Robinson, 1980). The role of prefrontal cortex is less well understood, but the studies in the monkey (Schiller, 1977; Schiller et al., 1980) suggest that its main influences on eye movements are mediated by pathways in parallel rather than in series with the deep layers of the tectum.

The sensory responses of the movement-related cells may have a variety of sources. In nonmammals, either direct projections from the retina or intracollicular projections may provide the primary source of visual sensory input, but in mammals there appears to be a shift to cortical input from nonprimary visual areas. The sensory responses to nonvisual stimuli that can be recorded in the deep layers may depend either on brainstem pathways (Edwards *et al.*, 1979; Killackey and Erzurumlu, 1981) or on projections from cortex (Kuypers and Lawrence, 1967; Wise and Jones, 1977). In the absence of evidence either for direct interconnections between the superficial and deep layers, or for shared sources of input, we must leave unanswered the question of the significance of the register of visual sensory and motor maps in the superior colliculus of mammals. Indeed, in view of the evidence for direct connections between these layers in nonmammals, it seems reasonable to propose that the register of maps is more a reflection of the premammalian organization of the structure than of any direct interrelationships in mammals.

The roles that the visual and nonvisual sensory inputs play in the initiation of the movement-related responses of the deep tectal cells also remain a puzzle. This puzzle is partly due to the apparent independence of the sensory and motor responses. For example, the movement-related responses of deep tectal cells can occur in the absence of a preceding sensory response, and many movement-related cells may not exhibit sensory responses (Mays and Sparks, 1980; Wurtz and Albano, 1980). Moreover, the motor responses of deep-layer cells in the monkey are still present after ablation of visual cortex, but the cells no longer have visual receptive fields (Schiller *et al.*, 1974). Finally, even if both responses occur in the same cells, as was the case for cells G and H in Fig. 3, the long time delay between visual and the movement-related responses suggests that they may not be causally related (Sparks and Mays, 1981). Similar arguments apply to the inputs to the deep tectum from other sensory modalities, since long temporal delays can also occur between the sensory responses to these stimuli and the eye movement-related responses of the deep tectal cells (Jay and Sparks, 1982).

Regardless of the contributions of the sensory responses to the movement-related activity, the pathways from the basal ganglia must play an important role in determining which deep tectal cells respond prior to a particular saccade. As we discussed earlier, both visual and nonvisual sensory inputs can be traced to substantia nigra pars reticulata via relays in the corpus striatum (Fig. 18). Indeed, these inputs are probably responsible for the finding that the decrease in discharge rate that can be recorded from a nigral neuron is specific for saccades toward targets that lie in the receptive field of the cell (Hikosaka and Wurtz, 1981a). Therefore, the distribution of activity from substantia nigra, rather than the more direct inputs from traditional sensory pathways, may determine the movement-related responses of the tectal output cells.

These conclusions may seem surprising. At one time, it was believed that unraveling the connectional relationships between the superficial and deep layers would provide the key to understandng the basis for sensorimotor transformations in the tectum. But orienting responses are not simply reflex saccades to visual stimuli. Other variables, such as eye position, competition among concur-

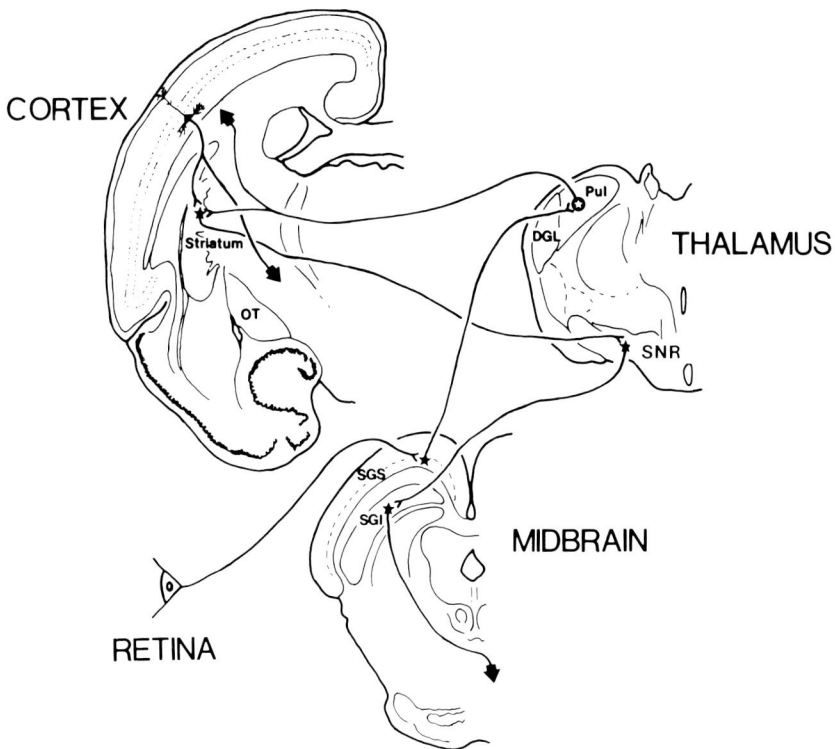

Fig. 18. Summary of pathways linking the basal ganglia with the deep tectal layers. The corpus striatum receives input directly from visual cortex and from the superficial layers of the superior colliculus by way of a relay in the pulvinar. The corpus striatum projects to substantia nigra pars reticulata, which, in turn, projects to the deep tectum. OT, Optic tract; SGS, stratum griseum superficiale; SGI, stratum griseum intermediale; DGL, dorsal lateral geniculate nucleus; Pul, pulvinar; SNR, substantia nigra pars reticulata.

rent stimuli, and past experience, influence the orienting response (Mays and Sparks, 1980; Sparks and Porter, 1983; Hikosaka and Wurtz, 1981b) and this complexity is probably reflected by the multiplicity of inputs—direct and indirect—to the deep layers. However, one important conclusion that has emerged from the studies described above is that pathways to the tectum from the basal ganglia are present and probably play a crucial role in determining the movement-related activity of tectal cells throughout vertebrates. Moreover, if the nigral input is indeed the critical determinant of the movement-related activity in the deep tectum, it is likely that the sensory inputs to the basal ganglia, rather than more direct tectal afferents, play the key role in the selection of an appropriate response. A final conclusion that emerges from this work is that the deep tectal layers—with respect to their connections with the basal ganglia, cerebellum, and cortical nonprimary sensory areas—are remarkably similar to the motor areas of the cortex. Therefore, the sensorimotor transformations mediated by these two diverse structures may eventually be understood in terms of the operation of similar mechanisms.

ACKNOWLEDGMENTS

We would like to thank Drs. M. Behan, J. P. Donoghue, C. S. Lin, J. T. McIlwain, and L. F. Schweitzer for their comments during the preparation of this article. We are especially grateful to Dr. N. B. Cant for her many helpful suggestions. We also thank Mrs. A. Boyd for typing and Ms. L. Klatt for her assistance with the figures.

This work was supported by Public Health Service Grant EY-04060 and by National Science Foundation Grant BNS-8109794.

REFERENCES

Abplanalp, P. (1970). Some subcortical connections of the visual system in tree shrews and squirrels. *Brain Behav. Evol.* **3**, 155–168.

Albano, J. E., Norton, T. T., and Hall, W. C. (1979). Laminar origin of projections from the superficial layers of the superior colliculus in tree shrew, *Tupaia glis*. *Brain Res.* **175**, 1–11.

Altman, J., and Carpenter, M. B. (1961). Fiber projections of the superior colliculus in the cat. *J. Comp. Neurol.* **116**, 157–178.

Angaut, P. (1969). The fastigio-tectal projections. An anatomical experimental study. *Brain Res.* **13**, 186–189.

Beckstead, R. M., and Frankfurter, A. (1982). The distribution and some morphological features of substantia nigra neurons that project to the thalamus, superior colliculus and pedunculopontine nucleus in the monkey. *Neuroscience* **7**, 2377–2388.

Beckstead, R. M., Edwards, S. B., and Frankfurter, A. (1981). A comparison of the intranigral distribution of nigrotectal neurons labelled with horseradish peroxidase in the monkey, cat and rat. *J. Neurosci.* **1**, 121–125.

Behan, M. (1981). Identification and distribution of retinocollicular terminals in the cat: An electron microscopic autoradiographic analysis. *J. Comp. Neurol.* **199**, 1–15.

Behan, M. (1983). An EM-autoradiographic analysis of the projection from cortical areas 17, 18 and 19 to the superior colliculus in the cat. In press.

Benevento, L. A., and Fallon, J. H. (1975). The ascending projections of the superior colliculus in the rhesus monkey (*Macaca mulatta*). *J. Comp. Neurol.* **160**, 339–362.

Bentivoglio, M., Van der Kooy, D., and Kuypers, H. G. J. M. (1979). The organization of the efferent projections of the substantia nigra in the rat. A retrograde fluorescent double labeling study. *Brain Res.* **174**, 1–17.

Berson, D. (1982). Inputs from visual cortex to deep layers of the cat's superior colliculus: The Y-indirect pathway. *Neurosci. Abstr.* **8**, 406.

Berson, D. M., and McIlwain, J. T. (1982). Retinal Y-cell activation of deep-layer cells in superior colliculus of the cat. *J. Neurophysiol.* **47**, 700–714.

Berson, D. M., and McIlwain, J. T. (1983). Visual cortical inputs to the deep layers of cat's superior colliculus. *J. Neurophysiol.* **50**, 1143–1155.

Brodal, P. (1972a). The corticopontine projection from the visual cortex of the cat. I. The total projection and the projection from area 17. *Brain Res.* **39,** 297–317.
Brodal, P. (1972b). The corticopontine projection from the visual cortex of the cat. II. The projection from areas 18 and 19. *Brain Res.* **39,** 319–335.
Butler, A. B., and Northcutt, R. G. (1971). Retinal projections in *Iguana iguana* and *Anolis carolinensis. Brain Res.* **26,** 1–13.
Casagrande, V. A., and Diamond, I. T. (1974). Ablation study of the superior colliculus in the tree shrew *(Tupaia glis). J. Comp. Neurol.* **156,** 207–238.
Chalupa, L. M., and Rhoades, R. W. (1977). Responses of visual, somatosensory and auditory neurons in the golden hamster's superior colliculus. *J. Physiol. (London)* **270,** 595–626.
Chevalier, G., Deniau, J. M., Thierry, A. M., and Feger, J. (1981). The nigro-tectal pathway. An electrophysiological reinvestigation in the rat. *Brain Res.* **213,** 253–263.
Crommelinck, M., Guitton, D., and Roucoux, A. (1977). Retinotopic versus spatial coding of saccades: Clues obtained by stimulating deep layers of cat's superior colliculus. *In* "Control of Gaze by Brain Stem Neurons" (R. Baker and A. Berthoz, eds.), pp. 425–435. Elsevier, Amsterdam.
Dacey, D. M. (1982). Neural organization of the optic tectum in the eastern garter snake, *Thamnophis sirtalis:* Structural analysis of a sensorimotor transformation. Ph.D. Thesis, University of Chicago.
Deniau, J. M., Chevalier, G., and Feger, J. (1978). Electrophysiological study of the nigro-tectal pathway in the rat. *Neurosci. Lett.* **10,** 215–220.
Dräger, U. C., and Hubel, D. H. (1975). Responses to visual stimulation and relationship between visual, auditory, and somatosensory inputs in mouse superior colliculus. *J. Neurophysiol.* **38,** 690–713.
Dray, A. (1979). The striatum and substantia nigra: A commentary on their relationships. *Neuroscience* **4,** 1407–1439.
Ebner, F. F. (1969). A comparison of primitive forebrain organization in metatherian and eutherian mammals. *Ann. N.Y. Acad. Sci.* **167,** 241–257.
Edwards, S. B. (1980). The deep cell layers of the superior colliculus: Their reticular characteristics and structural organization. *In* "The Reticular Formation Revisited: Specifying Functions for a Non-Specific System" (J. A. Hobson and M. A. Brazier, eds.), pp. 193–209. Raven, New York.
Edwards, S. B., Rosenquist, A. C., and Palmer, L. A. (1974). An autoradiographic study of ventral lateral geniculate projections in the cat. *Brain Res.* **72,** 282–287.
Edwards, S. B., Ginsburg, C. L., Henkel, C. K., and Stein, B. E. (1979). Sources of subcortical projections to the superior colliculus in the cat. *J. Comp. Neurol.* **184,** 309–330.
Faull, R. L. M., and Mehler, W. R. (1978). The cells of origin of nigrotectal nigrothalamic and nigrostriatal projections in the rat. *Neuroscience* **3,** 989–1002.
Finlay, B. L., Schneps, S. E., Wilson, K. G., and Schneider, G. E. (1978). Topography of visual and somatosensory projections to the superior colliculus of the golden hamster. *Brain Res.* **142,** 223–235.
Foster, R. E., and Hall, W. C. (1975). The connections and laminar organization of the optic tectum in a reptile *(Iguana iguana). J. Comp. Neurol.* **163,** 397–426.
Frankfurter, A., Beckstead, R. M., and Harting, J. K. (1982). Retinal projections to the deep layers of the superior colliculus in the rat and cat. *Anat. Rec.* **202,** 60.
Garey, L. J., Jones, E. G., and Powell, T. P. S. (1968). Interrelationships of striate and extrastriate cortex with the primary relay sites of the visual pathway. *J. Neurol. Neurosurg. Psychiatry* **31,** 135–157.
Giolli, R. A., and Guthrie, M. D. (1962). The primary optic projections in the rabbit: An experimental degeneration study. *J. Comp. Neurol.* **136,** 99–126.

Glendenning, K. K., Hall, J. A., Diamond, I. T., and Hall, W. C. (1975). The pulvinar nucleus of *Galago senegalensis*. *J. Comp. Neurol.* **161**, 419–458.

Goldberg, M. E., and Bushnell, M. C. (1981). Behavioral enhancement of visual responses in monkey cerebral cortex. II. Modulation in frontal eye fields specifically related to saccades. *J. Neurophysiol.* **46**, 773–787.

Goldman, P. S., and Nauta, W. J. H. (1976). Autoradiographic demonstration of a projection from prefrontal association cortex to the superior colliculus in the rhesus monkey. *Brain Res.* **116**, 145–149.

Gordon, B. (1973). Receptive fields in deep layers of cat superior colliculus. *J. Neurophysiol.* **36**, 157–178.

Graham, J., and Berman, N. (1981). Origins of the projections of the superior colliculus to the dorsal lateral geniculate nucleus and the pulvinar in the rabbit. *Neurosci. Lett.* **26**, 101–106.

Graham, J., and Casagrande, V. A. (1980). A light microscopic and electron microscopic study of the superficial layers of the superior colliculus of the tree shrew (*Tupaia glis*). *J. Comp. Neurol.* **191**, 133–151.

Graham, J., Lin, C.-S., and Kaas, J. H. (1979). Subcortical projections of six visual cortical areas in the owl monkey, *Aotus trivirgatus*. *J. Comp. Neurol.* **187**, 557–580.

Grantyn, A., and Grantyn, R. (1982). Axonal patterns and sites of termination of cat superior colliculus neurons projecting in the tecto-bulbo-spinal tract. *Exp. Brain Res.* **46**, 243–256.

Grantyn, A., Grantyn, R., Robiné, K.-P., and Berthoz, A. (1979). Electroanatomy of tectal efferent connections related to eye movements in the horizontal plane. *Exp. Brain Res.* **37**, 149–172.

Graybiel, A. M. (1974). Visuo-cerebellar and cerebello-visual connections involving the ventral lateral geniculate nucleus. *Exp. Brain Res.* **20**, 303–306.

Graybiel, A. M. (1975). Anatomical organization of retinotectal afferents in the cat: An autoradiographic study. *Brain Res.* **96**, 1–23.

Graybiel, A. M. (1978). Organization of the nigrotectal connection: An experimental tracer study in the cat. *Brain Res.* **143**, 339–348.

Harris, L. R. (1980). The superior colliculus and movements of the head and eyes in cats. *J. Physiol. (London)* **300**, 367–391.

Harris, J. F., and Gammow, I. R. (1971). Snake infrared receptors: Thermal or photochemical mechanism. *Science* **172**, 1252–1253.

Harting, J. K., and Noback, C. R. (1971). Subcortical projections from the visual cortex of the tree shrew (*Tupaia glis*). *Brain Res.* **25**, 21–33.

Harting, J. K., Hall, W. C., Diamond, I. T., and Martin, G. F. (1973). Anterograde degeneration study of the superior colliculus in *Tupaia glis:* Evidence for a subdivision between superficial and deep layers. *J. Comp. Neurol.* **148**, 361–386.

Hepp, K., Henn, V., and Jaeger, J. (1982). Eye movement related neurons in the cerebellar nuclei of the alert monkey. *Exp. Brain Res.* **45**, 253–264.

Hikosaka, O., and Wurtz, R. H. (1981a). The role of substantia nigra in the initiation of saccadic eye movements. *In* "Progress in Oculomotor Research" (A. F. Fuchs and W. Becker, eds.), Vol. 12, pp. 145–152. Elsevier, Amsterdam.

Hikosaka, O., and Wurtz, R. H. (1981b). Response of substantia nigra cells related to saccades to remembered targets. *Neurosci. Abstr.* **7**, 132.

Hoffman, K. P. (1973). Conduction velocity in pathways from retina to superior colliculus in the cat: A correlation with receptive field properties. *J. Neurophysiol.* **36**, 409–424.

Holcombe, V., and Hall, W. C. (1981a). Laminar origin of ipsilateral tectopontine pathways. *Neuroscience* **6**, 255–260.

Holcombe, V., and Hall, W. C. (1981b). The laminar origin and distribution of the crossed tectoreticular pathways. *J. Neurosci.* **1**, 1103–1112.

Holländer, H. (1970). The projection from the visual cortex to the lateral geniculate body (LGB): An experimental study with silver impregnation methods in the cat. *Exp. Brain Res.* **10,** 219–235.

Holländer, H. (1974). On the origin of the corticotectal projections in the cat. *Exp. Brain Res.* **21,** 433–439.

Horn, G., and Hill, R. M. (1966). Responsiveness to sensory stimulation of units in the superior colliculus and subjacent tectotegmental regions of the rabbit. *Exp. Neurol.* **14,** 199–223.

Hubbard, J. I., Llinás, R., and Quastel, D. M. J. (1969). "Electrophysiological Analysis of Synaptic Transmission," pp. 248–253. Williams & Wilkens, Baltimore, Maryland.

Hubel, D. H., LeVay, S., and Wiesel, T. N. (1975). Mode of termination of retinotectal fibers in Macaque monkey: An autoradiographic study. *Brain Res.* **96,** 25–40.

Humphrey, N. K. (1968). Responses to visual stimuli of units in the superior colliculus of rats and monkeys. *Exp. Neurol.* **20,** 312–340.

Ingle, D. J., and Quinn, S. (1982). Retrograde labelling of neurons of known behavioral function in frog tectum. *Neurosci. Abstr.* **8,** 406.

Jay, M. F., and Sparks, D. L. (1982). Auditory and saccade-related activity in the superior colliculus of the monkey. *Neurosci. Abstr.* **8,** 951.

Jayaraman, A., Batton, R. R., III, and Carpenter, M. B. (1977). Nigrotectal projections in the monkey: An autoradiographic study. *Brain Res.* **135,** 147–152.

Jones, E. G., and Powell, T. P. S. (1970). An anatomical study of converging sensory pathways within the cerebral cortex of the monkey. *Brain* **93,** 793–820.

Jones, E. G., Coulter, J. D., Burton, H., and Porter, R. (1977). Cells of origin and terminal distribution of corticostriatal fibers arising in the sensory-motor cortex of monkey. *J. Comp. Neurol.* **173,** 53–80.

Kass, L., Loop, M. S., and Hartline, P. H. (1978). Anatomical and physiological localization of visual and infrared cell layers in tectum of pit vipers. *J. Comp. Neurol.* **182,** 811–820.

Kawamura, K., and Hashikawa, T. (1978). Cell bodies of origin of reticular projections from the superior colliculus in the cat: An experimental study with the use of horseradish peroxidase as a tracer. *J. Comp. Neurol.* **182,** 1–16.

Kawamura, S., and Kobayashi, E. (1975). Identification of laminar origin of some tecto-thalamic fibers in the cat. *Brain Res.* **91,** 281–285.

Kawamura, S., Sprague, J. M., and Niimi, K. (1974). Corticofugal projections from the visual cortices to the thalamus, pretectum and superior colliculus in the cat. *J. Comp. Neurol.* **158,** 339–362.

Kawamura, S., Fukushima, N., Hattori, S., and Tashior, T. (1978). A ventral lateral geniculate nucleus projection to the dorsal thalamus and midbrain in the cat. *Exp. Brain Res.* **31,** 95–106.

Kawamura, S., Fukushima, N., Hattori, S., and Kudo, M. (1980). Laminar segregation of cells of origin of ascending projections from the superficial layers of the superior colliculus in the cat. *Brain Res.* **184,** 486–490

Kawamura, S., Hattori, S., Higo, S., and Matsuyama, T. (1982). The cerebellar projections to the superior colliculus and pretectum in the cat: An autoradiographic and horseradish peroxidase study. *Neuroscience* **7,** 1673–1689.

Keller, E. L. (1979). Colliculoreticular organization in the oculomotor system. *Prog. Brain Res.* **50,** 725–734.

Kemp, J. M., and Powell, T. P. S. (1970). The cortico-striate projection in the monkey. *Brain* **93,** 525–546.

Killackey, H. P., and Erzurumlu, R. S. (1981). Trigeminal projections to the superior colliculus of the rat. *J. Comp. Neurol.* **201,** 221–242.

Kuypers, H. G. J. M., and Lawrence, D. G. (1967). Cortical projections to the red nucleus and the brain stem in the rhesus monkey. *Brain Res.* **4,** 151–188.

Laties, A. M., and Sprague, J. M. (1966). The projection of optic fibers to visual centers in the cat. *J. Comp. Neurol.* **127,** 35–70.

Leichnetz, G. R. (1980). An anterogradely-labeled prefrontal cortico-oculomotor pathway in the monkey demonstrated with HRP gel and TMB neurohistochemistry. *Brain Res.* **198,** 440–445.

Leichnetz, G. R., Spencer, R. F., Hardy, S. G. P., and Astruc, J. (1981). The prefrontal corticotectal projection in the monkey; an anterograde and retrograde horseradish peroxidase study. *Neuroscience* **6,** 1923–1041.

Lin, C. S., and Hall, W. C. (1982). Visual pathways from the superficial superior colliculus to the basal ganglia. *Neurosci. Abstr.* **8,** 294.

Lund, R. D. (1966). The occipitotectal pathway of the rat. *J. Anat.* **100,** 51–62.

Lund, R. D. (1969). Synaptic patterns in the superficial layers of the superior colliculus of the rat. *J. Comp. Neurol.* **135,** 179–208.

Lund, R. D. (1972a). Synaptic patterns in the superficial layers of the superior colliculus of the monkey, *Macaca mulatta*. *Exp. Brain Res.* **15,** 194–211.

Lund, R. D. (1972b). Anatomic studies on the superior colliculus. *Invest. Ophthalmol.* **11,** 434–144.

Marchiafava, P. L., and Pepeu, G. C. (1966). Electrophysiological study of tectal responses to optic nerve volley. *Arch. Ital. Biol.* **104,** 406–420.

Mathers, L. H., and Mascetti, G. G. (1975). Electrophysiological and morphological properties of neurons in the ventral lateral geniculate nucleus of the rabbit. *Exp. Neurol.* **46,** 506–520.

May, P. J., and Hall, W. C. (1980). The morphology and ultrastructure of tectal neurons with known efferent projections. *Soc. Neurosci. Abstr.* **6,** 751.

May, P. J., and Hall, W. C. (1981). A relationship between nigrotectal and crossed tectoreticular pathways in the grey squirrel. *Soc. Neurosci. Abstr.* **7,** 776.

May, P. J., and Hall, W. C. (1982). Visual input to the intermediate grey layer of the optic tectum. *Invest. Ophthalmol. Visual Sci.* **22,** 245.

May, P. J., and Hall, W. C. (1983). Projections from motor structures to eye movement-related neurons in the superior colliculus. *Anat. Rec.* **205,** 127A.

Mays, E. L., and Sparks, D. L. (1980). Dissociation of visual and saccade-related responses in superior colliculus neurons. *J. Neurophysiol.* **43,** 202–232.

McIlwain, J. T., and Buser, P. (1968). Receptive fields of single cells in the cat's superior colliculus. *Exp. Brain Res.* **5,** 314–325.

Michael, C. R. (1972). Functional organization of cells in superior colliculus of the ground squirrel. *J. Neurophysiol.* **35,** 833–846.

Miles, F. A. (1983). Plasticity in the transfer of gaze. *Trends Neurosci.* **6,** 57–60.

Mohler, C. W., and Wurtz, R. H. (1976). Organization of monkey superior colliculus: Intermediate layer cells discharging before eye movements. *J. Neurophysiol.* **39,** 722–744.

Mower, G., Gibson, A., and Glickstein, M. (1979). Tectopontine pathway in the cat: Laminar distribution of cells of origin and visual properties of target cells in dorsolateral pontine nucleus. *J. Neurophysiol.* **42,** 1–15.

Nauta, H. J. W. (1979a). Projections of the pallidal complex: An autoradiographic study in the cat. *Neuroscience* **4,** 1853–1873.

Nauta, H. J. W. (1979b). A proposed conceptual reorganization of the basal ganglia and telencephalon. *Neuroscience* **4,** 1875–1881.

Nauta, W. J. H., and Mehler, W. R. (1966). Projections of the lentiform nucleus in the monkey. *Brain Res.* **1,** 3–42.

Niimi, K., Kanaseki, T., and Takimoto, T. (1963). The comparative anatomy of the ventral nucleus of the lateral geniculate body in mammals. *J. Comp. Neurol.* **121,** 313–323.

Nudo, R. J., and Masterton, R. B. (1983). Tectospinal tract in mammals. *Anat. Rec.* **205,** 145A.

Otpican, L. M., and Miles, F. A. (1979). Visually induced adaptive changes in oculomotor control signals. *Soc. Neurosci. Abstr.* **5,** 380.

Optican, L. M., and Robinson, D. A. (1980). Cerebellar-dependent adaptive control of primate saccadic system. *J. Neurophysiol.* **44,** 1058–1076.

Pandya, D. N., and Seltzer, B. (1982). Association areas of the cerebral cortex. *Trends Neurosci.* **5**(11), 386–390.

Raczkowski, D., Casagrande, V. A., and Diamond, I. T. (1976). Visual neglect in the tree shrew after interruption of the descending projections of the deep superior colliculus. *Exp. Neurol.* **50,** 14–29.

Ramón y Cajal, S. (1911). "Histologie du Système Nerveux de L'homme et des Vertébrés," Vol. II. Instituto Ramón y Cajal, Madrid.

Reale, R. A., and Imig, T. J. (1983). Auditory cortical field projections to the basal ganglia of the cat. *Neuroscience* **8,** 67–86.

Reiner, A., Brauth, S. E., Kitt, C. A., and Karten, H. J. (1980). Basal ganglionic pathways to the tectum: Studies in reptiles. *J. Comp. Neurol.* **193,** 565–589.

Reiner, A., Brecha, N. C., and Karten, H. J. (1982). Basal ganglia pathways to the tectum: The afferent and efferent connections of the lateral spiriform nucleus of pigeon. *J. Comp. Neurol.* **208,** 16–36.

Rhoades, R. W., Juo, D. C., Polcer, J. D., Fish, S. E., and Voneida, T. J. (1982). Indirect visual cortical input to the deep layers of the hamster's superior colliculus via the basal ganglia. *J. Comp. Neurol.* **208,** 239–254.

Rinvik, E., Grofová, I., and Ottersen, O. P. (1976). Demonstration of nigrotectal and nigroreticular projections in the cat by axonal transport of proteins. *Brain Res.* **112,** 388–394.

Robinson, D. A. (1972). Eye movements evoked by collicular stimulation in the alert monkey. *Vision Res.* **12,** 1795–1808.

Robson, J. A., and Hall, W. C. (1977). Organization of the pulvinar in the grey squirrel (*Sciurus carolinensis*). I. Cytoarchitecture and connections. *J. Comp. Neurol.* **173,** 355–388.

Roldan, M., and Reinoso-Suárez, F. (1981). Cerebellar projections to the superior colliculus in the cat. *J. Neurosci.* **1,** 827–834.

Schiller, P. H. (1977). The effect of superior colliculus ablation on saccades elicited by cortical stimulation. *Brain Res.* **122,** 154–156.

Schiller, P. H., and Koerner, F. (1971). Discharge characteristics of single units in superior colliculus of the alert rhesus monkey. *J. Neurophysiol.* **34,** 920–937.

Schiller, P. H., and Stryker, M. (1972). Single-unit recording and stimulation in superior colliculus of the alert rhesus monkey. *J. Neurophysiol.* **35,** 915–924.

Schiller, P. H., Stryker, M., Cynader, M., and Berman, N. (1974). Response characteristics of single cells in the monkey superior colliculus following ablation or cooling of visual cortex. *J. Neurophysiol.* **37,** 181–194.

Schiller, P. H., True, S. C., and Conway, J. L. (1980). Deficits in eye movements following frontal eye-field and superior colliculus ablations. *J. Neurophysiol.* **44,** 1175–1189.

Schneider, G. E. (1969). Two visual systems: Brain mechanisms for localization and discrimination are dissociated by tectal and cortical lesions. *Science* **163,** 895–902.

Schneider, G. E. (1973). Early lesions of superior colliculus: Factors affecting the formation of abnormal retinal projections. *Brain Behav. Evol.* **8,** 73–109.

Segal, R. L., Edwards, S. B., and Beckstead, R. M. (1982). Identification of visual cortical areas that project to the superficial or deep layers of the superior colliculus in cats. *Neurosci. Abstr.* **8,** 672.

Sereno, M. (1982). Axonal and dendritic morphology of tectoreticular cells in a turtle, *Pseudemys scripta*. *Neurosci. Abstr.* **8,** 951.

Sparks, D. L. (1978). Functional properties of neurons in the monkey superior colliculus: Coupling of neuronal activity and saccade onset. *Brain Res.* **156,** 1–16.

Sparks, D. L., and Mays, L. E. (1981). The role of the monkey superior colliculus in the control of

saccadic eye movements: A current perspective. *In* "Progress in Oculomotor Research" (A. F. Fuchs and W. Becker, eds.), Vol. 12, pp. 137–144. Elsevier, Amsterdam.
Sparks, D. L., and Pollack, J. G. (1977). The neural control of saccadic eye movements: The role of the superior colliculus. *In* "Eye Movements" (B. A. Brooks and F. J. Bajandas, eds.), pp. 179–219. Plenum, New York.
Sparks, D. L., and Porter, J. D. (1983). Spatial localization of saccade targets. II. Activity of superior colliculus neurons preceding compensatory saccades. *J. Neurophysiol.* **49**, 64–74.
Sparks, D. L., Mays, L. E., and Pollack, J. G. (1977). Saccade-related unit activity in the monkey superior colliculus. *In* "Control of Gaze by Brainstem Neurons" (R. Baker and A. Berthoz, eds.), pp. 437–444. Elsevier, Amsterdam.
Spear, P. D., Smith, D. C., and Williams, L. L. (1977). Visual receptive-field properties of single neurons in cat's ventral lateral geniculate nucleus. *J. Neurophysiol.* **40**, 390–409.
Sprague, J. M. (1975). Mammalian tectum: Intrinsic organization, afferent inputs, and integrative mechanisms. Anatomical substrate. *Neurosci. Res. Prog. Bull.* **13**(2), 204–213.
Sprague, J. M., and Meikle, T. H., Jr. (1965). The role of the superior colliculus in visually guided behavior. *Exp. Neurol.* **11**, 115–146.
Stein, B. E., and Gaither, N. S. (1981). Sensory representation in reptilian optic tectum: Some comparisons with mammals. *J. Comp. Neurol.* **202**, 69–87.
Sterling, P. (1971). Receptive fields and synaptic organization of the superficial gray layer of the cat superior colliculus. *Vision Res.* **11**, (Suppl. 3), 309–328.
Straschill, M., and Hoffmann, K. P. (1969). Functional aspects of localization in the cat's tectum opticum. *Brain Res.* **13**, 274–283.
Stryker, M. P., and Schiller, P. H. (1975). Eye and head movements evoked by electrical stimulation of monkey superior colliculus. *Exp. Brain Res.* **23**, 103–112.
Swanson, L. W., Cowan, W. M., and Jones, E. G. (1974). An autoradiographic study of the efferent connections of the ventral lateral geniculate nucleus in the albino rat and the cat. *J. Comp. Neurol.* **156**, 143–164.
Székely, G. (1973). Anatomy and synaptology of the optic tectum. *In* "Handbook of Sensory Physiology" (R. Jung, ed.), Vol. 7 (Part B). Central Processing, pp. 1–26. Springer-Verlag, Berlin and New York.
Székely, G., Sétáló, G., and Lázár, G. (1973). Fine structure of the frog's optic tectum: Optic fiber termination layers. *J. Hirnforsch.* **14**, 189–225.
Updyke, B. V. (1974). Characteristics of unit responses in superior colliculus of the cebus monkey. *J. Neurophysiol.* **37**, 896–909.
Wickelgren, B. G. (1971). Superior colliculus: Some receptive field properties of bimodally responsive cells. *Science* **173**, 69–72.
Wise, S. P., and Jones, E. G. (1977). Cells of origin and terminal distribution of descending projections of the rat somatic sensory cortex. *J. Comp. Neurol.* **175**, 129–158.
Wurtz, R. H., and Albano, J. E. (1980). Visual-motor function of the primate superior colliculus. *Annu. Rev. Neurosci.* **3**, 189–226.
Wurtz, R. H., and Goldberg, M. E. (1971). Superior colliculus cell responses related to eye movements in awake monkeys. *Science* **171**, 82–84.
Wurtz, R. H., and Goldberg, M. E. (1972). Activity of superior colliculus in behaving monkey. III. Cells discharging before eye movements. *J. Neurophysiol.* **35**, 575–586.
Yoshida, M., and Precht, W. (1971). Monosynaptic inhibition of neurons of the substantia nigra by caudatonigral fibers. *Brain Res.* **32**, 225–228.
Yoshida, M., Nakajima, N., and Niijima, K. (1981). Effect of stimulation of the putamen on the substantia nigra in the cat. *Brain Res.* **217**, 169–174.

Development of Layers in the Dorsal Lateral Geniculate Nucleus in the Tree Shrew

JUDY K. BRUNSO-BECHTOLD AND VIVIEN A. CASAGRANDE*

DEPARTMENT OF ANATOMY
BOWMAN GRAY SCHOOL OF MEDICINE
WAKE FOREST UNIVERSITY
WINSTON-SALEM, NORTH CAROLINA
AND *DEPARTMENT OF ANATOMY
VANDERBILT SCHOOL OF MEDICINE
NASHVILLE, TENNESSEE

I.	Introduction	41
II.	Features of Lamination in the Mature LGN	43
	A. What Is an LGN Layer?	43
	B. Laminar Organization of the Adult Tree Shrew LGN	44
III.	Development of LGN Layers	49
	A. Early Stages of LGN Development: Cell Proliferation and Migration	49
	B. Development of Cytoarchitectural and Cytological Features of Lamination	50
	C. Development of the Laminar Pattern of Afferent Projections	56
IV.	The Role of Retinogeniculate Fibers in the Development of Individual Features of Lamination	62
	A. Effect of Enucleation on the Development of the Cytological and Cytoarchitectural Features of Layers	63
	B. Effect of Enucleation on the Development of the Laminar Pattern of Afferent Terminations	69
V.	A Model of LGN Development	71
	References	74

I. INTRODUCTION

The heterogeneity in the microscopic anatomy of the vertebrate nervous system is readily apparent by looking at low-power magnifications of stained sections of the brain and spinal cord. Variations exist in cell distribution, size, morphology, and staining intensity. The variations are notably consistent between brains of a single species and in fact are remarkably consistent even between unrelated species. The consistency of these cellular variations suggests that predictable rules govern major developmental events such as proliferation, migration, differentiation, cell death, and formation of intercellular connections. A knowledge of the way these events interact and contribute to the formation of cellular patterns within the brain may shed light on general principles of nervous system development as well as on overall nervous system organization.

The cellular patterns in the nervous system reflect a functional organization in that they dictate the types of physiological interactions that can take place. One of the most obvious patterns of cellular distribution is that of stratification of cells into layers. Such layers are particularly striking in regions of cerebral and cerebellar cortex, hippocampus, superior colliculus, and certain thalamic nuclei such as the dorsal lateral geniculate nucleus. In these structures the layers segregate cells into groups that help determine their functional role. For example, in humans normal visual function depends upon normal development of layers in the dorsal lateral geniculate nucleus (LGN), the major relay of visual information from the eye to the visual cortex. In addition to humans, many other mammals, such as monkeys and tree shrews, have conspicuously laminated LGNs (Walls, 1953; Polyak, 1957; Hassler, 1964; Kaas et al., 1972, 1978; Casagrande et al., 1978; Guillery, 1979). The development of LGN layers forms an interesting set of complex ontogenetic problems. First of all, the layers of the LGN must segregate input into functionally distinct pathways. Not only is information typically segregated by left and right eye but by other parameters as well. For example, in species such as tree shrews such segregation involves laminar separation of input from ON-center and OFF-center ganglion cells (Conway et al., 1980). In other species LGN layers segregate input from classes of retinal ganglion cells in terms of X-, Y-, and W-functional characteristics (Norton and Casagrande, 1982). Second, each layer must develop in retinotopic register with every other layer. Finally, all other visual afferent pathways also terminate in the LGN in precise topographic alignment with the retinal terminations. The development of such a precise and complex organization presents a considerable challenge to the developing nervous system.

In this article we shall consider the ontogenetic sequence by which layers form in the LGN. In the first section we shall discuss what we mean by lamination, and shall use the tree shrew LGN as an example. In the next section we shall focus on the normal sequence of events involved in the process of laminar formation. With the normal sequence of LGN development in mind, we shall then discuss what manipulations of the system have revealed about mechanisms that produce the mature laminar organization. In the final section we shall suggest a working model to explain how each developmental event might contribute to the formation of LGN layers in the adult. Throughout the article we shall rely heavily on our own work on LGN development in the tree shrew (*Tupaia belangeri*). This species is particularly well suited for an ontogenetic investigation of LGN laminar development because the LGN layers in the adult are very distinct and form primarily postnatally.

II. FEATURES OF LAMINATION IN THE MATURE LGN

A. What Is an LGN Layer?

In order to understand how LGN layers form, one must first define what is meant by a layer. Typically what comes to mind at the mention of LGN layers is a textbook schematic drawing of stacked sheets of cells separated by relatively cell-free interlaminar spaces in the human LGN. Actually, this pattern of *cytoarchitectural* lamination is the hallmark of the LGN in relatively few mammals. Most of the species that are characterized by this feature of lamination are ones such as our own relatives, the primates, and a few other species that rely heavily on visual acuity. Such cytoarchitectural lamination into cell layers separated by interlaminar spaces presumably reflects selective pressure to segregate functionally distinct groups of cells. This feature of lamination is not present in such common laboratory mammals as rats, rabbits, and hamsters, which exhibit no cell layers within their LGN.

Another way that LGN layers can be defined is by *cytological* features. The most obvious example of this feature concerns the laminar differences in cell size between the magno- and parvocellular layers of primate LGN. Even in species that do not have as dramatic cytological differences between layers as do primates, there are some cytological features that distinguish individual layers. In cats and tree shrews, for example, there are subtle cytological differences between cells of individual layers enabling the layers to be distinguished by cell size and staining intensity (Guillery, 1970; Casagrande *et al.*, 1978).

Even in the absence of cytoarchitectural and cytological features of lamination, most mammals exhibit laminar segregation of retinal input to the LGN (Kaas *et al.*, 1972, 1978; Guillery, 1979). Such *afferent* lamination is easily revealed by injection of one eye with any one of a variety of neuronal tracers. Layers of retinogeniculate input exhibit remarkable variability; for example, certain marsupials (Royce *et al.*, 1976; Sanderson and Pearson, 1977, 1981; Sanderson, 1980) exhibit more than 10 layers of retinogeniculate input. In many species the LGN can be divided into more retinogeniculate input layers than cell layers (Kaas *et al.*, 1978; Sanderson and Pearson, 1981). In others, such as tree shrews, old world monkeys, and humans, the six layers of retinogeniculate input match six distinct cell layers (Casagrande and Harting, 1975; Hubel, 1975; Hickey and Guillery, 1978; Kaas *et al.*, 1978). Lamination of the other afferent systems projecting to the LGN is also present in many species. In the tree shrew, for example, extraretinal input tends to "laminate" into bands in the relatively cell-free interlaminar spaces of the nucleus (Casagrande, 1974; Brunso-Bechtold *et al.*, 1982, 1983).

The reason for distinguishing between the cytoarchitectural, cytological, and afferent features of LGN lamination is that studies of LGN development have shown that the ontogenetic sequence of each feature is somewhat distinct and that proper interaction between them is essential to normal laminar formation.

B. Laminar Organization of the Adult Tree Shrew LGN

To illustrate the ideas described above and to lay groundwork for our discussion of LGN laminar development, we will briefly review the organization of the LGN in an adult tree shrew, which has a distinctly laminated LGN. As in other mammals, the tree shrew LGN receives topographic projection from the ipsilateral temporal and contralateral nasal retina (Fig. 1). The visuotopic map within the LGN is organized with central vision represented at the caudomedial pole and peripheral vision represented in a surrounding crescent occupying principally the ventral portion and the rostral pole of the nucleus. In the LGN, upper and lower visual fields are represented roughly within rostral and caudal portions of the nucleus, respectively. In the tree shrew, as in other mammals, individual points in the visual field are represented by lines of cells that run perpendicular to the main axis of the LGN cell layers. These layers are best viewed in the horizontal plane (Fig. 2) and can be distinguished by the three criteria we mentioned earlier, namely, cytoarchitecture, cytology, and afferent innervation (Brunso-Bechtold and Casagrande, 1982). In addition, laminar distinctions can be made based upon differences in the projections of LGN cells to visual cortex and upon differences in their physiological properties.

Taking into account all of these criteria, the six LGN layers can be grouped into two matched pairs (layers 1 and 2 and layers 4 and 5) and two unpaired layers (layers 3 and 6). One member of each matched pair, layer 1 and layer 5, receives ipsilateral retinal input while the remaining four layers receive contralateral retinal input (Fig. 3). Cells in each of the layers are spindle shaped and oriented perpendicular to the axis of the interlaminar spaces except those in layer 6, which appear more scattered. Cells in layers 1 and 2 are medium sized, stain distinctly, respond almost exclusively to the ON-set of light, and project to the upper tier of layer IV of striate cortex (Harting *et al.*, 1973; Conway *et al.*, 1980; Conley *et al.*, 1982; Norton *et al.*, 1983). In contrast, cells in layers 4 and 5 are larger, stain darker, respond to the OFF-set of light, and project to the lower tier

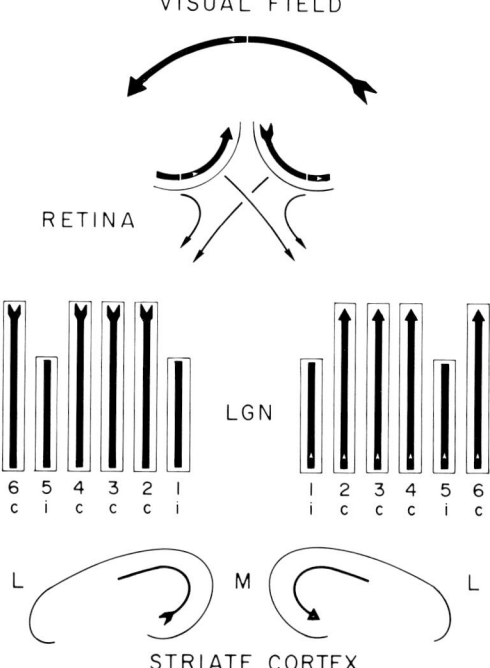

FIG. 1. A schematic drawing of the topographic organization of the retino-geniculo-cortical projection. The nasal portions of each retina project to the contralateral LGN layers 2, 3, 4, and 6 whereas the temporal portions project to the ipsilateral LGN layers 1 and 5. The peripheral or monocular portions of the visual field are represented only in the contralateral projection. Note that a single point in the visual field (white arrow) is represented in immediately adjacent parts of each layer through the nucleus. i, Ipsilateral; c, contralateral; M, medial; L, lateral.

of layer IV of striate cortex (Harting *et al.*, 1973; Conley *et al.*, 1982; Conway *et al.*, 1980; Norton *et al.*, 1983). Finally, cells in the unpaired layers 3 and 6 are smaller, stain paler than those in the other layers, receive predominantly fine-axon input from small ganglion cells, and project mainly to cortical layers above layer IV (Carey *et al.*, 1979; Conley *et al.*, 1982; DeBruyn and Casagrande, 1983).

The mature tree shrew LGN also receives a substantial input from striate cortex and superior colliculus. As can be seen from Fig. 4, this extraretinal input is laminated. Unlike the retinal input that terminates preferentially within the cell layers, the extraretinal input concentrates mainly in the interlaminar spaces (Casagrande, 1974; Brunso-Bechtold *et al.*, 1983), although layer 3 also receives a substantial projection from the superior colliculus. In the adult, the corticogeniculate input concentrates in all interlaminar spaces as well as within a

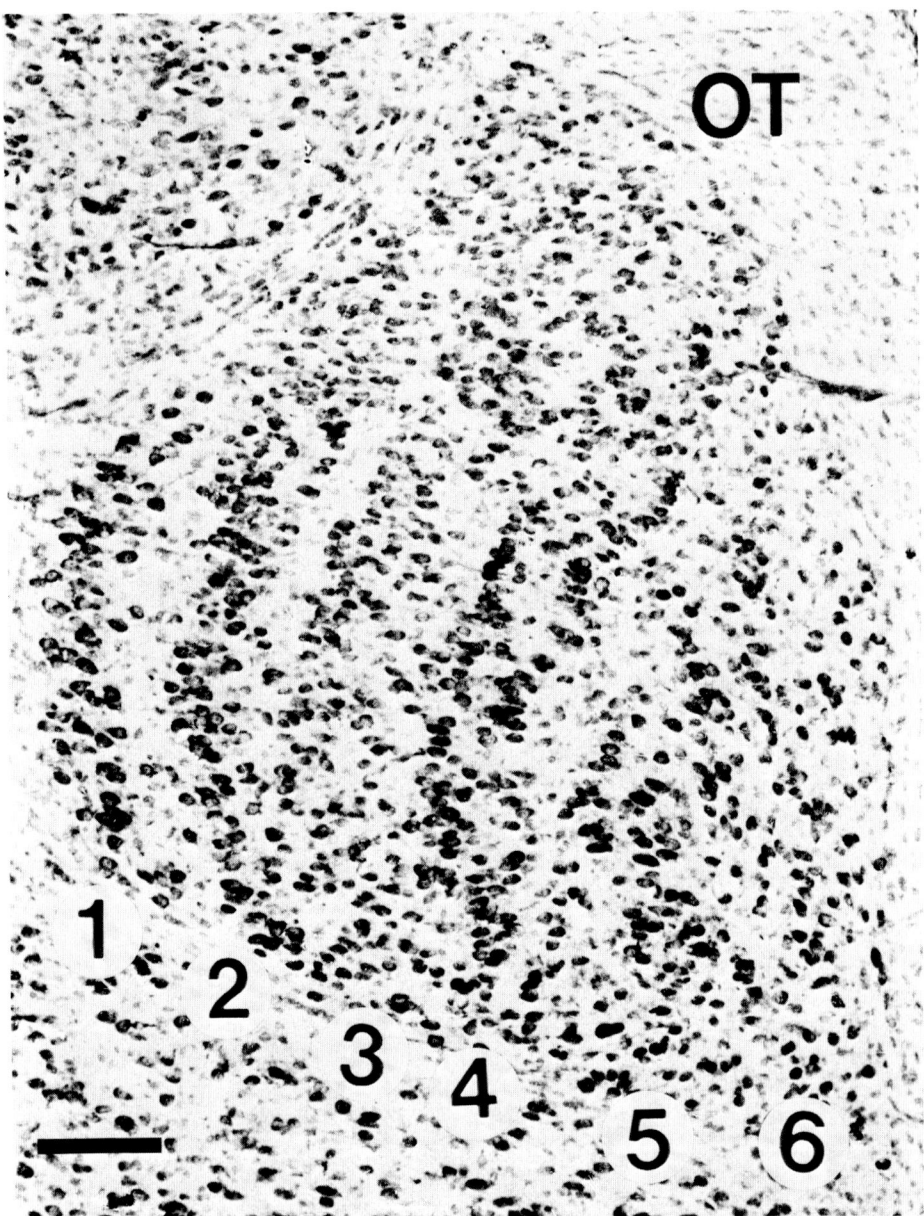

Fig. 2. A horizontal section through the LGN of an adult tree shrew. In this nucleus there are six cell layers separated by relatively cell-free interlaminar spaces and further distinguished by cytological criteria. Note, for example, that the cells in layer 3 are small and pale staining in comparison to those in other layers. The cells in layer 4 are particularly distinct; these large, dark-staining cells also tend to separate into a bilayer. In addition, all cells are clearly oriented perpendicular to the interlaminar spaces except those in layer 6, which tend to appear somewhat scattered. In this and all other photomicrographs, unless otherwise indicated, rostral is toward the top and medial is toward the left. OT, Optic tract. Bar = 0.1 mm.

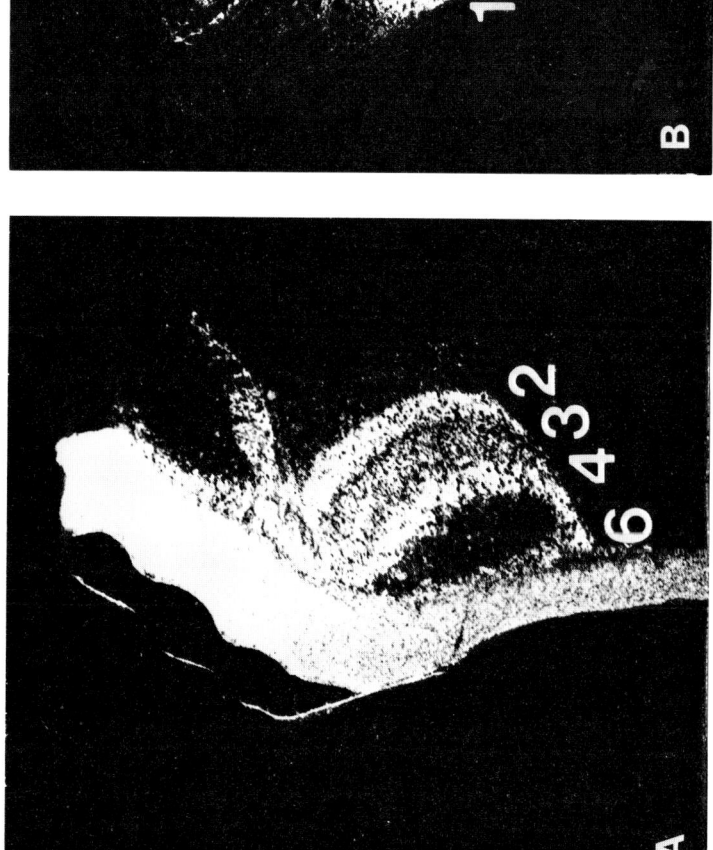

FIG. 3. Low-power dark-field photomicrograph of horizontal sections through the LGN of an adult tree shrew that received an injection of [³H]proline in the right eye. (A) Contralateral to the injected eye; (B) ipsilateral to the injected eye. Medial is at the right in (A) and at the left in (B). Note that all layers *except* 1 and 5 are filled with label and tracer in the contralateral LGN, whereas only layers 1 and 5 are filled with label in the ipsilateral nucleus. Bar = 0.5 mm.

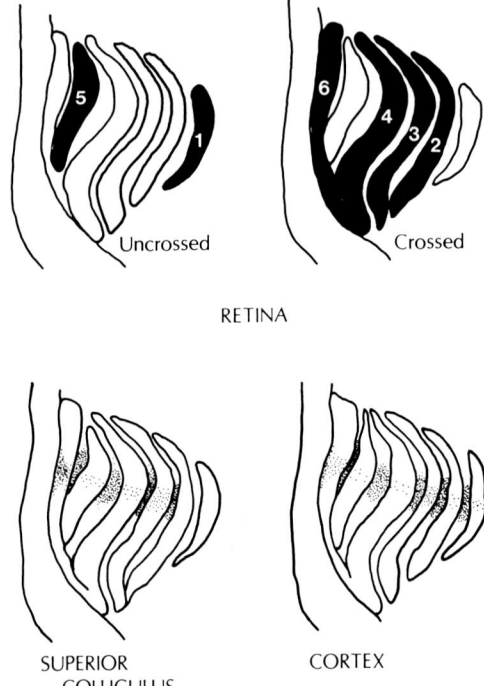

Fig. 4. Schematic drawing of horizontal sections through the LGN in an adult tree shrew, demonstrating the projection patterns of the major afferent pathways to the LGN. Note that each projection terminates in a laminar pattern. The fibers from the retina are laminated in that (1) the ipsilateral retina projects only to layers 1 and 5 and the contralateral retina projects only to layers 2, 3, 4, and 6, and (2) the retinal fibers terminate in the cell layers rather than in the interlaminar spaces. The fibers from the visual cortex and superior colliculus both project predominantly to the interlaminar spaces. The corticogeniculate projection, however, terminates in all of the interlaminar spaces whereas the colliculogeniculate projection does not extend as far medially. In these sections medial is toward the right and rostral is toward the bottom.

band of cells surrounding the nucleus (possibly the equivalent of the perigeniculate nucleus of the cat) (Ide, 1982). In contrast, afferents from the superior colliculus remain restricted to the lateral part of the nucleus and appear to avoid layers 1 and 2 and the interlaminar space between them.

The ultrastructure of the mature tree shrew LGN shares a number of features in common with that of the LGN in other species (Szentagothai, 1963; Wong-Riley, 1972; Casagrande, 1974; Guillery, 1979; Hajdu et al., 1982). The optic terminals are large and contain round vesicles and pale mitochondria, whereas the nonoptic terminals from the visual cortex and superior colliculus are small and contain round vesicles and dark mitochondria (when present). In the tree shrew, optic terminals commonly establish synapses with dendritic shafts and spines and occur most often in large, complex synaptic regions within the cell layers. In contrast, nonoptic terminals are more commonly found in simpler synaptic zones in the interlaminar spaces (Casagrande, 1974; Guillery and Casagrande, unpublished observations).

In general, the basic organization and connections of the tree shrew LGN apply to other species with well-developed, laminated lateral geniculate nuclei. Details, of course, differ with species specialization. For example, lamination of extraretinal inputs appears either to be unique to, or at least more distinct in, some species such as the tree shrew. Also, individual features of lamination vary between species. However, such differences do not obscure basic cross-species similarities in structure as well as in the ontogenetic sequence by which LGN layers develop.

III. DEVELOPMENT OF LGN LAYERS

Having defined the various features of LGN lamination and described the laminar organization in the mature LGN, we will now consider the development of that lamination. In this section, we will briefly describe what is known about the earliest developmental events of proliferation and migration in the LGN. We will then focus specifically on the development of cytoarchitectural and cytological features of lamination and, finally, on the development of laminar patterns of afferent input.

A. Early Stages of LGN Development: Cell Proliferation and Migration

Thus far, our work on the tree shrew has not addressed the timing of LGN cell proliferation. However, several studies in different species have addressed this early ontogenetic event. In all mammalian species studied, cells destined for the LGN are generated quite early, i.e., well before birth (e.g., Rakic, 1977c; Altman and Bayer, 1979). In the rhesus monkey these neuroblasts are generated near the surface of the third ventricle during the first half of gestation and subsequently migrate to the edge of the diencephalon, with first-born cells ending up at the lateral-most edge of the nucleus and cells born last ending up at the medial-most edge, resulting in an "outside-in" pattern of cell birthdates (Rakic, 1977c). In contrast Shatz (1983) has reported an "inside-out" pattern of cell birthdates in the cat. It is noteworthy that in mammals with laminated LGNs the layers tend to run parallel to the optic tract, which at all early stages of development lies in a lateral position. Either an outside-in (lateral to medial) or an inside-out (medial to lateral) pattern of cellular proliferation would then suggest that the cells within individual cell layers are born at roughly the same time. An equally interesting observation is that, according to Rakic (1977b), lines of cells in the adult monkey LGN that represent the same point in the visual field appear to originate from the same stem cell population within the germinal epithelium. These observations may relate to data suggesting that the cytological features of individual layers as well as topographic organization can develop independent of retinal input (Brunso-Bechtold and Casagrande, 1981; Brunso-Bechtold et al., 1983).

B. Development of Cytoarchitectural and Cytological Features of Lamination

As the postmitotic LGN cells migrate to their positions in the anlage of the nucleus, a stratified organization is not initially present. At this early time in development, Nissl-stained LGN sections reveal a nucleus that is undifferentiated and homogeneous, both cytoarchitecturally as well as cytologically. This absence of laminar differentiation has been reported in numerous species, including humans, monkeys, tree shrews, cats, ferrets, and squirrels (Rakic, 1977a,c; Hitchock and Hickey, 1980; Brunso-Bechtold and Casagrande, 1981, 1982; Linden et al., 1981; Cusick and Kaas, 1982; Shatz, 1983; G. Rager, personal communication). Because the tree shrew is born at a relatively early stage of LGN development (when LGN layers are undifferentiated), all subsequent stages can easily be followed postnatally. Thus, we will describe our own studies on development of LGN lamination in this species (Brunso-Bechtold and Casagrande, 1982) as an example of subsequent events in LGN laminar formation.

In marked contrast to the obvious LGN lamination in the adult tree shrew (Fig. 2) is the lack of LGN lamination in the neonatal tree shrew shown in Fig. 5A. This is a photomicrograph of a Nissl-stained horizontal section through the middle of the LGN in a tree shrew sacrificed within the first 6 hours of life (PND 0[1]). Not only are the regional differences in cytology not present at birth, but at that time the cells are extremely immature. The cell bodies at this stage of development have indistinct nuclear borders, multiple nucleoli, and scant cytoplasm and are in contrast to those in the adult, which have clear nuclear

---

[1]We refer to the first 24 hours of life as postnatal day (PND) 0, the second full day of life as PND 1, and so on. It should also be noted that the developmental stage of the animal may vary at birth. Consequently, our emphasis is not on the absolute time of occurrence of a developmental event but rather on the time of occurrence of events relative to each other, e.g., the beginning of lamination of afferent projections relative to interlaminar space formation.

borders, single or double nucleoli, and abundant, well-staining cytoplasm. At the electron microscopic level the cells also appear quite immature, with scant cytoplasm, and are often present in clusters of as many as seven contiguous cell bodies. One such group is shown in the montage of electron micrographs shown in Fig. 6. Although synaptic profiles are not abundant in this part of the tree shrew LGN at birth, the one shown in Fig. 7A demonstrates that mature synapses are present at that age. The afferent source of synapses present at this stage is not yet clear. However, because the retinal input is at a more advanced stage of development at birth than is the extraretinal input, it seems reasonable to suppose that at least some of the profiles we see at birth are retinogeniculate terminals. Other studies support this view (Hendrickson and Rakic, 1977). The LGN on PND 0 is further characterized by the presence of numerous dendritic growth cones as defined by the criteria of Skoff and Hamburger (1974). An example of a growth cone is shown in Fig. 7B. Such growth cones are characterized by a dendrite filled with neurotubules that fan out into a large terminal swelling. The terminal swellings of the growth cones are filled with a flocculent material and occasional mitochondria, but otherwise are quite free of organelles.

The first of the laminar features to become apparent in Nissl-stained material is the formation of interlaminar spaces. These do not all form at the same time, however. The first interlaminar spaces to become evident in the tree shrew are those between layers innervated by opposite eyes. Hints of these spaces can first be seen between layers 1 and 2 and layers 4 and 5 by PND 2–4. These spaces are marked by arrows in the section through the middle of the nucleus on PND 3 shown in Fig. 5B. Several days after interlaminar space formation has begun between layers innervated by opposite eyes, the cell distribution in the block of layers innervated by the same eye (i.e., layers 2, 3, and 4) begins to change subtly (PND 5–8). Figure 5C shows a section through the LGN of a tree shrew sacrificed on PND 7 as incipient interlaminar spaces between those layers (i.e., borders of layer 3) are beginning to be evident. In Fig. 3D (PND 8), interlaminar spaces are clearly present, although they are still considerably narrower than those seen in the adult (cf. Fig. 2). Another cytoarchitectural feature that develops during the first postnatal week is the formation of a dense line of cells that can be seen just medial to the lateral-most interlaminar space in Fig. 5B and C. This line of cells is destined to form the outer segment of a split of layer 4 into a bilayer that can be seen by PND 8 (Fig. 5D).

The period of maturation of cytological characteristics overlaps the time during which the interlaminar spaces are forming. During the time of interlaminar space formation between layers innervated by opposite eyes, the cells are becoming more spindle shaped and oriented, although they otherwise appear quite immature. It is during the period of interlaminar space formation between layers innervated by the same eye that the cells are developing the specific features characteristic of individual layers. At the electron microscopic level, cells at this

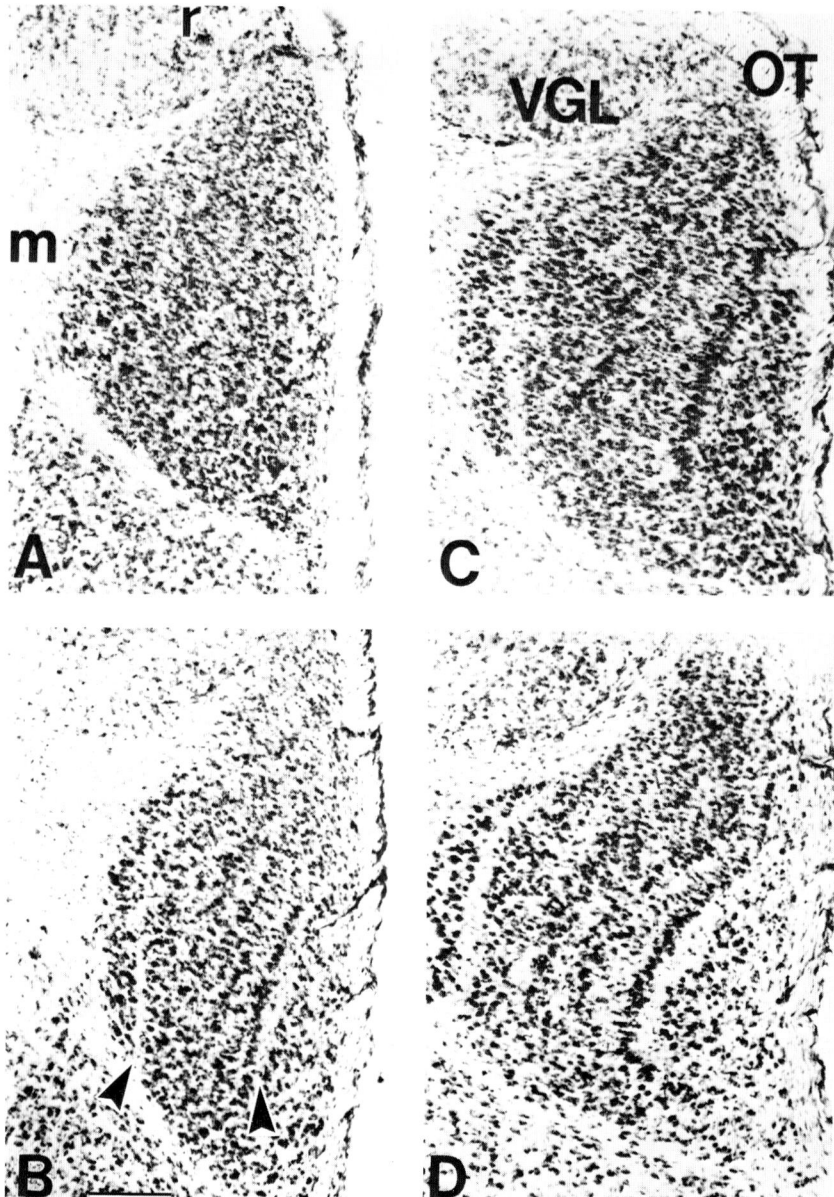

FIG. 5. Horizontal sections through the LGN of tree shrews at various stages of laminar development. (A) PND 0, prior to any cytoarchitectural or cytological lamination. (B) PND 3, during the period of formation of interlaminar spaces between layers innervated by opposite eyes. The arrows indicate the beginnings of interlaminar spaces between layers 1 and 2 and layers 4 and 5. In addition to interlaminar spaces, other cytoarchitectural features, such as the increase in cell density at the outer

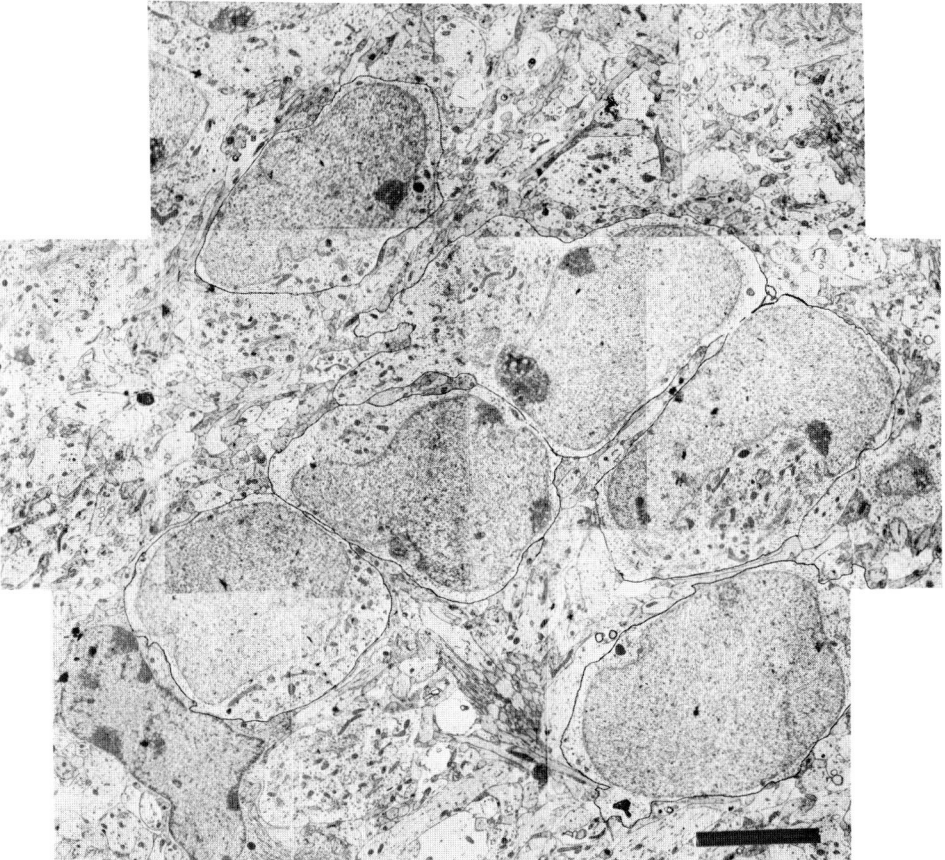

Fig. 6. Montage of electron micrographs from layer 1 of a tree shrew on PND 0, in which the neuronal outlines have been enhanced. Note the immature appearance and scant cytoplasm of the somata. Many cells at this stage of development are in groups with immediately adjacent somata. Bar = 5 μm.

stage are clearly more mature than on PND 0; they are spaced farther apart and show many indications of being in a highly active metabolic state. Nuclei are clearly eccentric and there is abundant cytoplasm rich in rough endoplasmic reticulum, free ribosomes, and Golgi apparatus. Interestingly, the neurons at this stage have dendritic outgrowths that tend to be oriented in the same direction.

By the second postnatal week cytological features that characterize the adult

---

edge of presumptive layer 4, begin to appear at this time. (C) PND 6, during the period of formation of interlaminar spaces between layers innervated by the same eye. (D) PND 8, later in the same developmental period as (C). m, Medial; r, rostral; OT, optic tract; VGL, ventral lateral geniculate nucleus. Bar = 0.1 mm. (From Brunso-Bechtold and Casagrande, 1982.)

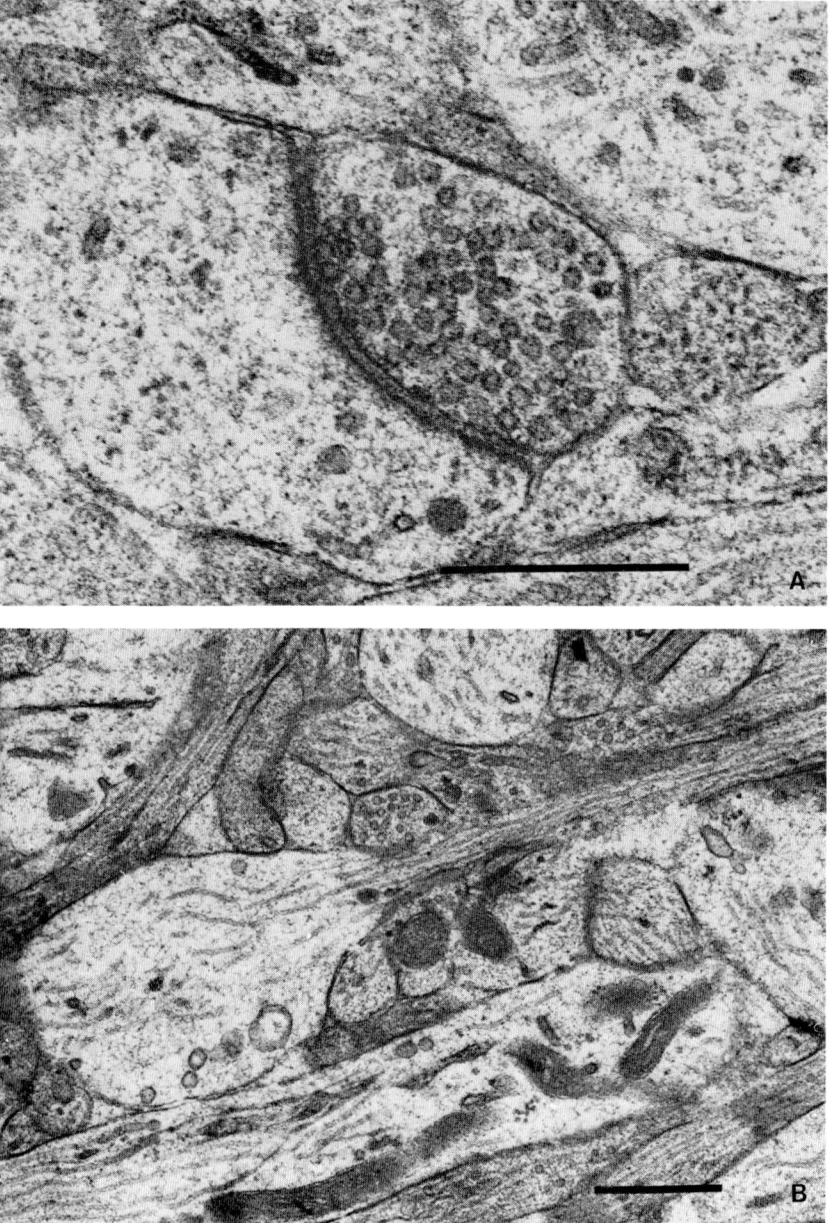

FIG. 7. (A) Synaptic profile from presumptive layer 1 on PND 0. This is a small-type synaptic terminal that is quite mature in appearance. Note the distinct vesicles and well-defined pre- and postsynaptic membranes. Bar = 0.5 μm. (B) Dendritic growth cone from presumptive layer 1 on

nucleus are clearly recognizable at the light microscopic level. However, ultrastructural details such as the presence of dendritic growth cones suggest that maturation is not complete. In addition, the interlaminar spaces continue to widen even after this time. In fact, the nucleus continues to grow in volume with a peak at PND 39, after which it decreases until PND 82 or close to adulthood (3 months) (Zilles, 1978).

Studies in other species confirm various aspects of the cytological and cytoarchitectural development of layers described for the tree shrew. Birth is obviously an arbitrary point in development, and despite the fact that monkeys (Rakic, 1977c), cats (Kalil, 1978), and humans (Hitchock and Hickey, 1980) are born with clearly laminated LGNs and other species such as the tree shrew (Brunso-Bechtold and Casagrande, 1982; G. Rager, personal communication), gray squirrel (Cusick and Kaas, 1982), and ferret (Linden *et al.*, 1981) develop layers postnatally, in each example the cytological and cytoarchitectural features develop from an apparently undifferentiated cell mass in the approximate location of the adult LGN. In addition, studies in the ferret (Linden *et al.*, 1981), human (Hitchcock and Hickey, 1980), and cat (Kalil, 1978) indicate that the formation of interlaminar spaces begins when the somata are quite immature. For example, although cell layers have begun to form prenatally in the cat, during the first 8 postnatal weeks the cells triple in size, show tremendous dendritic growth, and the entire nucleus shows a sevenfold increase in volume (Kalil, 1978; Mason, 1981).

Less information is available about the time individual interlaminar spaces appear relative to each other. However, in humans, as in tree shrews, the first interlaminar space appears between layers innervated by opposite eyes, i.e., between magnocellular layers 1 and 2 (Hitchock and Hickey, 1980). In addition, preliminary observations of the human LGN (T. L. Hickey, personal communication) suggest that the one interlaminar space between adjacent layers innervated by the same eye, namely, between layers 2 and 3, begins forming slightly later than all of the other interlaminar spaces. Finally, Hickey (1977) observed in humans that LGN cells in parvo- and magnocellular layers have differential growth rates such that parvocellular neurons reach full size by 6 postnatal months, whereas magnocellular neurons require 2 years to develop fully. The latter observation not only demonstrates that functionally and cytologically distinct cells in different layers mature at different rates but also reinforces the idea that final maturation of cytological features of LGN lamination is a protracted process.

PND 0. The neck of the growth cone opens into a terminal swelling. The swelling contains flocculent material, a few microtubules, and, in some other examples, mitochondria; but it is otherwise relatively free of organelles. Bar = 0.5 μm.

C. Development of the Laminar Pattern of Afferent Projections

We will now turn to a consideration of the development of projection patterns of the major LGN afferents—those from the retina, visual cortex, and superior colliculus. We will begin by considering the retinogeniculate fibers, which arrive in the LGN and begin to segregate by eye prenatally in all animals studied thus far, with the possible exception of the opossum (e.g., Rakic, 1977; Cavalcante and Rocha-Mirana, 1978; So *et al.*, 1978; Frost *et al.*, 1979; Brunso-Bechtold and Casagrande, 1981, 1982; Linden *et al.*, 1981; Shatz, 1983). At this time, the LGN is still cytologically and cytoarchitecturally immature (Brunso-Bechtold and Casagrande, 1981, 1982; Linden *et al.*, 1981; Shatz, 1983).

The arrival of the retinogeniculate fibers from the right and left eyes does not occur simultaneously. In the animals such as hamster, rat, ferret, and cat (So *et al.*, 1978; Bunt and Lund, 1981; Cucchiaro and Guillery, 1982; Shatz, 1983; Bunt *et al.*, 1983), data suggest that the crossed afferents arrive in the LGN prior to uncrossed afferents. These are later joined by uncrossed retinogeniculate fibers, which either project to their adult location immediately (e.g., hamster; So *et al.*, 1978), overlapping the preexisting crossed projection, or which spread beyond their adult location, partially (cat; Shatz, 1983) or completely (monkey; Rakic, 1976, 1977a) overlapping with the crossed projection. Whether these differences really reflect species differences or a problem in quantifying overlap in animals with widely differing ranges of binocular vision remains to be determined. In any case it seems clear that afferents from the right and left retinas overlap for a period of time prior to their segregation.

The initiation of segregation of crossed and uncrossed retinogeniculate fibers has been studied closely by Shatz (1983) in the cat. That study indicates that although the first retinogeniculate fibers arrive in the nucleus prior to the completion of retinal ganglion cell or LGN neuronal proliferation, the main period of retinogeniculate fiber segregation into layers occurs after LGN cells are in place and after the last retinal cells have been added (Shatz, 1983). This suggests that direct interactions between developing fibers and migrating LGN neuroblasts are not solely responsible for the final lamination of the retinogeniculate projection.

It has been popular to assume that this final phase of retinogeniculate lamination involves binocular competition for synaptic space, much as has been described for the development of ocular dominance columns in the visual cortex (LeVay *et al.*, 1980; Rakic, 1981). Although such competition may indeed exist, it does not explain the formation of adjacent layers innervated by the same eye. For example, in the tree shrew, layers 2, 3, and 4 of the LGN are innervated by the contralateral eye (see Fig. 3). Similarly, in the monkey LGN, adjacent layers 2 and 3 are innervated by the ipsilateral eye. Presumably other differences between retinogeniculate fibers or their targets, or both, allow them to segregate into layers when they originate from the same retina.

With respect to the segregation of retinogeniculate fibers it is also noteworthy that in many species there is a dramatic loss of ganglion cells rather late in ontogeny, well after axons have reached the LGN (Lam et al., 1982; Ng and Stone, 1982; Potts et al., 1982; Rakic and Riley, 1982; Sengelaub and Finlay, 1982; Stone et al., 1982). Rakic and Riley (1982) suggested that the loss of optic axons in the monkey is synchronized in time with the segregation of retinogeniculate fibers. Thus, it may be that the segregation of optic fibers within the LGN may be due, in part at least, to ganglion cell loss and to the related loss of axons of those neurons.

In the tree shrew, the segregation of the retinogeniculate fibers is well underway at birth. In fact, the retinogeniculate projection at that time looks quite mature (Brunso-Bechtold and Casagrande, 1981, 1982; G. Rager, personal communication) in comparison with the less mature stage of cytological and cytoarchitectural development present at birth. Figure 8A and B illustrates the results of a monocular injection of [^{3}H]proline on PND 0. In Fig. 8A, showing the LGN contralateral to the injection site, four bands of label can be seen representing presumptive layers 2, 3, 4, and 6; in Fig. 8B, showing the LGN ipsilateral to the injection, two bands of label can be seen representing presumptive layers 1 and 5. The contrasting lack of cytological and cytoarchitectural features of lamination in the LGN at this age is demonstrated in Fig. 8C, a lightfield photomicrograph of the same nucleus shown in Fig. 8B.

Although autoradiographic background is generally high in neonatal tissue, close inspection of Fig. 8A and B suggests that there is label outside the normal adult projection pattern, indicating that at this time retinogeniculate segregation is not entirely complete. A similar conclusion can be drawn from the results of bilateral [^{3}H]proline eye injections in infant tree shrews. Following such eye injections on PND 0, the gaps in label at the laminar borders appear narrower than they are in the adult (Casagrande and Brunso-Bechtold, 1983). Even at PND 5, binocular [^{3}H]proline injections reveal that the retinogeniculate fibers are still present in the interlaminar spaces. The retinogeniculate fibers continue to withdraw from the interlaminar spaces during the period that cytoarchitectural and cytological lamination is occurring. Whether they actually finish segregating before or after the interlaminar spaces are fully formed is difficult to determine. The problem is twofold; first, quantification involves precise definition of the boundaries of layers and spaces between them. Such criteria are difficult to establish and depend on a variety of parameters, including the region of the nucleus, histological tracer, and plane of section, among others. Second, in available light microscopic material, especially that labeled with tritiated or histochemical tracers from the eye, it is often impossible to be certain whether

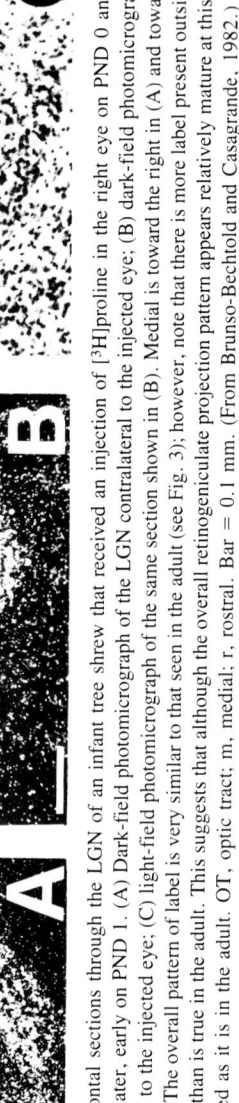
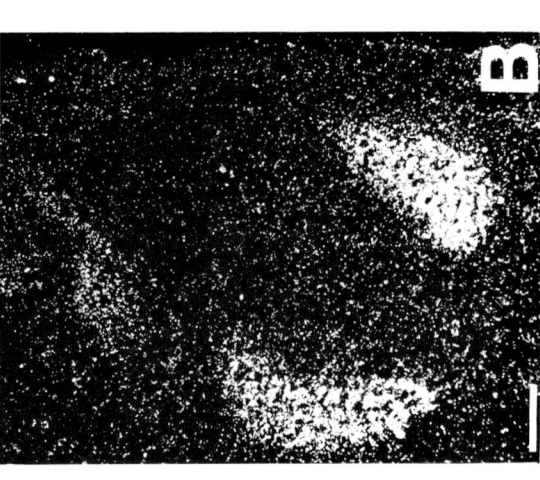
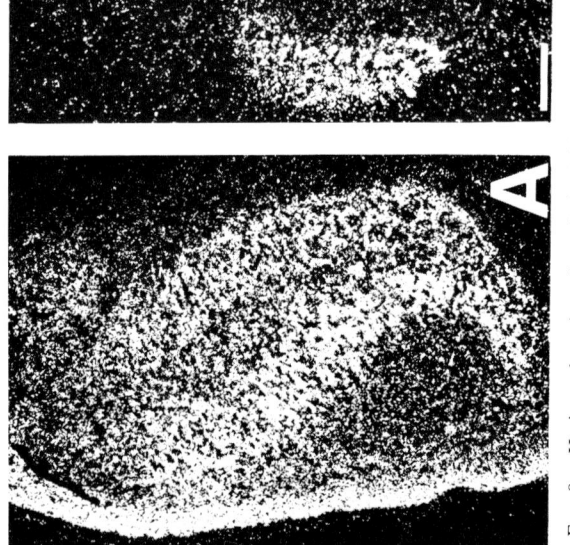

FIG. 8. Horizontal sections through the LGN of an infant tree shrew that received an injection of [³H]proline in the right eye on PND 0 and was perfused 12 hours later, early on PND 1. (A) Dark-field photomicrograph of the LGN contralateral to the injected eye; (B) dark-field photomicrograph of the LGN ipsilateral to the injected eye; (C) light-field photomicrograph of the same section shown in (B). Medial is toward the right in (A) and toward the left in (B) and (C). The overall pattern of label is very similar to that seen in the adult (see Fig. 3); however, note that there is more label present outside the normal target zone than is true in the adult. This suggests that although the overall retinogeniculate projection pattern appears relatively mature at this time, it is not as restricted as it is in the adult. OT, optic tract; m, medial; r, rostral. Bar = 0.1 mm. (From Brunso-Bechtold and Casagrande, 1982.)

the label reflects the terminal points of developing axons, growth cones, fibers of passage, or general background problems encountered with fetal or neonatal tissue. Regardless, evidence in the tree shrew as well as in other species suggests that some overlap of retinogeniculate input destined for individual layers may still be present after LGN cells have begun to separate into those layers.

At birth, the stage of development of the retinogeniculate projection in the tree shrew is considerably advanced in comparison with that of the corticogeniculate projection. At that time the corticogeniculate fibers not only do not demonstrate a laminated projection pattern, but they have only reached the medial extreme of

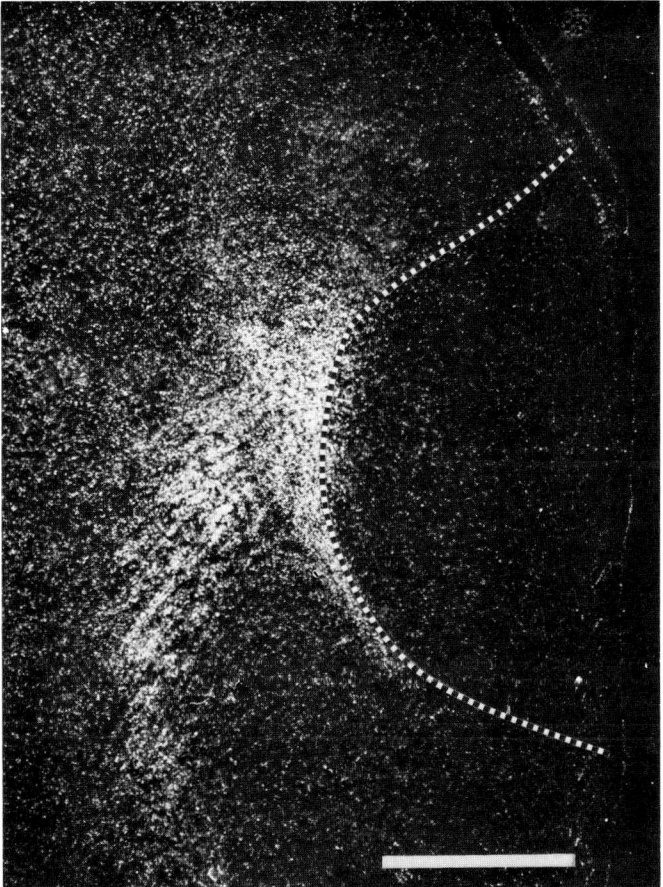

FIG. 9. Dark-field photomicrograph of the pattern of label in the LGN of a tree shrew that received an injection of [^{3}H]proline into the ipsilateral visual cortex on PND 0. Note that although the retinogeniculate projection appears laminated at this stage of development (Fig. 8) the corticogeniculate projection has only reached the medial extreme of the nucleus. Bar = 0.5 mm.

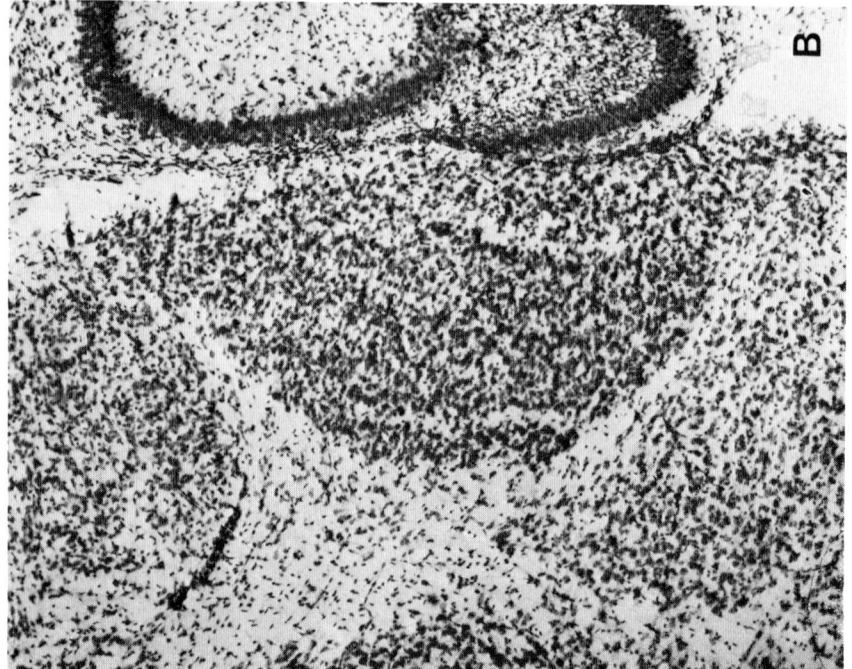
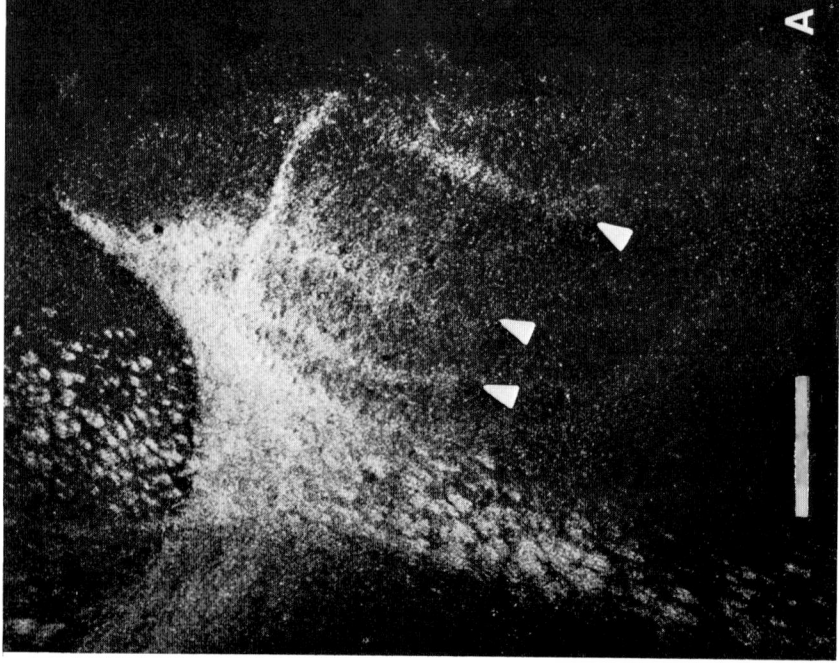

the nucleus (Brunso-Bechtold et al., 1982). This is demonstrated in Fig. 9, which shows the pattern of ^{3}H labeling in the LGN following an injection of [^{3}H]proline into striate cortex on PND 0; significant labeling is only found in the region of presumptive layer 1. During the same period, when the interlaminar spaces form, the corticogeniculate projection also begins to terminate in the interlaminar spaces (Brunso-Bechtold et al., 1982). Figure 10A shows the results of a cortical injection of [^{3}H]proline on PND 5. Three bands of ^{3}H label are apparent; the left and right arrows indicate ^{3}H label in the interlaminar spaces between layers 1 and 2 and layers 4 and 5, respectively. The band of label indicated by the middle arrow is in the position of the border between presumptive layers 2 and 3. A light-field photomicrograph of an adjacent section is shown in Fig. 10B. A comparison between Fig. 10A and B suggests that the corticogeniculate projection concentrates at the laminar borders, either just as the interlaminar spaces are beginning to form or shortly before. It is of particular interest that the retinogeniculate fibers establish a laminar projection pattern by withdrawing from a more extensive innervation, whereas the majority of the corticogeniculate fibers appear to establish a laminar projection pattern immediately upon entering the nucleus.

The rhesus monkey is the only other species for which data are available on the development of the corticogeniculate pathway (Shatz and Rakic, 1981). These data suggest that some corticogeniculate fibers are present prior to the segregation of retinogeniculate fibers by eye and before the formation of cell layers. The corticogeniculate projection appears to be mature by embryonic day 95, which is also when laminar formation is taking place in the monkey LGN. These results, however, are difficult to relate to similar developmental events in the tree shrew LGN for three reasons. First, in the rhesus monkey, the adult corticogeniculate projection is not laminated. Second, Shatz and Rakic (1981) make no temporal distinction between the beginning and end of retinogeniculate fiber segregation by eye. Finally, as is true in most prenatal experiments, the experimental time intervals are rather large, making it difficult to determine the temporal relationships of all events.

At present, the only information available on the development of the col-

---

FIG. 10. (A) Dark-field photomicrograph of the pattern of label in the LGN of a tree shrew that received an ipsilateral cortical injection of [^{3}H]proline on PND 5. There are three clear bands of label indicated by the arrows. The one on the left is between presumptive layers 1 and 2, the one on the right is between layers 4 and 5, and the middle one appears to be in the general location of the border between presumptive layers 2 and 3. Compare this pattern with the pattern of interlaminar spaces in (B), a light-field photomicrograph of an adjacent section. In (B) clear interlaminar spaces are present between layers 1 and 2 and layers 4 and 5, but within presumptive layers 2, 3, and 4 there are only slight irregularities in packing density, indicative of the beginnings of interlaminar spaces. This suggests that these corticogeniculate fibers concentrate as the interlaminar spaces are just beginning to form. Bar = 0.2 mm.

liculogeniculate pathway comes from our own work in the tree shrew (Brunso-Bechtold *et al.*, 1982). These data suggest that at birth the colliculogeniculate projection is more mature than the corticogeniculate projection but less developed than the retinogeniculate pathway. At birth the colliculogeniculate fibers are present within the nucleus and, as in adults, are retinotopically restricted. However, unlike in the adult, the colliculogeniculate pathway at birth appears unlaminated. So far, attempts to follow the development of the colliculogeniculate projection have met with difficulties related to the generally high background that is present in autoradiographs in the neonate. The corticogeniculate projection, however, does appear to concentrate in the developing interlaminar zones slightly ahead of the colliculogeniculate projection. Although these results are preliminary, they suggest two interesting points: (1) Corticogeniculate fibers enter the LGN after arrival of colliculogeniculate afferents, but upon entry immediately concentrate at the site of their mature location; (2) at birth, colliculogeniculate fibers are uniformly distributed across the LGN layers and only later, perhaps after the corticogeniculate fibers have entered the nucleus, concentrate in appropriate interlaminar spaces.

Thus, the timing of lamination of the afferent pathways to the LGN reveals some interesting relationships. The beginning of retinogeniculate fiber segregation begins first, well before other aspects of afferent lamination have begun to develop, and continues after all other features of lamination have begun to form. Although a few fibers may be present earlier, the majority of the corticogeniculate fibers appear to enter the nucleus and immediately form a laminar projection pattern at the approximate time the interlaminar spaces are beginning to form. In contrast, the colliculogeniculate fibers, which are present in a topographic projection column within the LGN prior to the entry of the corticogeniculate fibers, are like the retinogeniculate fibers in that they withdraw from a broad projection into their mature, laminated projection pattern.

IV. THE ROLE OF RETINOGENICULATE FIBERS IN THE DEVELOPMENT OF INDIVIDUAL FEATURES OF LAMINATION

As we have described in the tree shrew, there is a recognizable sequence of development of certain features of LGN layers. The existence of this sequence raises the possibility that the development of an initial feature is a prerequisite for the development of subsequent features. For example, in all species the laminar segregation of retinogeniculate fibers is the first feature of lamination to begin to develop; what, if any, significance does that event have for the development of later features of lamination, such as other afferent projections, cytology, or cytoarchitecture?

Beyond the fact that the primary visual fibers in the LGN begin to laminate before the other features of lamination appear, there are other reasons for suspecting that their presence plays a critical role in the development of the nucleus in which they terminate. Studies in other species in the somatosensory (Woolsey and Wann, 1976; Killackey and Belford, 1980) and auditory systems (Levi-Montalcini, 1949; Parks, 1979), as well as work in the visual system (see Cowan, 1970), have demonstrated that early removal of primary sense organs has dramatic effects on the subsequent development of the central sensory structures relating to those systems. Those effects relate to changes in cytological features such as cell number and morphology as well as to changes in cytoarchitecture. Thus, one might suspect that removing the retinogeniculate fibers would also have an effect on LGN laminar development.

Studies of early enucleation have, for the most part, either focused on the development of an unlaminated visual structure, such as rat LGN, or have removed one eye, which only partially denervates the LGN and does not rule out subsequent axonal and dendritic sprouting within the nucleus. Bilateral enucleation prior to laminar formation, on the other hand, provides an excellent way to approach the issue of the role of the primary sensory fibers in laminar formation. Thus, the remainder of this article will address some of these questions by reviewing our experiments employing bilateral enucleation in the tree shrew. We will also consider how the answers to those questions, together with data from similar experiments in other species, provide support for a proposed model for laminar development.

A. Effect of Enucleation on the Development of the Cytological and Cytoarchitectural Features of Layers

Bilateral enucleation just after birth in the tree shrew removes the retinogeniculate fibers after they have begun to segregate by eye but before any other laminar features have formed. Thus, we can ask whether the initial segregation of retinogeniculate fibers into their laminar projection pattern is the critical event for the subsequent formation of LGN layers. The data from such bilaterally enucleated tree shrews suggest that this is not the case. Figure 11 shows the LGN from an adult animal bilaterally enucleated within the first 6 hours of birth. The most obvious difference between the LGN in this animal and that in a normal adult is that no interlaminar spaces are present in the bilaterally enucleated animal. As in the LGN of a normal tree shrew sacrificed on PND 0, there are occasional variations in packing density but these do not align among sections in a laminar pattern.

Nevertheless, the LGN in the adult tree shrew that was bilaterally enucleated

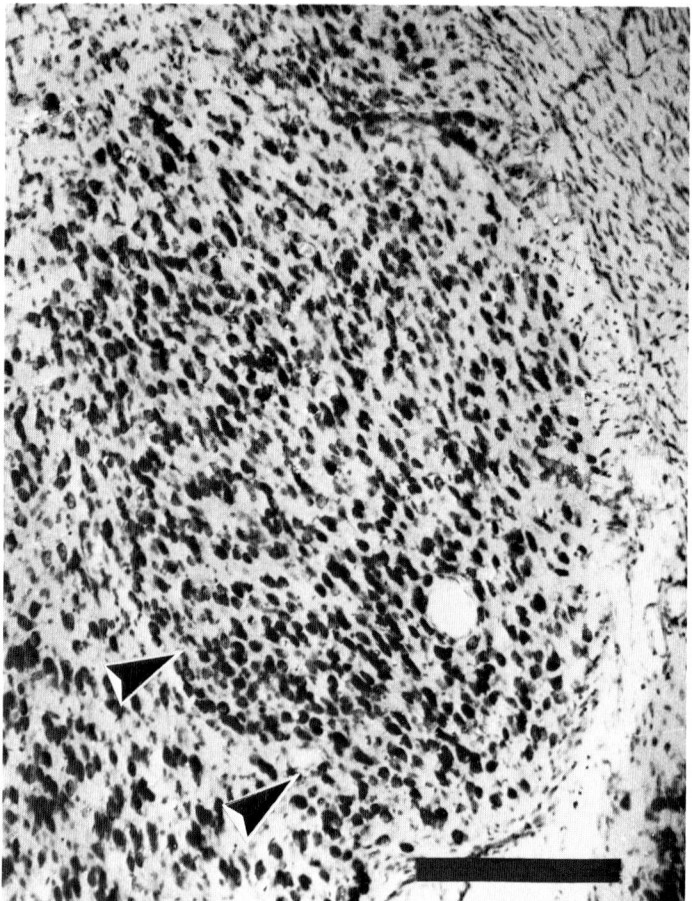

FIG. 11. A horizontal section through the LGN of an adult tree shrew enucleated on PND 0. Note that although interlaminar spaces are absent, indications of laminar borders can be distinguished on the basis of cytological characteristics. For example, the arrows indicate the borders of presumptive layer 4 on the basis of its large, dark-staining cells, which seem to segregate slightly into a bilayer at its rostal end. In addition, the cells just medial to it are somewhat smaller and more pale staining, common characteristics of layer 3. Bar = 0.2 mm.

at birth does not have the same homogeneous appearance as does the LGN in the normal animal sacrificed on PND 0. In several sections throughout the LGN, and exemplified by the one in Fig. 11, other laminar features within the nucleus can be seen. For example, cells in the location of presumptive layer 4 in the bilaterally enucleated animal (indicated by arrows in Fig. 11) are darkly stained and relatively large, as is the case in the LGN of normal animals. Furthermore, the cells in presumptive layer 3, just medial to the left arrow, are more palely stained and smaller. Both of these features are characteristics of cells in the normal layer 3. In addition, as in normal animals, most of the LGN cells are oriented perpendicular to the laminar borders. Finally, hints of the normal segregation of layer 4 into a bilayer can also be seen in the bilaterally enucleated animal. Thus, in the absence of retinogeniculate fibers, the interlaminar spaces do not form although other cytoarchitectural and cytological features of LGN layers do develop.

Understanding the developmental role of the retinogeniculate fibers depends on knowing whether the lack of interlaminar spaces is due to a failure to form or to a deterioration after formation. Our results in animals bilaterally enucleated at birth and sacrificed at various times during the normal period of interlaminar space formation indicate that they simply do not form (Brunso-Bechtold and Casagrande, 1981). Figure 12 shows the LGN from an enucleated animal sacrificed on PND 7, just after all interlaminar spaces normally can be distinguished. In addition to the absence of interlaminar spaces the nucleus in this animal appears quite immature cytologically. Unlike the cells in the normal LGN at PND 7, which are clearly differentiating, the cells in the LGN of the bilaterally enucleated animal appear quite uniform in size and staining intensity, suggesting a retarded maturation. This observation is difficult to relate to data from the visual system of other species because, in most cases, the rate of cellular maturation following enucleation has not been discussed. Peusner and Morest (1977), however, have reported the timetable of development in nucleus vestibularis tangentialis of the chick to be unchanged following deafferentation.

It is, of course, possible that the presence of the retinogeniculate fibers is essential only for the process of interlaminar space formation to begin. If this were true, bilateral enucleation after the first interlaminar spaces had begun to form would have no effect on the formation of the remaining interlaminar spaces. However, our data show that the continued presence of the retinogeniculate fibers is essential. The LGN from an adult tree shrew that was bilaterally enucleated on PND 3 during the formation of interlaminar spaces between layers innervated by opposite eyes (i.e., between layers 1 and 2 and layers 4 and 5) is shown in Fig. 13A. The LGN from a normal littermate that was sacrificed when the experimental animal was enucleated is shown in Fig. 13B. Although the nucleus shown in Fig. 13A somewhat resembles that of a mature tree shrew bilaterally enucleated at birth, interlaminal spaces are clearly more apparent. Interestingly, the interlaminar spaces that are present are those between layers 1 and 2 and layers 4 and 5, suggesting development was arrested at the time of enucleation. Rakic (1981) has reported a similar phenomenon when rhesus monkeys are unilaterally enucleated during laminar development.

The effect of removing retinal input during LGN development has also been described in mice, ferrets, and humans (Duckworth and Cooper, 1966; Cullen and Kaiserman-Abramof, 1976; LaMantia and Guillery, 1982). Although the

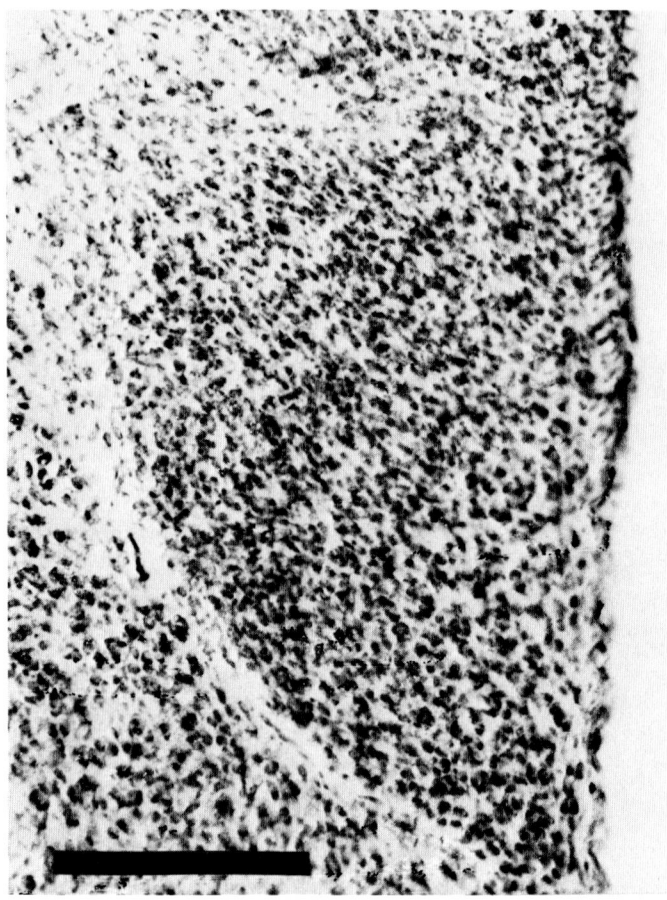

FIG. 12. A horizontal section through the LGN of a tree shrew bilaterally enucleated on PND 0 and perfused on PND 7. In contrast to sections through the LGN in a normal tree shrew at this age, the nucleus in this case is very homogeneous in appearance with no indications of cytological maturation, thus suggesting that the enucleation may result in a slowdown in development. Bar = 0.2 mm.

studies on congenitally anophthalmic and neonatally enucleated mice do not pertain to the issue of laminar development, because LGN layers are absent in those animals, Cullen and Kaiserman-Abramof (1976) do report normal development of cytological characteristics such as size, shape, and dendritic configuration in the LGN of anophthalmic mice. Unlike mice, the mature ferret has a laminated LGN. In the ferret, as in the tree shrew (Brunso-Bechtold and Casagrande, 1981), a preservation of normal cytological characteristics of layers in the absence of interlaminar spaces has been reported following bilateral enuclea-

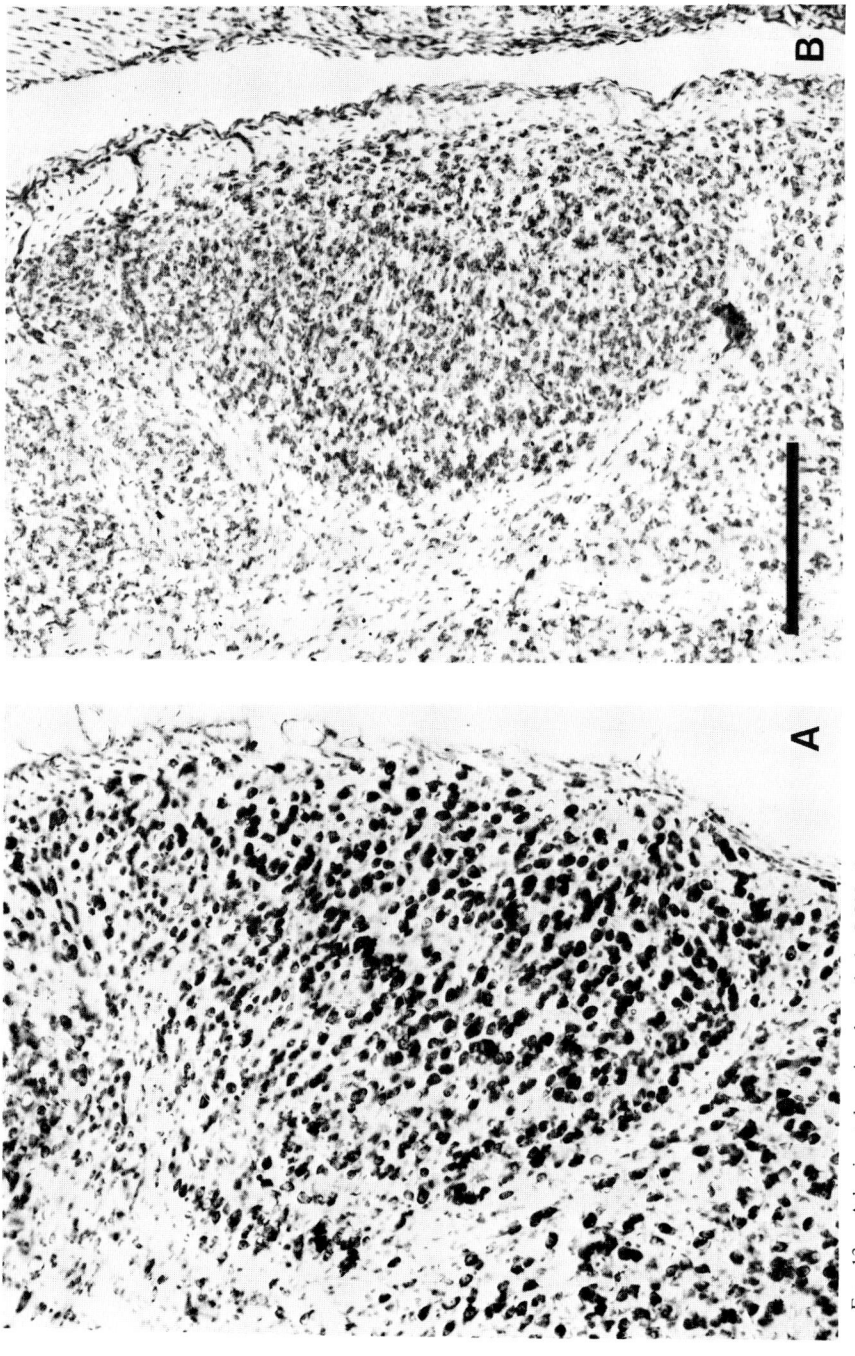

FIG. 13. A horizontal section through the LGN of an adult tree shrew that was bilaterally enucleated on PND 3 (A) at which time its littermate [LGN shown in (B)] was perfused. Note that the only interlaminar spaces present in (A) are those between presumptive layers 1 and 2 and between 4 and 5, which had begun to form at the time of enucleation (B). Bar = 0.2 mm.

tion at a time in development when retinogeniculate fibers have begun to segregate by eye but when no other features of LGN lamination are yet apparent (LaMantia and Guillery, 1982). In congenitally anophthalmic humans, an absence of any laminar formation has been reported (Duckworth and Cooper, 1966). Although the authors do not comment on the cytological characteristics of the nucleus it is apparent from a low-power photomicrograph that interlaminar spaces are absent.

It is important to emphasize that our evaluation of the effect of bilateral enucleation on cytological development is, thus far, based solely on Nissl-stained material. Consequently, although it would not be surprising for bilateral enucleation to affect dendritic, axonal, or other features of cytological development, our present results do not address this point. Studies in other systems, however, indicate that although some cells (e.g., Mauthner cells) begin differentiation prior to arrival of afferents (Piatt, 1947; Kimmel *et al.*, 1977) and other cells (e.g., cells in the chick vestibular system) begin initial dendritic development in the absence of afferents (Peusner and Morest, 1977), attainment of normal, mature dendritic morphology is generally dependent upon the presence of afferent input (e.g., Kelly and Cowan, 1972; Hamori, 1973; Peusner and Morest, 1977).

The formation of spaces between cell layers in the LGN can be compared to the formation of other cytoarchitectural features in different systems. An example in the somatosensory cortex of the rat is that the formation of cellular rings or the barrel fields does not take place completely when the sense organs, the vibrissae, or the thalamic inputs are removed prior to barrel formation (Woolsey and Wann, 1976; Wise and Jones, 1978). Similarly, the superficial layers of the chick optic tectum do not develop if retinal input is removed before the layers have formed (Kelly and Cowan, 1972). As is true for the LGN, the main afferent input to these areas is normally present before cytoarchitectural differentiation takes place (Woolsey and Wann, 1976; Killackey and Belford, 1979; LaVail and Cowan, 1971).

In some other instances, cytoarchitectural differentiation occurs in spite of the absence of the major afferent projection. For example, cellular aggregation into layers can be distinguished in somatosensory cortex in the mature rat thalamotomized at birth (Wise and Jones, 1978). Studies of rat cortical development (Wise and Jones, 1976; Lund and Mustari, 1977) report that laminar differentiation in the cortex takes place while thalamocortical afferents essentially wait in the adjacent white matter, prior to the arrival of callosal afferents (Wise and Jones, 1978). This does not prove that the differentiation of these structures is wholly independent of afferent input. The cytoarchitectural differentiation could be under the control of fibers that may arrive well before the majority of the afferents that have been studied or, as suggested by Wise and

Jones (1976), other extrinsic or intrinsic connections could be playing the critical role.

B. Effect of Enucleation on the Development of the Laminar Pattern of Afferent Terminations

The primary sensory fibers play a potentially important role not only in the formation of characteristic cytological and cytoarchitectural features of structures but also in the formation of the afferent and efferent connections of these structures. For example, the interlaminar spaces that fail to form as a result of bilateral enucleation of tree shrews at birth are also the predominant termination sites of the projection from the visual cortex to the LGN. The obvious question then is, what effect does the absence of interlaminar spaces have on the termination pattern of the corticogeniculate projection which, in normal animals, develops after the time that the experimental animals were bilaterally enucleated?

There are two possible answers to this question. First, there could be no effect on the corticogeniculate termination pattern, resulting in the densest termination of the corticogeniculate fibers at the cytologically defined laminar borders. In that case the projection might resemble that seen between presumptive layers 2 and 3 on PND 5 (Fig. 10), in which the corticogeniculate projection forms a band but in which no interlaminar space is apparent. Second, in the absence of interlaminar spaces, the corticogeniculate projection could simply terminate throughout the cell layers.

This question can be resolved by comparing autoradiographs through the LGN after injections of [^{3}H]proline into the visual cortex of a normal adult tree shrew (Fig. 14A) and into the visual cortex of one that was bilaterally enucleated at birth (Fig. 14B) (Brunso-Bechtold *et al.,* 1983). As can be seen in Fig. 14A, the pattern of LGN label following [^{3}H]proline injections into the cortex of a normal animal is arranged in a discrete column that is densest and broadest in the interlaminar spaces. In contrast, similar injections in enucleated animals result in a restricted column of label stretching across the nucleus but not concentrated at the laminar borders.

Thus, in the absence of retinogeniculate fibers the predominant synaptic site of the corticogeniculate fibers is no longer the laminar borders. The change in termination pattern is probably due to two factors acting together, (1) a synaptic reorganization and (2) incomplete dendritic development. First, in the absence of retinogeniculate fibers, the ingrowing corticogeniculate fibers may occupy the synaptic sites that are normally occupied by fibers from the retinas. These sites appear to be located more proximally on the dendrites and such a shift in synaptic location would result in a denser than normal projection of the corticogeniculate fibers to the central part of the cell layers. Such synaptic reorganization follow-

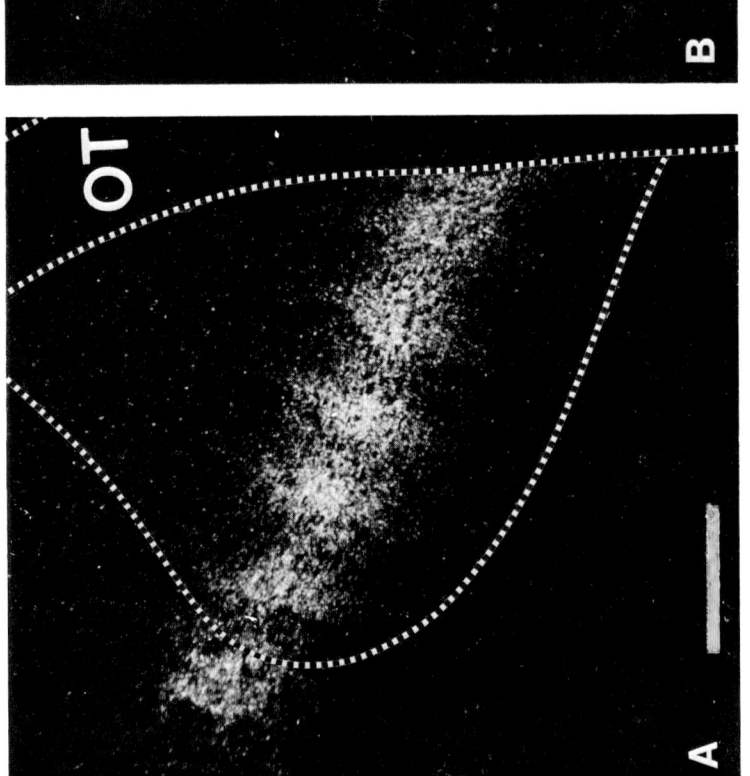

FIG. 14. Dark-field photomicrographs demonstrating the pattern of labeling in horizontal LGN sections following ipsilateral cortical injections of [³H]proline in (A) a normal adult tree shrew and in (B) an adult that was bilaterally enucleated at birth. In the normal animal (A), the concentration of labeled corticogeniculate fibers is densest and broadest in the interlaminar spaces. In contrast, in the animal bilaterally enucleated at birth (B), the corticogeniculate labeling does not concentrate at the laminar borders but instead spreads through the cell layers. In both cases, however, the projection column is topographically restricted. Bar = 0.2 mm.

ing partial deafferentation has been reported in several systems. For example, Cullen and Kaiserman-Abramof (1976) report that in anophthalmic and postnatally enucleated mice the synaptic sites that are normally occupied by retinogeniculate terminals are instead occupied by terminals with a very different morphology. Second, in the absence of retinogeniculate fibers, there may be insufficient ''trophic'' stimulation to produce normal dendritic development of the LGN cells. Consequently, the distal dendrites, which are the predominant synaptic targets of the corticogeniculate projection in normal animals, may never develop, thus providing additional impetus for these fibers to terminate elsewhere. As we have described earlier, the dependence of dendritic development on afferent input has been well documented; however, the degree to which enucleation actually affects the dendritic development of LGN cells will necessarily await the results of ongoing Golgi studies. These two ways in which the absence of retinogeniculate fibers might relate to the absence of a laminated projection pattern of the corticogeniculate fibers are obviously closely interrelated in that one enhances the effect of the other. They further closely relate to a working model of LGN laminar development that we have proposed on the basis of the work we have described.

V. A MODEL OF LGN DEVELOPMENT

Our working model of LGN development represents what we feel to be the most reasonable scenario of developmental events that can be deduced from the known facts. Although additional issues obviously must be explored before a firm model of laminar development can be proposed, it is useful to have a working hypothesis of the mechanisms underlying these developmental events in order to provide direction for further inquiry.

The facts consist of the following: first, the sequence of events in the laminar development in the normal LGN and, second, the response of the developmental events to bilateral enucleation in the neonatal tree shrew. Briefly, the sequence of development of individual features of LGN layers is as follows. Initially, the crossed and uncrossed retinogeniculate fibers begin to segregate. Then, the interlaminar spaces between layers innervated by opposite eyes begin to form. The corticogeniculate fibers enter the nucleus and begin to concentrate in the newly forming interlaminar spaces while the interlaminar spaces between layers innervated by the same eye begin to form. During this latter period, cytological features of individual layers become apparent. Also at this stage of development, the retinogeniculate fibers still are not fully segregated into their mature laminar pattern of termination.

Several changes in the development of laminar features following bilateral enucleation in the neonatal tree shrew may be summarized. Following bilateral enucleation on PND 0, the LGN interlaminar spaces fail to form. Nevertheless, the cell bodies appear to differentiate normally but at a somewhat slower rate. Thus, laminar boundaries in many sections may be distinguished on the basis of cytological differences in the absence of interlaminar spaces. The absence of primary visual afferents also affects the pattern of termination of corticogeniculate fibers. In bilaterally enucleated animals lacking interlaminar spaces these fibers do not terminate at the laminar borders, but instead terminate evenly across the layers. The termination of the fibers, however, remains topographically restricted.

Based on these facts, we make several assumptions. First, we assume that the retinogeniculate fibers have a "trophic" influence on the differentiation and maintenance of LGN cells. This statement is reinforced not only by our own evidence of massive LGN cell death in cases with very short survivals following neonatal enucleation (Brunso-Bechtold and Casagrande, unpublished observations) and the apparently slowed maturation of LGN cells following bilateral enucleation at birth (Brunso-Bechtold and Casagrande, 1981), but also by numerous investigations in other systems (Cowan, 1970). Second, we assume that there is a specificity of connections between target areas (e.g., proximal or distal dendrites) and the afferents that normally innervate them such that any competition between afferents will result in innervation by the type of input that normally innervates that target area.

On the basis of our observations and assumptions we have constructed the following model of LGN development. At birth, a competition between the retinogeniculate fibers from the right and left eyes for synaptic space has resulted in the beginning of segregation of the retinogeniculate projection. At that time, the LGN cells appear undifferentiated. The retinogeniculate fibers have a "trophic" effect on the LGN cells, stimulating dendritic growth and perhaps other features of differentiation. The cells are already organized in appropriate, laminar groups by birth order and/or by initial migration patterns and there is some mechanism of cell-to-cell communication or interaction that helps maintain that organization. Subsequently, as dendritic development takes place, the dendrites from adjacent layers grow toward the laminar borders. As the dendrites are developing the corticogeniculate fibers grow in. Because the synaptic sites on the proximal LGN cell dendrites are occupied by terminals from the retina, the corticogeniculate fibers terminate more distally on the LGN dendrites. This may also provide trophic stimulation for additional dendritic growth which, in turn, provides more synaptic space for later arriving corticogeniculate terminals. The retinogeniculate fibers are prevented from occupying the newly formed synaptic territory by competition with the corticogeniculate fibers that normally terminate on those synaptic sites. The combination of dendritic growth of cells in adjacent layers and the dense projection of the corticogeniculate fibers on the distal LGN cell dendrites thus result in the formation of the interlaminar spaces and the laminar projection pattern of the corticogeniculate fibers. The specificity of retinogeniculate fibers for particular layers plus their competition with the corticogeniculate fibers for synaptic space on the newly forming dendrites result in the segregation of retinogeniculate fibers into their appropriate laminar pattern. This segregation may, of course, partly result from the loss of retinal ganglion cells and/or their fibers in the optic nerve and by other factors that are not yet apparent.

According to this scenario of LGN development, the absence of interlaminar spaces following bilateral enucleation at birth is due to a combination of (1) a reduction of dendritic growth at the laminar borders due to a lack of trophic stimulation by the retinogeniculate fibers and (2) the shift in termination of the corticogeniculate fibers from the laminar borders to the synaptic sites within the cell layers normally occupied by the retinogeniculate terminals. The development of cytological features characteristic of individual layers, in the absence of retinogeniculate fibers, is presumably due to a combination of intrinsic cellular differentiation independent of afferent input and, perhaps to some degree of "trophic" stimulation by intact afferent systems such as the late-arriving corticogeniculate projection. This latter possibility is supported by the retarded but eventual differentiation of the LGN cells in cases lacking retinogeniculate fibers but with intact corticogeniculate fibers.

On the basis of this working model several predictions can be made. For example, the model would predict a temporal correlation between LGN dendritic development and interlaminar space formation. In addition, the model would predict a rearrangement of the synaptic sites of the remaining afferent projections following bilateral enucleation. These and numerous other topics remain to be addressed by Golgi studies and additional ultrastructural studies presently underway. Our current knowledge of the normal development of LGN laminar features and the effect of prior removal of primary visual afferents on the development of those features has provided the framework of a basic model whereby we can begin to explore and understand some of the essential developmental interactions that are taking place in a central nervous system structure with a clearly layered organization.

ACKNOWLEDGMENTS

The authors wish to thank Drs. Robert Bechtold, Ed DeBruyn, Lance Durden, Sherre Florence, Ray Guillery, Ron Oppenheim, and Mike Sesma for editorial comments, Vera Henley for expert typing of the manuscript, and Donna Moore Smith for help in all phases of preparation of this article. The research on the developing tree shrew LGN was supported by the following grants from the National Institutes of Health: EY03881, EY01778, IF32N-526206, and K04-EY00223.

REFERENCES

Altman, J., and Bayer, S. A. (1979). Development of the diencephalon in the rat. IV. Quantitative study of the time of origin of neurons and the internuclear chronological gradients in the thalamus. *J. Comp. Neurol.* **188,** 455–472.

Brunso-Bechtold, J. K., and Casagrande, V. A. (1981). Effect of bilateral enucleation on the development of layers in the dorsal lateral geniculate nucleus. *Neuroscience* **6,** 2579–2586.

Brunso-Bechtold, J. K., and Casagrande, V. A. (1982). Early postnatal development of laminar characteristics in the dorsal lateral geniculate nucleus of the tree shrew. *J. Neurosci.* **2,** 589–597.

Brunso-Bechtold, J. K., Florence, S. L., and Casagrande, V. A. (1982). The development of laminar patterns of extraretinal projections in the dorsal lateral geniculate nucleus. *Neurosci. Abstr.* **8,** 814.

Brunso-Bechtold, J. K., Florence, S.L., and Casagrande, V. A. (1983). The role of retinogeniculate afferents in the development of connections between visual cortex and the dorsal lateral geniculate nucleus. *Dev. Brain Res.* **10,** 33–39.

Bunt, S. M., and Lund, R. D. (1981). Development of a transient retino-retinal pathway in hooded and albino rats. *Brain Res.* **211,** 399–404.

Bunt, S. M., Lund, R. D., and Land, P. W. (1983). Prenatal development of the optic projection in albino and hooded rats. *Dev. Brain Res.* **6,** 147–168.

Carey, R. G., Fitzpatrick, D., and Diamond, I. T. (1979). Layer I of striate cortex of *Tupaia glis* and *Galago senegalensis:* Projections from the thalamus and claustrum revealed by retrograde transport of horseradish peroxidase. *J. Comp. Neurol.* **186,** 393–438.

Casagrande, V. A. (1974). The laminar organization and connections of the lateral geniculate nucleus in tree shrew (*Tupaia glis*). *Anat. Rec.* **178,** 323.

Casagrande, V. A., and Brunso-Bechtold, J. K. (1983). The relationship between afferent laminar development and cell layer formation in the lateral geniculate nucleus (LGN). *Neurosci. Abstr.* **9,** 25.

Casagrande, V. A., and Harting, J. K. (1975). Transneuronal transport of tritiated fucose and proline in the visual pathways of the tree shrew, *Tupaia glis*. *Brain Res.* **96,** 367–373.

Casagrande, V. A., Guillery, R., and Harting, J. K. (1978). Differential effects of monocular deprivation seen in different layers of the lateral geniculate nucleus. *J. Comp. Neurol.* **179,** 469–486.

Cavalcante, L. A., and Rocha-Miranda, C. E. (1978). Postnatal development of retinogeniculate, retinopretectal, and retinotectal projections in the opossum. *Brain Res.* **146,** 231–248.

Conley, M., Fitzpatrick, D., and Diamond, I. T. (1982). Projections of individual lateral geniculate layers to the striate cortex in the tree shrew (*Tupaia glis*). *Neurosci. Abstr.* **8,** 260.

Conway, J., Schiller, P. H., and Misler, L. (1980). Functional organization of the tree shrew lateral geniculate nucleus. *Neurosci. Abstr.* **6,** 583.

Cowan, W. M. (1970). Anterograde and retrograde transneuronal degeneration in the central and peripheral nervous system. *In* "Contemporary Research Methods in Neuroanatomy" (W. J. M. Nauta and S. O. E. Ebbeson, eds.), pp. 217–249. Springer-Verlag, Berlin and New York.

Cucchiaro, J., and Guillery, R. W. (1982). The structure and development of the dorsal lateral geniculate nucleus and its retinal afferents in the albino ferret (*Mustela putorius furo*). *Soc. Neurosci. Abstr.* **8,** 814.

Cullen, M. J., and Kaiserman-Abramof, I. R. (1976). Cytological organization of the dorsal lateral geniculate nuclei in mutant anophthalmic and postnatally enucleated mice. *J. Neurocytol.* **5,** 407–424.

Cusick, C. G., and Kaas, J. H. (1982). Retinal projections in the adult and newborn grey squirrels. *Dev. Brain Res.* **4,** 275–284.

DeBruyn, E. J., and Casagrande, V. A. (1983). Morphological differences in retinal ganglion cells projecting to different layers of the dorsal lateral geniculate nucleus in the tree shrew. *Neurosci. Abstr.* **9,** 2512.

Duckworth, T., and Cooper, E. R. A. (1966). A study of anophthalmia in an adult. *Acta Anat.* **63,** 509–522.

Frost, P. D., So, K. F., and Schneider, G. E. (1979). Postnatal development of retinal projections in Syrian hamsters: A study using autoradiographic and anterograde degeneration techniques. *Neuroscience* **4,** 1649–1677.

Guillery, R. W. (1970). Laminar distribution of retinal fibers in the dorsal lateral geniculate nucleus of the cat: A new interpretation. *J. Comp. Neurol.* **138,** 339–368.

Guillery, R. W. (1979). A speculative essay on geniculate lamination and its development. *In* "Progress in Brain Research: Development and Chemical Specificity of Neurons" (M. Cuenod, G. W. Kreutzberg, and F. E. Bloom, eds.), Vol. 51, pp. 403–418. Elsevier, Amsterdam.

Hajdu, F., Hassler, R., and Wagner, A. (1982). The distribution of crossed and uncrossed optic fibers in the different layers of the lateral geniculate nucleus in the tree shrew (*Tupaia glis*). *Anat. Embryol.* **164,** 1–8.

Hamori, J. (1973). The inductive role of presynaptic axons in the development of post-synaptic spines. *Brain Res.* **62,** 337–344.

Harting, J. K., Hall, W. C., Diamond, I. T., and Martin, G. F. (1973). Anterograde degeneration study of the superior colliculus in *Tupaia glis:* Evidence for a subdivision between superficial and deep layers. *J. Comp. Neurol.* **148,** 361–386.

Hassler, R. (1964). Die zentralen Systeme des Sehens. *In* "Bericht ueber die 66te Zusammenkunft der Deutschen Opthalmologischen Geselschaft, Heidelberg," pp. 229–251. Bergman, Munich.

Hendrickson, A., and Rakic, P. (1977). Histogenesis and synaptogenesis in the dorsal lateral geniculate nucleus (LGd) of the fetal monkey brain. *Anat. Rec.* **187,** 602.

Hickey, T. L. (1977). Postnatal development of the human lateral geniculate nucleus: Relationship to a critical period for the visual system. *Science* **198,** 836–838.

Hickey, T. L., and Guillery, R. W. (1978). Variability of laminar patterns in the human lateral geniculate nucleus. *J. Comp. Neurol.* **183,** 221–246.

Hitchcock, P. F., and Hickey, T. L. (1980). Prenatal development of the human lateral geniculate nucleus. *J. Comp. Neurol.* **194,** 395–412.

Hubel, D. H. (1975). An autoradiographic study of the retinocortical projections in the tree shrew (*Tupaia glis*). *Brain Res.* **96,** 41–50.

Ide, L. S. (1982). The fine structure of the perigeniculate nucleus in the cat. *J. Comp. Neurol.* **210,** 317–335.

Kaas, J. H., Guillery, R. W., and Allman, J. M. (1972). Some principles of organization in the dorsal lateral geniculate nucleus. *Brain Behav. Evol.* **6,** 253–299.

Kaas, J. H., Huerta, M. F., Weber, J. T., and Harting, J. K. (1978). Patterns of retinal terminations and laminar organization of the lateral geniculate nucleus of primates. *J. Comp. Neurol.* **182,** 517–554.

Kalil, R. (1978). Development of the dorsal lateral geniculate nucleus in the cat. *J. Comp. Neurol.* **183,** 265–292.

Kelly, J. P., and Cowan, W. M. (1972). Studies on the development of the chick optic tectum. III. Effects of early eye removal. *Brain Res.* **42,** 263–288.

Killackey, H. P., and Belford, G. R. (1979). The formation of afferent patterns in the somatosensory cortex of the neonatal rat. *J. Comp. Neurol.* **183,** 285–304.

Killackey, H. P., and Belford, G. R. (1980). Central correlates of peripheral pattern alterations in the trigeminal system of the rat. *Brain Res.* **183,** 205–210.

Kimmel, C. D., Skabtach, E., and Kimmel, R. J. (1977). Developmental interactions in the growth and branching of the lateral dendrite of Mauthner's cell (*Amblystoma mexicanum*). *Dev. Biol.* **55,** 244–259.

Lam, K., Sefton, A. J., and Bennett, M. R. (1982). Loss of axons from the optic nerve of the rat during early postnatal development. *Dev. Brain Res.* **3,** 487–491.

LaMantia, A.-S., and Guillery, R. W. (1982). The effects of binocular enucleation on the development of the dorsal lateral geniculate nucleus (DLGN) of the ferret. *Neurosci. Abstr.* **8,** 814.

LaVail, J. H., and Cowan, W. M. (1971). The development of the chick optic tectum. II. Autoradiographic studies. *Brain Res.* **28,** 321–441.

LeGros Clark, W. E. (1959). "The Antecedents of Man." Edinburgh Univ. Press, Edinburgh.

LeVay, S., Wiesel, T., and Hubel, D. (1980). The development of ocular dominance columns in normal and visually deprived monkeys. *J. Comp. Neurol.* **191,** 1–52.

Levi-Montalcini, R. (1949). The development of the acoustico-vestibular centers in the chick embryo in the absence of the afferent root fibers and of descending fiber tract. *J. Comp. Neurol.* **91,** 209–241.

Linden, D. Card, Guillery, R. W., and Cucchiaro, J. (1981). The dorsal lateral geniculate nucleus of the normal ferret and its postnatal development. *J. Comp. Neurol.* **203,** 189–212.

Lund, R. D., and Mustari, M. J. (1977). Development of the geniculocortical pathway in rat. *J. Comp. Neurol.* **173,** 289–306.

Mason, C. A. (1981). Postnatal maturation of lateral geniculate neurons in relation to developing retinal afferents in kitten. *Neurosci. Abstr.* **7,** 675.

Ng, A. Y. K., and Stone, J. (1982). The optic nerve of the cat: Appearance and loss of axons during normal development. *Dev. Brain Res.* **5,** 263–271.

Norton, T. T., and Casagrande, V. A. (1982). Laminar organization of receptive field properties in lateral geniculate nucleus of bushbaby (*Galago crassicaudatus*). *J. Neurophysiol.* **47,** 715–741.

Norton, T. T., Kretz, R., and Rager, G. (1983). On and off regions in layer IV of tree shrew striate cortex. *Invest. Ophthalmol. Visual Sci. Suppl.* **24,** 265.

Parks, T. N. (1979). Afferent influences on the development of the brain stem auditory nuclei of the chicken: Otocyst ablation. *J. Comp. Neurol.* **183,** 665–677.

Peusner, K. D., and Morest, D. K. (1977). Neurogenesis in the nucleus vestibularis tangentialis of the chick embryo in the absence of the primary afferent fibers. *Neuroscience* **2,** 253–270.

Piatt, J. (1947). A study of the factors controlling the differentiation of Mauthner's cell in *Amblystoma*. *J. Comp. Neurol.* **86,** 199–236.

Polyak, S. (1957). "The Vertebrate Visual System." Univ. of Chicago Press, Chicago, Illinois.

Potts, R. A., Dreher, B., and Bennett, M. R. (1982). The loss of ganglion cells in the developing retina of the rat. *Dev. Brain Res.* **3,** 481–486.

Rakic, P. (1976). Prenatal genesis of connections subserving ocular dominance in the rhesus monkey. *Nature (London)* **261,** 467–471.

Rakic, P. (1977a). Prenatal development of the visual system in the rhesus monkey. *Philos. Trans. R. Soc. London Ser. B* **278,** 245–260.

Rakic, P. (1977b). Effect of prenatal unilateral eye enucleation on the formation of layers and retinal connections in the dorsal lateral geniculate nucleus (LG_d) of the rhesus monkey. *Neurosci. Abstr.* **3,** 573.

Rakic, P. (1977c). Genesis of the dorsal lateral geniculate nucleus in the rhesus monkey: Site and time of origin, kinetics of proliferation, routes of migration and pattern of distribution of neurons. *J. Comp. Neurol.* **176,** 23–52.

Rakic, P. (1979). Genesis of visual connections in the rhesus monkey. *In* "Developmental Neurobiology of Vision" (R. D. Freeman, Ed.), pp. 249–276. Plenum, New York.

Rakic, P. (1981). Development of visual centers in the primate brain depends on binocular competition before birth. *Science* **214,** 928–930.

Rakic, P., and Riley, K. P. (1982). Number of axons in the optic nerve of the developing rhesus monkey: Overproduction and elimination before birth. *Neurosci. Abstr.* **8,** 814.

Romer, A. S. (1967). Major steps in vertebrate evolution. *Science* **158,** 1629–1637.

Royce, G. J., Ward, J. P., and Harting, J. K. (1976). Retinofugal pathways in two marsupials. *J. Comp. Neurol.* **170,** 391–414.

Sanderson, K. J. (1980). Binocular segregation in the lateral geniculate nucleus. *Aust. J. Optom.* **63,** 220–226.

Sanderson, K. J., and Pearson, L. J. (1977). Retinal projections in the native cat, *Dasyurus viverrinus*. *J. Comp. Neurol.* **174,** 347–358.

Sanderson, K. J., and Pearson, L. J. (1981). Retinal projections in the hairy-nosed wombat *Lasiorhinus latifrons* (Marsupialis: Vombatidae). *Aust. J. Zool.* **29,** 473–481.

Sengelaub, D. R., and Finlay, B. L. (1982). Cell death in the mammalian visual system during normal development. I. Retinal ganglion cells. *J. Comp. Neurol.* **204,** 311–317.

Shatz, C. J. (1981). Inside-out pattern of neurogenesis in the cat's lateral geniculate nucleus. *Neurosci. Abstr.* **7,** 140.

Shatz, C. J. (1983). The prenatal development of the cat's retinogeniculate pathways. *J. Neurosci.* **3,** 482–499.

Shatz, C. J., and Rakic, P. (1981). The genesis of efferent connections from the visual cortex of the fetal rhesus monkey. *J. Comp. Neurol.* **196,** 287–307.

Skoff, R. P., and Hamburger, V. (1974). Fine structure of dendritic and axonal growth cones in embryonic chick spinal cord. *J. Comp. Neurol.* **153,** 107–148.

So, K. F., Schneider, G. E., and Frost, P. D. (1978). Postnatal development of retinal projections to the lateral geniculate body in Syrian hamsters. *Brain Res.* **142,** 343–352.

Stone, J., Rapaport, D. H., Williams, R. W., and Chalupa, L. (1982). Uniformity of cell distribution in the ganglion cell layer of prenatal cat retina: Implications for mechanisms of retinal development. *Dev. Brain Res.* **2,** 231–242.

Szentagothai, J. (1963). The structure of the synapse in the lateral geniculate body. *Acta Anat. Basel* **55,** 166–185.

Tigges, J. (1966). Ein experimentellet Beitrag zum sub-korikalen optischen System von *Tupaia glis*. *Folia Primat.* **4,** 103–151.

Walls, G. L. (1953). The lateral geniculate nucleus and visual histophysiology. *Physiology* **9,** 1–100.

Wise, S. P., and Jones, E. G. (1976). The organization and postnatal development of the commissural projection of the rat somatic sensory cortex. *J. Comp. Neurol.* **168,** 313–344.

Wise, S. P., and Jones, E. G. (1978). Developmental studies of thalamocortical and commissural connections in the rat somatic sensory cortex. *J. Comp. Neurol.* **178,** 187–208.

Wong-Riley, M. T. (1972). Terminal degeneration and glial reactions in the lateral geniculate nucleus of the squirrel monkey after eye removal. *J. Comp. Neurol.* **144,** 61–92.

Woolsey, T. A., and Wann, J. R. (1976). Areal changes in mouse cortical barrels following vibrissal damage at different postnatal ages. *J. Comp. Neurol.* **170,** 53–66.

Zilles, K. J. (1978). Ontogenesis of the visual system. *Adv. Anat. Embryol. Cell Biol.* **54,** 5–138.

2-Deoxyglucose Studies of Stimulus Coding in the Brainstem Auditory System of the Cat

RANDOLPH J. NUDO AND R. BRUCE MASTERTON

DEPARTMENT OF PSYCHOLOGY
FLORIDA STATE UNIVERSITY
TALLAHASSEE, FLORIDA

I.	Introduction	79
II.	Interpretation of 2-DG Autoradiographs	81
III.	Effects of Variations in Sound Onset	85
IV.	Effects of Variations in Frequency	89
V.	Effects of Variations in Intensity	93
VI.	Summary	95
	References	96

I. INTRODUCTION

The development of the radioactively labeled [1-^{14}C]2-deoxy-D-glucose (or 2-DG) technique for mapping neural activity in the central nervous system provides a new approach to some of the questions surrounding stimulus coding in the central auditory system (Sokoloff et al., 1977). Its application derives from the demonstration that alterations in neuronal activity are accompanied by alterations in glucose consumption (Kennedy et al., 1975). For the 2-DG method, a structural analog of glucose, 2-deoxyglucose, begins to be metabolized within a neuron by the same mechanism as glucose. However, intracellular glycolysis ceases following the initial phosphorylation step and the 2-DG is trapped within the cell. Therefore, serial sections of the brain of an animal injected with radioactively labeled 2-DG can be exposed to X-ray film and the resulting image will indicate the relative uptake of 2-DG and, hence, differentiate between more active and less active sites within the brain. Autoradiographs obtained by this method have already been used to show specific functional activity in a wide variety of neural systems, including each of the sensory systems (e.g., see review by Hand, 1981; Plum et al., 1976).

However, the use of the 2-DG method for visualizing the distribution of activity over wide areas of the neuraxis has been slowed by the relatively high cost of $[^{14}C]$2-DG (\$15/100 g of body weight) and the publication of systematic experiments has been discouraged by the very high cost of printing the autoradiographs in journals. Nevertheless, 2-DG materials of the auditory system can now be found in several laboratories and, in a few, they can be found in some numbers.[1]

In our laboratory, the number of 2-DG cases focused on the mammalian auditory system alone has now risen to over 150. Most of these cases are 2-DG records of the response of the central auditory system of 6- to 8-week-old cats to sounds varying either in onset, frequency, intensity, or azimuth or to electrical stimulation applied directly to one or another auditory structure. Several cases have also been prepared in combination with unilateral or bilateral ablations and still others have investigated the structural variations in the auditory system of mice, rats, kangaroo rats, and prosimian primates.

The present article is restricted to the neural effects of variations either in the onset, frequency, or intensity of single, pure tones delivered through a speaker 40 cm from the head of the animal. For these cases, care was taken to assure the purity, amplitude, and frequency of the tones reaching the vicinity of the ear; but the distortions of the sound wave induced by the pinna or external auditory meatus were not controlled. Thus, the variations in neural activity seen in the 2-DG autoradiographs presented here are the result of the totality of physical, mechanical, and neurological transformations taking place in the auditory system from the pinna inward, together with any intrinsic and descending influences generated by the awake nervous system itself.

This article is necessarily restricted to auditory structures up to the inferior colliculus but not beyond. Although autoradiographs from sections throughout the thalamus and cerebrum of these same cases were routinely obtained and thoroughly studied, our technique yielded inconsistent labeling of the medial geniculate and auditory cortex. This is not to say that no cases displayed vivid labeling in the medial geniculate (MG)[2] or cortex; many of them did. But in our hands, the stimulation yielding good 2-DG marking in one case did not neces-

---

[1]For example, systematic 2-DG studies of the cochlea have been performed by Frank Ryan, Department of Otolaryngology, University of California, San Diego; of the avian central auditory system by Edwin Rubel and William Lippe, Department of Otolaryngology, University of Virginia; of the cat central auditory system by William Webster, Department of Psychology, Monash University, Australia.

[2]The following abbreviations are used in the figures and text: AVCN, anteroventral cochlear nucleus; DCN, dorsal cochlear nucleus; DLL, dorsal nucleus of the lateral lemniscus; IC, inferior

sarily show exactly the same marking in a replicating case and this variation could not be immediately explained on the basis of variations in materials or handling. It is not unlikely that there are factors other than the strictly physical parameters of sound affecting the activity of auditory units above the level of the inferior colliculus in awake animals and that these factors might eventually explain this inconsistency of 2-DG marking. But at present we can say only that the forebrain auditory system seems to require a wider ranging, more elaborate set of studies before anything more than a crude demonstration of its tonotopicity can be faithfully illustrated by the 2-DG techniques used here.

Each of the autoradiographs shown here was obtained in the same manner. After light anesthetization with halothane, tracheal and venous cannulas were fixed in place. Lidocaine was liberally applied to the wounds and the incisions closed. Following recovery from the anesthesia (as indicated by the onset of voluntary movements), gallomine triethiodide was injected via the venous cannula and artificial ventilation was begun. The preparation was then placed in a sound-treated chamber, auditory stimulation begun, and [^{14}C]2-DG (15 μCi/100 g) injected via the venous cannula. A stable state was maintained throughout the remainder of the procedure by occasional, brief injections of gallomine with a motor-driven pump.

After 45 minutes of continuous exposure to the sound and the 2-DG, sacrifice was accomplished with an overdose of pentothal administered through the venous cannula. The brain was quickly removed, frozen in precooled methylbutane, and cut in 30-μm sections either in a transverse or horizontal plane. The sections were dried under a jet of warm nitrogen, glued onto a cardboard sheet, and exposed to X-ray film in a light-tight cassette. After exposure and development the autoradiographs were mounted along with the Nissl-stained tissue for study and photodensitometry measurements (Fig. 1).

II. INTERPRETATION OF 2-DG AUTORADIOGRAPHS

Before turning to a systematic analysis of the resulting autoradiographs, it is important to note that despite our current knowledge of 2-DG chemistry, the glucose metabolism pathway, and the energy demands of neurons it is not yet

---

colliculus; ILL, intermediate nucleus of the lateral lemniscus; LSO, lateral superior olive; LTB, lateral nucleus of the trapezoid body; MSO, medial superior olive; MTB, medial nucleus of the trapezoid body; PVCN, posteroventral cochlear nucleus; SOC, superior olivary complex; VLL, ventral nucleus of the lateral lemniscus; VTB, ventral nucleus of the trapezoid body.

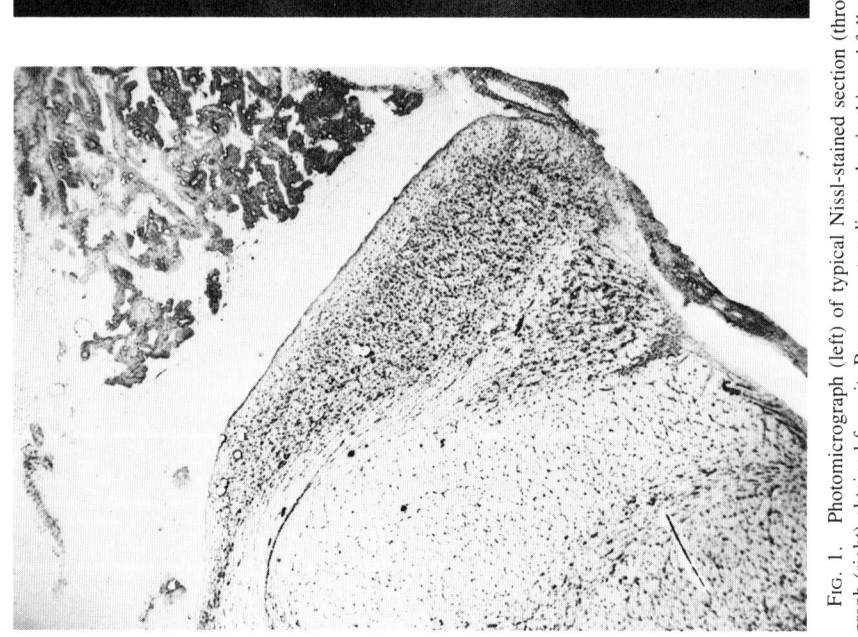
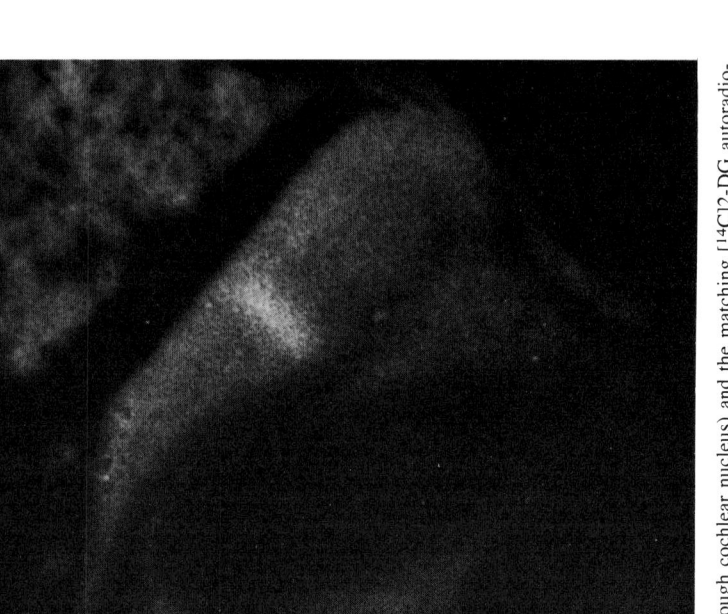

FIG. 1. Photomicrograph (left) of typical Nissl-stained section (through cochlear nucleus) and the matching [^{14}C]2-DG autoradiograph (right) obtained from it. Because autoradiographs, in this and following figures, have been printed in negative directly from X-ray film, high-activity zones appear white, low-activity zones black.

entirely clear just what 2-DG marks. Although there is no question that the presence of high levels of 2-DG means high levels of metabolic activity and little question that in the nervous system this usually means high levels of neural activity, the contribution of glial activity in the vicinity of neural activity, for example, is not known (Lippe et al., 1980). Still more important for the present purpose, it is not yet known to what degree the several components of neural activity contribute to 2-DG marking. That is, it is often tacitly assumed that 2-DG marking means heightened unit discharge rates. There is growing reason to believe that this interpretation is probably not entirely correct (e.g., see Schwartz et al., 1979).

For example, Fig. 2 shows the distribution of 2-DG-labeled activity in the auditory nuclei of the medulla in four separate cases: one with both cochleae destroyed (Fig. 2A), another with one cochlea destroyed (Fig. 2B), and a third with both ears intact (Fig. 2C), each stimulated with white noise; a fourth case with one cochlea destroyed is also included but this one was stimulated with a 32-kHz tone (Fig. 2D). The interpretation of these cases depends on the results of prior electrophysiology by others. For example, from electrophysiological studies we know that in the cases with one deafened ear (Fig. 2B and D) the lateral superior olive (LSO) on the right side (ipsilateral to the deafened ear) received only inhibitory input, whereas the left LSO received only excitatory input (Boudreau and Tsuchitani, 1968). The difference in marking between the left and right LSO is obvious in Fig. 2B and, at first glance, suggests that the difference in discharge rates of the excited units in the left LSO and the inhibited units in the right LSO accounts for the difference in 2-DG labeling. However, the comparison that suggests otherwise is between the right (inhibited) LSO in this case (Fig. 2B) and either LSO in the case with two deafened ears (Fig. 2A). This comparison shows that the inhibited (right) LSO in the case with only one deafened ear had a higher level of 2-DG marking than either LSO in the case with two deafened ears. A second example of this same phenomenon can be seen in Fig. 2D, a case with one deafened ear stimulated with a 32-kHz tone. In this case, 2-DG marking appears in the high-frequency (ventromedial) zone of both LSOs even though the left LSO was excited and the right LSO was inhibited.

Because LSO neurons receive very few if any descending afferents and, as the case with both ears deafened (Fig. 2A) shows, they also have low levels of spontaneous activity the 2-DG marking in the inhibited (right) LSO in Fig. 2B and D probably occurred in the absence of significant LSO cell discharge. In seeking a physiological basis for the presence of 2-DG marking in the absence of either spontaneous or sound-driven cell discharge, one is led to the idea that 2-DG marking, including the light but not negligible 2-DG marking in the right LSO in Fig. 2B and D, probably results from the presence of heightened *synaptic activity*. If this reasoning is correct, it follows that 2-DG labels synaptic activity (including inhibitory synaptic activity) even in the absence of cell discharge.

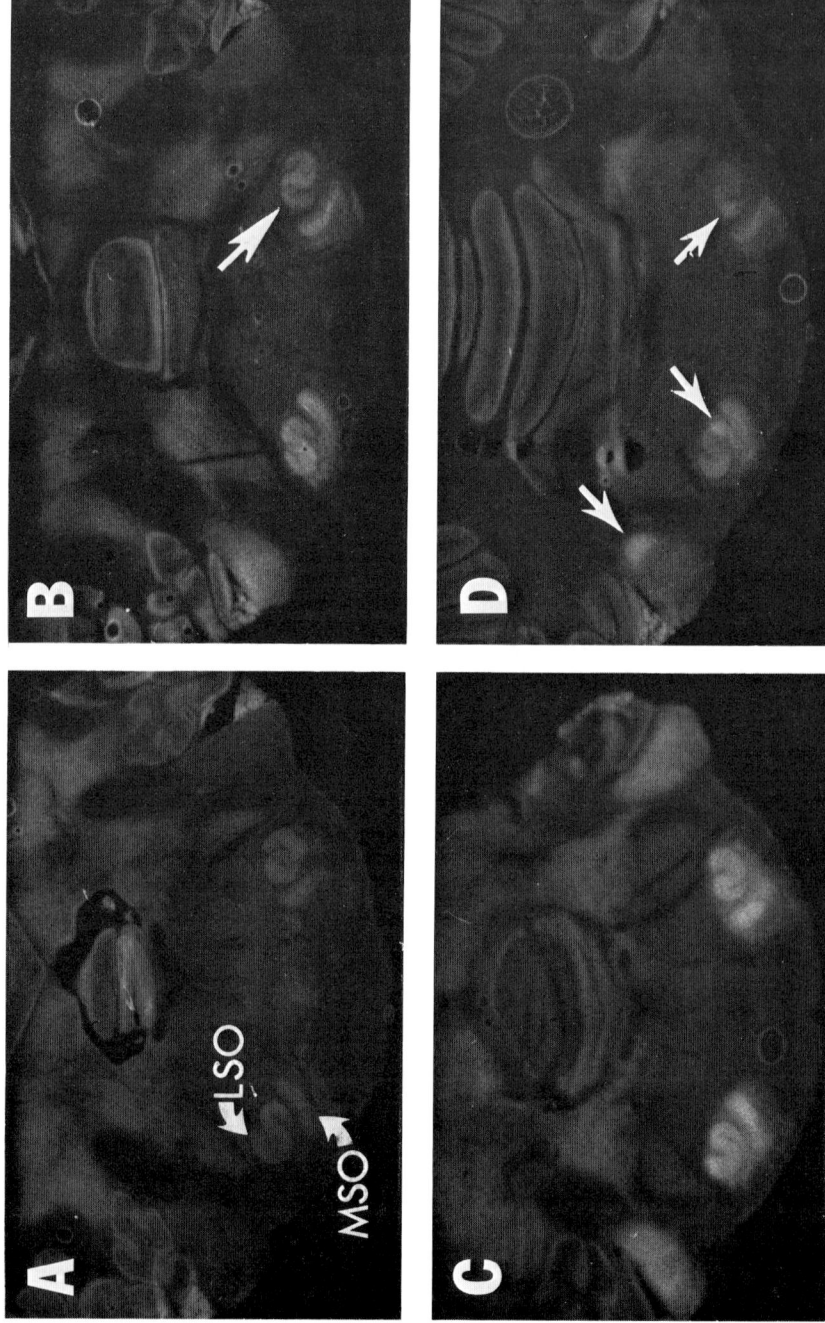

As a contrapositive example, every 2-DG autoradiograph shows very low levels of marking over fiber tracts regardless of the level of their impulse traffic (see absence of marking in the trapezoid body, Fig. 2). This observation also suggests that significant impulse propagation does not necessarily result in the presence of significant 2-DG marking. Finally, we have observed that antidromic stimulation also results in very little 2-DG marking of neural somata.

Examples such as these suggest, though they do not prove, that 2-DG probably marks synaptic activity, whether excitatory or inhibitory, more than it marks unit discharge. This point is important in interpreting the following autoradiographs because it means that 2-DG marking of a central nucleus probably illustrates the distribution of the *afferent terminals* in the nucleus instead of the discharges (and efferent activity) generated by the cells within the nucleus itself. Thus, a sharp line of 2-DG labeling in, say, the inferior colliculus illustrates the precision of afferent projections onto the inferior colliculus from other structures without necessarily revealing the intrinsic organization or input–output transformations of the colliculus itself. This point arises in each section below.

III. EFFECTS OF VARIATIONS IN SOUND ONSET

Unlike most other sensory stimuli, tones with abrupt onsets contain atonal transients easily heard by a listener. (This physical difference in a sound wave resulting from the rapidity of its onset is the difference between staccato and legato.) In most experiments in hearing, these physical transients are carefully eliminated by means of electronic switching that allows a tone to begin gradually over several of its sinusoidal cycles. But in addition to this physical difference accompanying the abrupt onset of sound, central auditory neurons (like most sensory neurons elsewhere) respond to all but the most gradual onsets with an "onset transient" of their own. That is, they often respond with an onset discharge even to sounds that have had their physical onset transients electronically removed. This neural onset discharge is usually at a higher rate, and in many cases at a considerably higher rate, than the steady discharge rate to a continuing

---

FIG. 2. Autoradiographs of frontal sections through comparable levels of hindbrain showing ventral cochlear nucleus, superior olivary complex, and trapezoid body in four separate cases: (A) with both cochleae destroyed; (B) with right cochlea destroyed, stimulated with white noise; (C) with both cochleae intact, stimulated with white noise; (D) with right cochlea destroyed, stimulated with 32-kHz tone. Arrow in (B) points to 2-DG labeling of the LSO receiving predominantly inhibitory synaptic input. Arrows in (D) point to frequency-specific labeling in the left AVCN and both left and right LSOs. Labeling in inhibited (right) LSOs in one-eared cases, (B) and (D), suggests that 2-DG marks synaptic activity even in the absence of local cell discharge.

sound. Furthermore, this transient, onset, or phasic response of central auditory neurons is less well tuned or frequency specific than the tonic response of the same neuron to a steady sound. One consequence of this characteristic is that the tonotopic map of a nucleus based on the transient responses of its constituent units might show little tonotopicity at all. A second consequence is that a continuous sound (or a pulsed sound with a very gradual onset of each pulse) is a poor stimulus for identifying auditory units in the nervous system. For these reasons, one might expect that a pulsed tone evokes more neural activity and, thus, wider marking in 2-DG studies whereas a continuous tone evokes less neural activity and, thus, narrower 2-DG marking. As it turns out, each brainstem auditory structure fulfills this expectation except one.

Figure 3 shows 2-DG autoradiographs from two cases: one stimulated by a continuous tone (16 kHz) at 90 dB SPL (Fig. 3, left) and the second (Fig. 3, right) stimulated by a tone of the same frequency and intensity, but pulsed at 4 tone pips per second. Each tone pip was stripped of *physical* onset transients by virtue of a 5-msec stimulus rise (and fall) time (i.e., the onset and offset of the individual tone pips each spanned 5×16, or 80 cycles of the stimulating 16-kHz tone).

As Fig. 3 shows, the dorsal cochlear nucleus (DCN) yields a discrete band of 2-DG marking under either condition. In contrast, the LSO and each of the other hindbrain nuclei show obvious marking to the continuous tone but little discrete marking to the pulsed tone. Further, it can be seen that pulsing the tone greatly enhanced the 2-DG marking throughout the medial superior olive (MSO).

Although one is tempted to explain this difference in labeling by reference to the phasic vs tonic discharge characteristics of units in the dorsal cochlear nucleus (DCN), LSO, and MSO, we have already suggested that it is synaptic activity, not cell discharge, that probably dominates 2-DG autoradiographs. For the LSO and MSO this means that what is seen as a difference in 2-DG marking must be explained by reference to the neurons contributing their afferents [anteroventral cochlear nucleus (AVCN) for MSO; AVCN and the medial nucleus of the trapezoid body (MTB) for LSO] or, in turn, to their afferents. For this reason we conclude that it is probably these lower level nuclei or structures at still more peripheral levels (e.g., spiral ganglion neurons, hair cells, basilar membrane, etc.) that are the source of the broadened or frequency-nonspecific responses seen in the LSO and MSO and in the other hindbrain auditory nuclei as well.

Turning to the response of the DCN under the same conditions, however, we see that each stimulus, whether pulsed or continuous, results in a discrete band of 2-DG label superimposed on widespread activity in its outer layers. Therefore, unlike other hindbrain nuclei, at least part of the response of the DCN reflects the frequency of the stimulating tone even in the face of onsets that the other nuclei find atonal.

Because the peculiar discharge characteristics of the efferent cells of the DCN

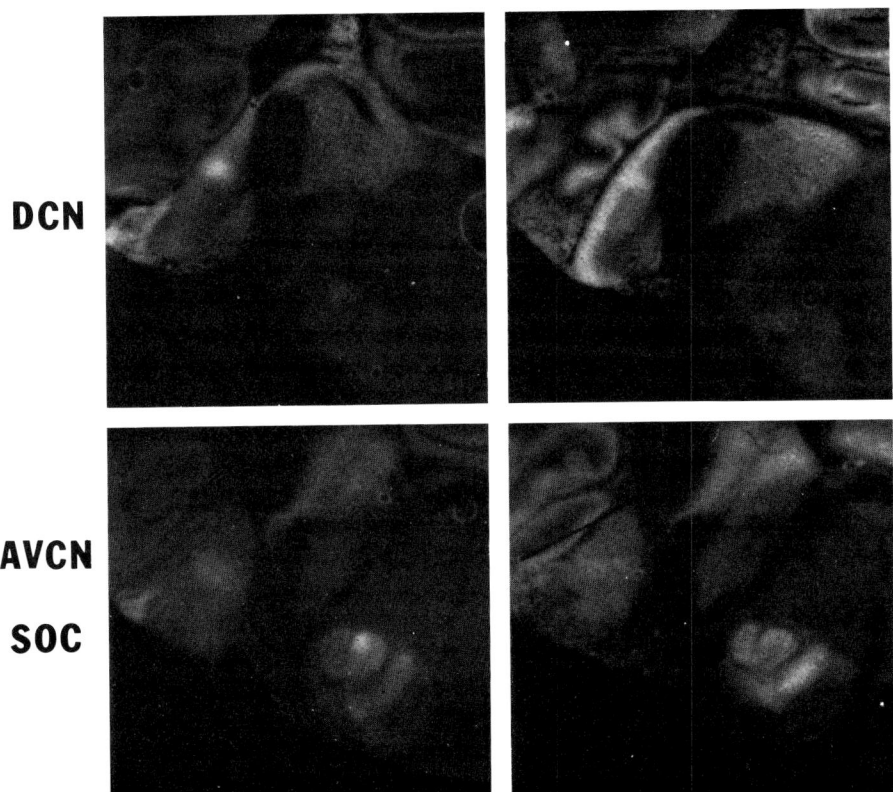

FIG. 3. Effect of sound onset on activity in cochlear nucleus and superior olives. Both cases were stimulated with a 16-kHz tone, continuously for case on left; pulsed at 4 tone pips/second for case on right. Although each tone pip was electronically gated with a rise and fall time of 5 msec (i.e., over 80 cycles of the 16-kHz tone), nonspecific recruitment of activity is widespread in each hindbrain nucleus excepting only the deeper layers of the DCN. In particular, note high levels of activity in the outer layers of the DCN and throughout the MSO and ventral nucleus of the trapezoid body.

(i.e., the pyramidal cells with their inhibitory side bands, for example) are probably *not* relevant to the observed 2-DG marking within the DCN, the cause of the relatively sharp-bordered band of 2-DG is not obvious. That is, if one assumes that the relatively nonspecific marking of the pulsed tone in the AVCN, posteroventral cochlear nucleus (PVCN), LSO, MSO, etc., is probably a secondary result of nonspecificity for transients at the cochlea and, further, that the cochlear nerve fibers terminating in the DCN are faithful conductors of this transient nonspecificity, then the sharpness of the 2-DG markings with pulsating tones in the DCN but not in the AVCN (or PVCN) seems mutually contradictory.

Although this unique response of the DCN obviously requires further study, we see at least two interesting possibilities. First, the cochlear input to the DCN may differ from that to the AVCN or PVCN—this suggestion has been made before on anatomical grounds (e.g., see Kane, 1974). Second, the response of the DCN may differ from the other nuclei because of its very large number of intrinsic connections. The DCN is known to contain a wealth of small cells, making a vast number of synaptic contacts throughout its molecular, granular, and principal cell layers. It is possible that the synaptic activity of these intrinsic connections, which far outnumber the primary connections, makes a larger contribution to the total 2-DG uptake in the DCN than does the synaptic activity of the primary auditory fibers from the cochlea. Therefore, what is seen as a band of activity in the DCN may well be evidence of the local intrinsic synapses differentiating the primary input and not necessarily a sign of some different kind of input from the cochlea itself.

As already mentioned, each hindbrain auditory nucleus *except the DCN* shows a wide broadening of its 2-DG marking when stimulated with a pulsing tone instead of a continuous tone. Because the efferents of these several nuclei converge on the inferior colliculus (IC), it is of interest to consider the distribution of activity there. Figure 4 shows that the IC displays broad marking with the pulsing tone—much like the majority of hindbrain nuclei. But the IC also shows a frequency-specific band under both conditions—much like the DCN. Thus, the IC shows both kinds of response: the result that would be expected on the basis of

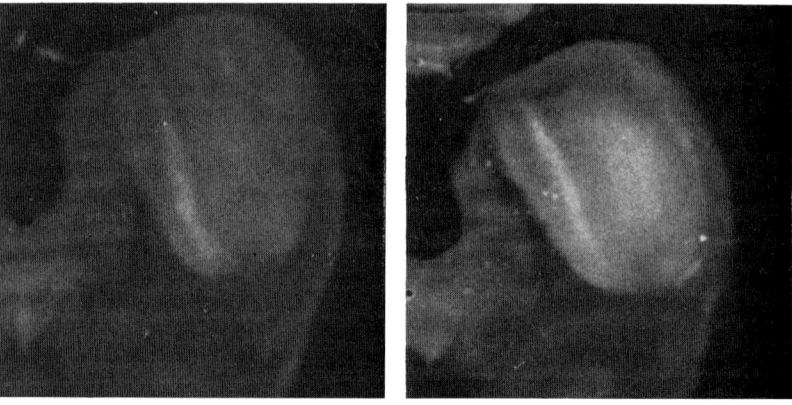

FIG. 4. Effect of sound onset on activity in the IC. Stimulation with 16-kHz tone, continuous on left, pulsed on right. Note that nonspecific activity evoked by pulsing tone almost obscures frequency-specific activity. Activity in hindbrain nuclei of the same cases (Fig. 3) suggests that frequency-specific marking may derive from direct DCN projections to colliculus, nonspecific marking from projections of other nuclei.

the overlap of its afferents converging both from the contralateral DCN and also from the superior olivary nuclei.

Furthermore, the idea that the frequency-specific band in the IC is probably transmitted from the contralateral DCN implies, in turn, that the frequency-specific band seen in the DCN probably includes its pyramidal cells, the major source of DCN efferents to the IC.

IV. EFFECTS OF VARIATIONS IN FREQUENCY

The tonotopic organization of the cat brainstem auditory system is clearly demonstrable by the 2-DG method, and examples of 2-DG labeling in the cochlear nuclei and IC have been illustrated before (e.g., see Webster *et al.*, 1978). However, possibly because of the depressive effects of anesthesia or because of the nonspecific 2-DG marking that accompanies stimulation by pulsed tones, frequency-specific labeling in the superior olivary nuclei has rarely been published (Ryan *et al.*, 1982). Figure 5 shows frequency-specific 2-DG marking in the cat's AVCN, PVCN, DCN, LSO, and MSO and Fig. 6 shows it in the IC. In general, each of these results and the tonotopic maps that can be derived from them are entirely consistent with those obtained electrophysiologically.[3]

In none of our materials (whether in frontal or horizontal sections or from cat, rat, mouse, kangaroo rat, or bushbaby) were clear frequency-specific bands of 2-DG found either in the lateral nucleus of the trapezoid body (LTB), the medial nucleus of the trapezoid body (MTB), the ventral nucleus of the lateral lemniscus (VLL), the intermediate nucleus of the lateral lemniscus (ILL), or the dorsal nucleus of the lateral lemniscus (DLL).[4] This is not to say that these nuclei are not tonotopically organized also. To begin with, the resolution of [^{14}C]2-DG probably excludes visualization of the necessarily compact frequency maps that may be present in small nuclei such as the LTB, MTB, ILL, and DLL. Therefore, only in the VLL is the absence of clear frequency-specific marking possibly indicative of the absence of strong tonotopicity. Even in this case, however, it is possible either that an overlap of nonspecific synapses with specific synapses

---

[3]This agreement between the two methods of mapping is not as trivial as it may first appear. Because 2-DG marks synaptic activity and, thus, afferent activity, whereas electrophysiology localizes discharging units and, thus, usually efferent activity, the equation of 2-DG and electrophysiological results is tantamount to the equation of input to output. This equation, in turn, suggests that there may be little or no integrative activity or analytical transformation of this particular stimulus dimension at these nuclei.

[4]Although an obscure gradient of activity can be educed from autoradiographs of the VLL and DLL with low frequencies more dorsal and high frequencies more ventral, frequency specificity is far less clear and systematic in these nuclei than in the cochlear nuclei, LSO, MSO, or IC.

obscures frequency-specific marking or that another plane of section might reveal it (cf. Aitkin *et al.*, 1970).

Turning to the nuclei with clear frequency-specific marking (Fig. 5), the DCN shows a continuous rostral–caudal band of marking for each frequency, with low frequencies ventral and high frequencies dorsal, as shown electrophysiologically (cf. Rose *et al.*, 1960). Once more, these bands are superimposed on a nonspecific background of lighter marking confined mostly to the molecular and granular layers.

The AVCN and PVCN show broader but much less heavy bands of labeling for each tone. Nevertheless, the activity bands in the AVCN and PVCN progress from rostral, lateral, and ventral to caudal, medial, and dorsal with each increment in stimulus frequency (cf. Rose *et al.*, 1960; Bourk *et al.*, 1981).

Also in Fig. 5, the LSO and MSO reveal their tonotopicity with rostral–caudal bands of 2-DG labeling. As demonstrated electrophysiologically by others, the labeled band shifts from dorsal to ventral in the MSO and from dorsolateral to ventromedial in the LSO as the frequency of the stimulation is raised (cf. Tsuchitani, 1977; Guinan *et al.*, 1972). It is of some interest to note that whereas the LSO shows a localized 2-DG mark for each frequency from 1 kHz to at least 32 kHz, the MSO shows 2-DG marking only up to 8 kHz. Thus, the presence of neurons in the MSO with characteristic frequencies above this range, as occasionally demonstrated electrophysiologically in cats, may be a rare occurrence. The present 2-DG materials suggest that the tonotopic map of the MSO in the cat is even more restricted to low frequencies than was once thought (cf. Guinan *et al.*, 1972).

It can also be seen in Fig. 5 that the dorsal (low-frequency) tip of the MSO is marked even for a tone of relatively high frequency. This result is not idiosyncratic; it is seen in every case in which the stimulating tone is low enough in frequency to mark the MSO elsewhere (i.e., 8 kHz or lower). Apparently, the dorsal-most cells in the MSO either receive frequency-nonspecific endings or are a site of converging frequency-specific endings whether from the MSO itself or elsewhere.

In the ventrolateral division of the central nucleus of the IC, frequency-specific sheets of activity have been shown before (Silverman *et al.*, 1977; Webster *et al.*, 1978; Serviere and Webster, 1981; Ryan *et al.*, 1982). As expected from electrophysiological studies once again, the sheets progress from dorsolateral to ventromedial as the frequency of the stimulating tone is raised (Fig. 6) (e.g., Merzenich and Reid, 1974). However, there are four variations to this general rule that may be of interest.

To begin with, Fig. 6 shows that the sheets of frequency-specific activity twist from nearly vertical in rostral IC to oblique in caudal IC. Second, from rostral to caudal, each sheet shifts progressively more dorsolateral. As a result, high frequencies (>16 kHz) are not represented in rostral IC, whereas low frequencies

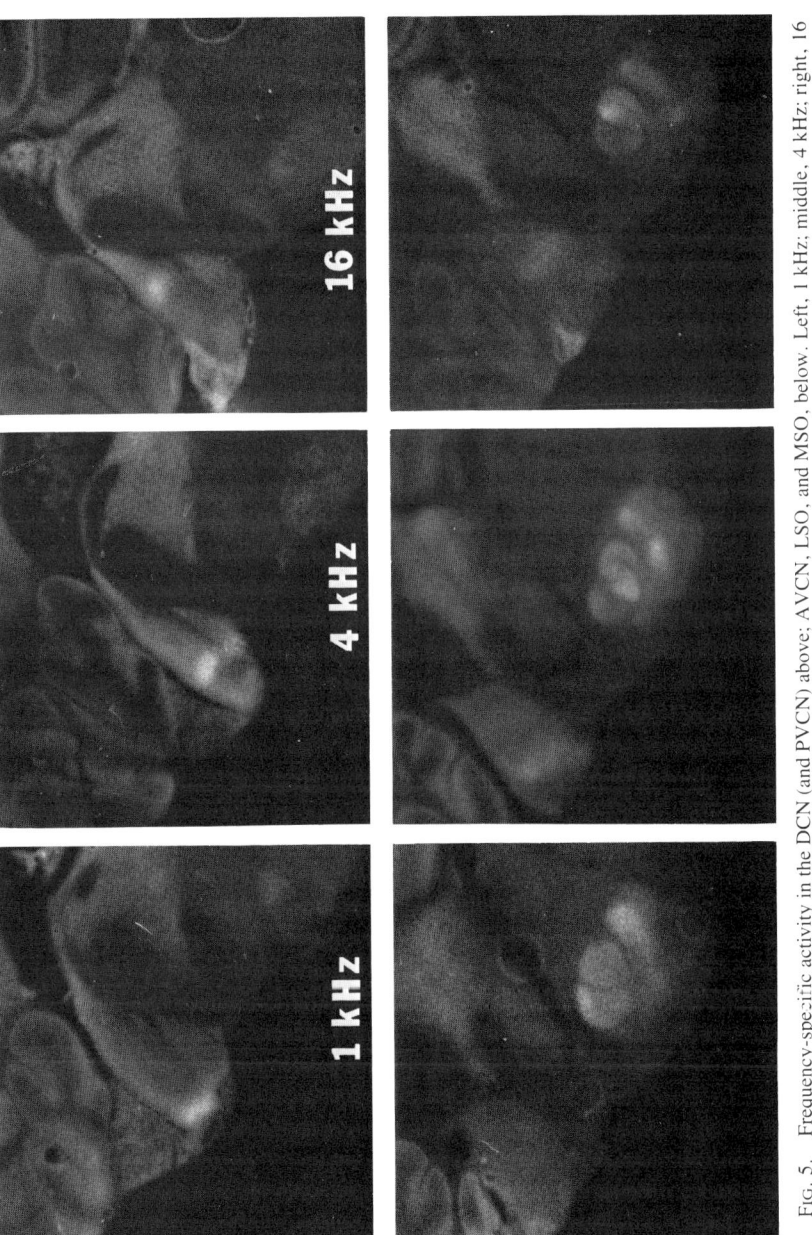

FIG. 5. Frequency-specific activity in the DCN (and PVCN) above; AVCN, LSO, and MSO, below. Left, 1 kHz; middle, 4 kHz; right, 16 kHz. As frequency increases, activity in cochlear nuclei progresses from ventrolateral to dorsomedial; in the LSO, from dorsolateral to ventromedial; in the MSO, from dorsal to ventral (1-kHz marking in the AVCN appears in more rostral sections). Note second zone of activity in the dorsal MSO in 4-kHz case and absence of MSO marking in 16-kHz case.

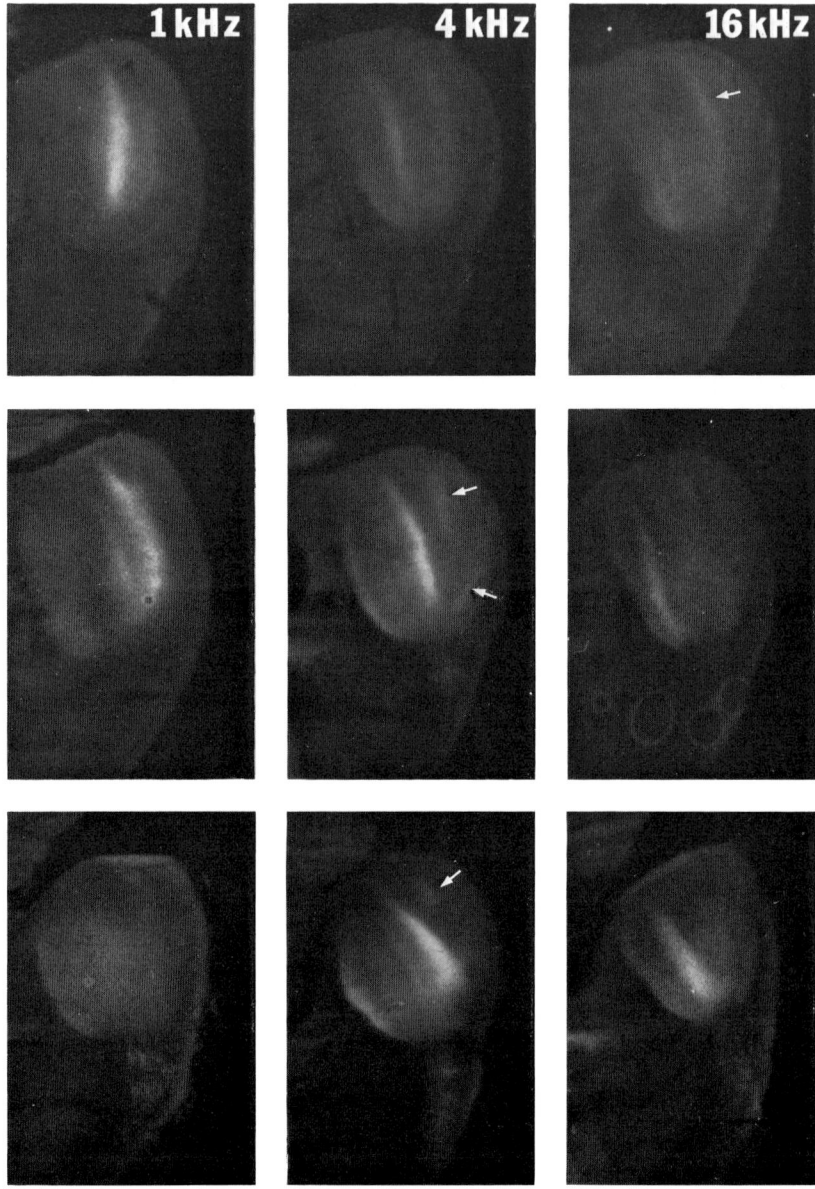

FIG. 6. Frequency-specific activity at three rostral–caudal levels of the IC. Top, rostral; bottom, caudal; left, 1 kHz; middle, 4 kHz; right, 16 kHz. As frequency increases, location of sheet of activity through the IC progresses from dorsolateral to ventromedial. Note absence of low-frequency activity caudally, absence of high-frequency activity rostrally. Arrows mark frequency-nonspecific activity in the IC.

(< 4 kHz) are not represented in caudal IC. Third, the frequency-specific sheets become progressively broader from rostral to caudal IC. Fourth, the frequency-specific sheets of 2-DG marking dissipate as the borders of either the dorsomedial division of the central nucleus or the pericentral or external nuclei of the IC are crossed. No clear evidence of frequency-specific marking could be found within either of these nuclei. Finally, there is a considerable amount of nonspecific marking within the IC. Part of this marking probably arises from intrinsic connections within the IC (Kuwada *et al.*, 1980). But another part may also arise from nucleus-specific terminal fields of the hindbrain nuclei (see arrows in Fig. 6).

The clear tonotopicity of each brainstem auditory nucleus large enough to show it (excepting only the VLL), as demonstrated by 2-DG, together with the virtually complete agreement of the 2-DG maps with electrophysiologically derived maps, allow several general conclusions. First, there is no evidence for, and mounting evidence against, the idea that frequency coding is "sharpened" as the central auditory system is ascended. The 2-DG evidence is in agreement with recent electrophysiological evidence that, if anything, the opposite is true—the proportion of frequency-nonspecific tissue and the proportion of neurons with broad tuning curves *increase* as the system is ascended. Furthermore, neither the 2-DG materials nor electrophysiological studies provide any support for the idea that tones with frequencies too low to be place encoded by the cochlea ever become place encoded at a higher level. In general, then, there is little reason to believe that the tonotopic maps seen in central auditory nuclei reflect anything more than a relatively passive preservation of the cochleotopicity seen in the auditory nerve.

V. EFFECTS OF VARIATIONS IN INTENSITY

Both von Bekesy's model of basilar membrane mechanics and the asymmetry of the tuning curves of primary fibers imply that the response of auditory nerve fibers increases with increase in tone intensity; impulse rate can be expected to increase for each active fiber and the recruitment of new fibers can be expected to progress from those with characteristic frequencies (CFs) equal to that of the stimulating tone to those mostly with CFs successively *higher* than that of the stimulating tone.

Figure 7 shows the response of the DCN and IC to three different intensities of a 16-kHz tone. The line graphs show that in the DCN the 16-kHz frequency band becomes denser and broader as intensity increases. Furthermore, the broadening of the band is more toward the (dorsal) high-frequency representation. Because, qualitatively at least, this is the same response as would be seen in the auditory

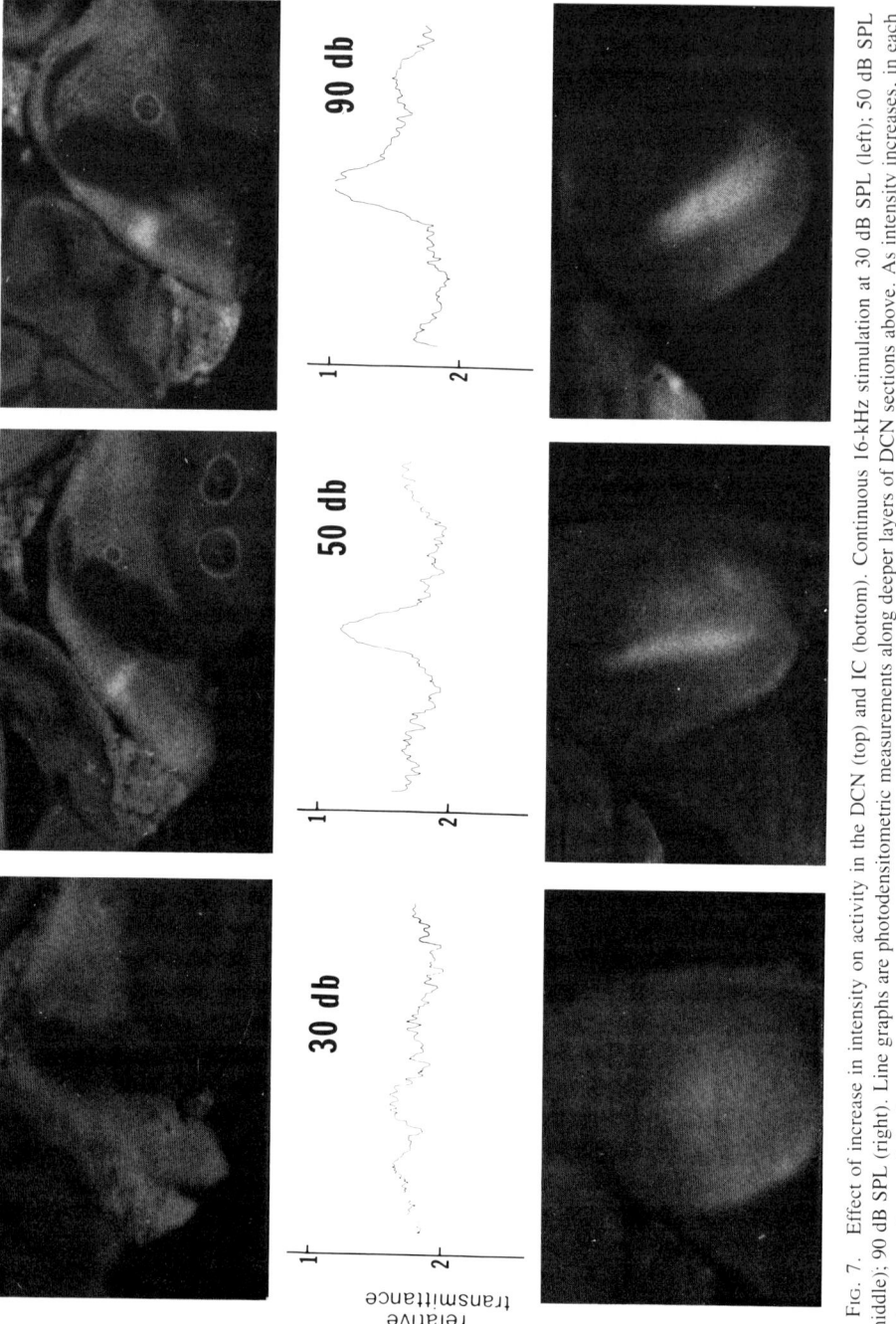

FIG. 7. Effect of increase in intensity on activity in the DCN (top) and IC (bottom). Continuous 16-kHz stimulation at 30 dB SPL (left); 50 dB SPL (middle); 90 dB SPL (right). Line graphs are photodensitometric measurements along deeper layers of DCN sections above. As intensity increases, in each brainstem nucleus activity increases and broadens mostly into higher frequency representation.

nerve, 2-DG provides no evidence that either the intrinsic or descending connections of the DCN significantly alter the representation of intensity in the primary input. In the IC, the same result obtains. The higher intensities result in a broader, higher density band of 2-DG marking. And again, the band broadens mostly into the region representing higher frequencies.

Parenthetically, it should be noted that many electrophysiological studies and a few 2-DG studies have shown a nonmonotonic relationship between central neural activity and sound intensity (e.g., Rose et al., 1971; Ryan and Miller, 1977; Sharp et al., 1981). At high-intensity levels (>90 dB SPL) many central auditory neurons seem to reduce their discharge rate. In our materials we have *not* seen a reduction in 2-DG marking at levels of stimulation up to 100 dB SPL. But we hasten to add that our use of an anticholinergic paralytic agent may be the causative factor. Middle ear reflexes are probably entirely absent in our animals whereas they may not be entirely absent in the anesthetized preparations usually used either in electrophysiological or in other 2-DG procedures.

Returning to intensity coding, the same result as shown in Fig. 7 for the DCN and IC is also obtained in the MSO, LSO, AVCN, and PVCN. Without exception, for more intense tones the 2-DG-labeled activity becomes denser and broadens preferentially into the higher frequency representation. This result suggests that each brainstem auditory nucleus responds to changes in intensity in the manner predicted by cochlear mechanics. Thus, once encoded by the cochlea and represented in the auditory nerve, intensity, much like frequency, does not seem to be reencoded by the brainstem nuclei, at least not over the part of their dynamic range suitable for 2-DG study.

VI. SUMMARY

In this article we have attempted to illustrate the variations in response of hindbrain and midbrain auditory nuclei in awake cats to variations in onset, frequency, and intensity of tones. Although most of these variations are easily predictable from prior electrophysiological studies, others are not. Part of this divergence of 2-DG and electrophysiological results can be accounted for by noting that 2-DG locates sites of high afferent activity whereas electrophysiology locates sites of high cell discharge, which usually means high efferent activity. Thus, the similarity of the two kinds of results, where it does exist, suggests an input–output relationship of some theoretical importance; it suggests that a reencoding of the stimulus parameter (other than possibly amplification and distribution) is *not* taking place. This conclusion seems to hold for frequency and intensity throughout the larger brainstem auditory nuclei at least, and also for sound onset at each nucleus except the lower layers of the DCN and, possibly, the MSO.

ACKNOWLEDGMENT

The preparation of this article was supported, in part, by Grants NDS NS07726-16 and NDS NS18877-01 from the National Institutes of Health.

REFERENCES

Aitkin, L. M., Anderson, D. J., and Brugge, J. F. (1970). Tonotopic organization and discharge characteristics of single neurons in nuclei of the lateral lemniscus of the cat. *J. Neurophysiol.* **33,** 421–440.

Boudreau, J. C., and Tsuchitani, C. (1968). Binaural interaction in the cat superior olive S-segment. *J. Neurophysiol.* **31,** 442–454.

Bourke, T. R., Mielcary, J. P., and Norris, B. E. (1981). Tonotopic organization of the anteroventral cochlear nucleus of the cat. *Hear. Res.* **4,** 215–241.

Guinan, J. J., Jr., Norris, B. E., and Guinan, S. S. (1972). Single auditory units in the superior olivary complex. II. Locations of unit categories and tonotopic organization. *Int. J. Neurosci.* **4,** 147–166.

Hand, P. (1981). The 2-deoxyglucose method. *In* "Neuroanatomical Tract Tracing Methods" (L. Heimer and M. J. Robards, eds.), pp. 511–538. Plenum, New York.

Kane, E. C. (1974). Synaptic organization in the dorsal cochlear nucleus of the cat: A light and electron microscopic study. *J. Comp. Neurol.* **155,** 301–330.

Kennedy, C., DesRosiers, M. H., Jehle, J. W., Reivich, M., Sharpe, F., and Sokoloff, L. (1975). Mapping of functional neural pathways by autoradiographic survey of local metabolic rate with [^{14}C]deoxyglucose. *Science* **187,** 850–853.

Kuwada, S., Yin, T. C. T., Haberly, L. B., and Wickesberg, R. E. (1980). Binaural interaction in the cat inferior colliculus: Physiology and anatomy. *In* "Psychophysical, Psychological and Behavioral Studies in Hearing." Delft Univ. Press, Delft, The Netherlands.

Lippe, W. R., Steward, O., and Rubel, E. W. (1980). The effect of unilateral basilar papilla removal upon nuclei laminaris and magnocellularis of the chick examined with [^{3}H]2-deoxy-D-glucose autoradiography. *Brain Res.* **196,** 43–58.

Merzenich, M. M., and Reid, M. D. (1974). Representation of the cochlea within the inferior colliculus of the cat. *Brain Res.* **77,** 397–415.

Plum, F., Gjedde, A., and Samson, F. E. (1976). Neuroanatomical functional mapping by the radioactive 2-deoxy-D-glucose method. *Neurosci. Res. Prog. Bull.* **14,** 457–518.

Rose, J. E., Galambos, R., and Hughes, G. (1960). Organization of frequency sensitive neurons in the cochlear nuclear complex of the cat. *In* "Neural Mechanisms of the Auditory and Vestibular Systems" (G. L. Rasmussen and W. F. Windle, Eds.), pp. 116–136. Thomas, Springfield, Illinois.

Rose, J. E., Hind, J. E., Anderson, D. J., and Brugge, J. F. (1971). Some effects of stimulus intensity on response of auditory nerve fibres in the squirrel monkey. *J. Neurophysiol.* **34,** 685–699.

Ryan, A., and Miller, J. (1977). Effects of behavioral performance on single-unit firing patterns in inferior colliculus of the rhesus monkey. *J. Neurophysiol.* **40,** 943–955.

Ryan, A. F., Woolf, N. K., and Sharp, F. R. (1982). Tonotopic organization in the central auditory pathway of the Mongolian gerbil: A 2-deoxyglucose study. *J. Comp. Neurol.* **207,** 369–380.

Schwartz, W. J., Smith, C. B., Davidsen, L., Savaki, H., Sokoloff, L., Mata, M., Fink, D. J., and Gainer, H. (1979). Metabolic mapping of functional activity in the hypothalamo-neurohypophysial system of the rat. *Science* **205,** 723–725.

Serviere, J., and Webster, W. R. (1981). A combined electrophysiological and [^{14}C]2-deoxyglucose study of the frequency organization of the inferior colliculus of the cat. *Neurosci. Lett.* **27,** 113–118.

Sharp, F. R., Ryan, A. F., Goodwin, P., and Woolf, N. K. (1981). Increasing intensities of wide band noise increase [^{14}C]2-deoxyglucose uptake in gerbil central auditory structures. *Brain Res.* **230,** 87–96.

Silverman, M. S., Hendrickson, A. E., and Clopton, B. M. (1977). Mapping of the tonotopic organization of the auditory system by uptake of radioactive metabolites. *Neurosci. Abstr.* **3,** 11.

Sokoloff, L., Reivich, M., Kennedy, C., Des Rosiers, M. G., Patlak, C. S., Pettigrew, K. D., Sakurada, O., and Shinohara, M. (1977). The [^{14}C]deoxyglucose method for the measurement of local cerebral glucose utilization: Theory, procedure, and normal values in the conscious and anesthetized albino rat. *J. Neurochem.* **28,** 897–916.

Tsuchitani, C. (1977). Functional organization of lateral cell groups of cat superior olivary complex. *J. Neurophysiol.* **40,** 296–318.

Webster, W. R., Serviere, J., Batini, C., and LaPlante, S. (1978). Autoradiographic demonstration with 2-[^{14}C]deoxyglucose of frequency selectivity in the auditory system of cats under conditions of functional activity. *Neurosci. Lett.* **10,** 43–48.

Axonal Organization in the Cat Medial Superior Olivary Nucleus

ILSA R. SCHWARTZ

HEAD AND NECK SURGERY
UNIVERSITY OF CALIFORNIA, LOS ANGELES SCHOOL OF MEDICINE
LOS ANGELES, CALIFORNIA

I.	History of Multiple Classes of Axons	99
II.	Classical Approaches to Identifying Axonal Populations	100
	A. Methods	101
	B. Results	101
	C. Discussion	113
III.	Differential Amino Acid-Labeling Studies	119
	A. Rationale	119
	B. Methods	120
	C. Results	121
	D. Discussion	124
	References	127

I. HISTORY OF MULTIPLE CLASSES OF AXONS

Although most pictures of the medial superior olivary nucleus (MSO) emphasize the bilateral principal input first described by LaVilla (1898) and Ramón y Cajal (1909) and now generally held responsible for the binaural interactions occurring in this nucleus (Goldberg and Brown, 1968, 1969), investigators have always recognized additional classes of axons within the MSO.

LaVilla mentioned a group of beaded axons at the periphery of the MSO surrounding the marginal cells and associated with the tips of the perpendicular dendrites of principal cells. LaVilla and Ramón y Cajal illustrated collaterals of kitten and mouse MSO axons that arborized within the MSO. Scheibel and Scheibel (1974) described a rostrocaudally oriented axon with many branches in the cat MSO. Lindsey (1975) demonstrated two classes of flat vesicle endings in the cat MSO that survived cochlear nucleus (CN) lesions, one with large and one with small vesicles. In the chinchilla, Perkins (1973) showed two classes of

MSO endings that survived CN lesions, one containing small vesicles and one containing intermediate-sized vesicles. In a preliminary report, Schwartz and Wittebort (1976) presented Golgi evidence for at least three extrinsic and one intrinsic MSO input in addition to the principal input in the cat. In the normal adult cat, Schwartz (1980a,b) demonstrated a higher percentage of small endings with symmetrical junctions and pleiomorphic and small vesicles on marginal cells as opposed to central cells.

The presence of several classes of axon terminals in the MSO is not surprising in light of its presumed role in auditory–visual interactions (Harrison and Irving, 1965) and the variety of MSO neuronal types that have been demonstrated anatomically (Schwartz, 1977) and physiologically. In addition to monaurally driven units, there are three types of bilaterally driven units, and units that display a variety of discharge patterns (see Guinan *et al.*, 1972, for a review of physiological studies). Recent intracellular recording studies in the gerbil and chinchilla have shown that binaurally driven units that are normally inhibited by simultaneous stimulation of the contralateral ear can be reversibly inhibited by strychnine, a potent inhibitor of glycine (Moore *et al.*, 1981; Moore and Caspary, 1983). It has always been important to understand the anatomical relationships of neural elements in the MSO because of its role as a major relay nucleus and as a major processor of information from the two ears. Our increasing understanding of differences in the functional capabilities of different classes of neurons in the MSO has made it imperative that we develop a complete picture of the different classes of axons that project to this nucleus, how they are distributed, how they relate to one another, and how they differ chemically.

In this article we will present data from studies with classical light and electron microscopic methods, as well as those from newly developed selective marking techniques that utilize radiolabeled compounds and autoradiographic procedures, to provide a picture of the axonal populations of the MSO as we now understand them.

II. CLASSICAL APPROACHES TO IDENTIFYING AXONAL POPULATIONS

The data in this section come from a systematic survey of axon classes in the cat MSO as identified by Golgi and electron microscopic methods. The data suggest that there is a morphological basis for a variety of interactions between MSO neurons and other elements in the auditory pathway, especially certain periolivary cell groups.

A. Methods

The MSO was studied in material from 24 normal adult cats and 92 kittens ranging in age from about the sixtieth day of gestation (estimated from the size at sacrifice) to the fifty-sixth postnatal day. The material was prepared for light microscopic examination with a variety of Golgi, Nissl, and reduced silver staining methods and for electron microscopic examination by perfusion with a variety of mixed aldehyde fixatives (Schwartz, 1977). To explore vesicle pleiomorphism, a variety of fixation procedures and osmotic conditions were employed. Following perfusion with 1% glutaraldehyde and 1% paraformaldehyde in $0.12\ M$ phosphate buffer, pH 7.2 (Sotelo and Palay, 1968), material from one animal was immersed for 60 minutes in $0.24\ M$ phosphate buffer (240 mOsm), in buffer plus 7% sucrose (345 mOsm), or buffer plus 25% sucrose (1000 mOsm), postfixed in the same solution containing 1% osmium tetroxide, dehydrated in ethanol and propylene oxide, and embedded in Epon. Material from another animal, similarly perfused, was immersed for 60 minutes in a solution containing two drops of 30% hydrogen peroxide to 33 ml of fixative (Perrachia and Mittler, 1972), postfixed in 1% osmium tetroxide in $0.12\ M$ phosphate buffer, uranyl block stained (Karnovsky, 1967), dehydrated, and embedded. Material was also prepared from six cats with ablation lesions of the CN made under visual control. The cerebellum was retracted and the anterior portion of the CN was removed with a suction pipette. No histology was performed on the lesions, but inspection of the brains after perfusion and removal from the skull showed that in all cases the anterior ventral cochlear nucleus (AVCN) had been completely removed. In some cases, portions of the eighth nerve, the posterior ventral cochlear nucleus (PVCN), and the dorsal cochlear nucleus (DCN) had also been removed. Stotler's (1953) study indicated that only the principal input to the MSO was lost following massive CN lesions and no attempt was made to restrict the lesion to any cellular subpopulation or area within the ventral cochlear nucleus (VCN); rather, we attempted complete removal of the AVCN. The lesioned animals were sacrificed 2, 4, or 6 days postoperatively by perfusion with mixed aldehyde fixative in phosphate buffer, postfixed in 1% osmium tetroxide in $0.12\ M$ phosphate buffer, dehydrated, and embedded in Epon.

B. Results

Golgi studies of axons in the MSO of adult cats and kittens reveal at least three extrinsic and one intrinsic input to the cat MSO in addition to the principal input to the MSO from the AVCN described by other authors (LaVilla, 1898; Ramón y Cajal, 1909; Stotler, 1953). Ultrastructural studies distinguish at least four classes of axon terminals and suggest a possible subpopulation in the AVCN input based on variations in vesicle morphology, in contrast to earlier electron microscopic studies (Lindsey, 1975, in the cat; Perkins, 1973, in the chinchilla) that recognized only three classes. Correlation of the Golgi and ultrastructural findings has so far been possible only for the major input to the MSO, the axons of AVCN spherical cells.

1. THE PRINCIPAL INPUT

These axons enter the MSO from the concave lateral and convex medial surfaces and distribute along the dendrites perpendicular to the plane of the nucleus and over the perikaryon. Along the dendrites, terminal specializations may occur as boutons en passant or as elongated finger-like processes. Broader terminal expansions sometimes occur in the vicinity of the perikaryon. Figure 1 illustrates these axons in a 5-day-old kitten brain impregnated with the rapid Golgi–Cox procedure of Ramon-Moliner (1970). Axons entering the medial surface arise as collaterals of axons crossing the trapezoid body. In a typical transverse section the spread of these axons includes only a few principal cells. In horizontal sections it becomes clear that these arbors actually have a candelabra-like rostrocaudal spread (Fig. 2). Morest (1973) has suggested that CN axons distribute in horizontal sheets through the MSO. Our data confirm this and further suggest that single axons that branch at the periphery of the nucleus in transverse sections probably contribute to more than one rostrocaudally oriented sheet with a thickness of several hundred micrometers.

Figure 3 illustrates the typical features of the principal input (PI) terminals, referred to by Lindsey (1975) as spherical vesicle (SV) endings. PI endings have multiple regions of synaptic membrane specialization. Intercellular substance (ICS), coated vesicles, neurofilaments, glial ensheathment, and round agranular synaptic vesicles are characteristic of these endings. The endings appear as elongated processes up to 20 μm in length and from 1 to 2 μm in thickness, or as boutons generally about 2 μm in diameter. Appearance as boutons is consistent with a cross-sectional view of an elongated terminal. Smaller boutons are consistent with cross-sections of small extensions connected to elongated terminals by a thin neck. The elongated terminals make repeated synaptic contacts with the MSO neurons but are separated from the neurons and adjacent terminals by a space up to 100 μm wide that contains ICS and small glial processes (Schwartz, 1972). The region of synaptic contact is curved, indenting the terminal surface. Densities associated with the synaptic area are asymmetric, with the postsynaptic surface associated with the greater density. The portion of the terminal not adjacent to the MSO neurons is ensheathed by glial processes. There is no indication that PI endings receive any synaptic inputs. The vesicles are round, agranular, homogeneous in size, and about 52 nm in diameter. Coated vesicles are abundant and preferentially located at or near membrane abutting ICS. Neurofilaments are present in longitudinal or circular arrays. These neurofilaments

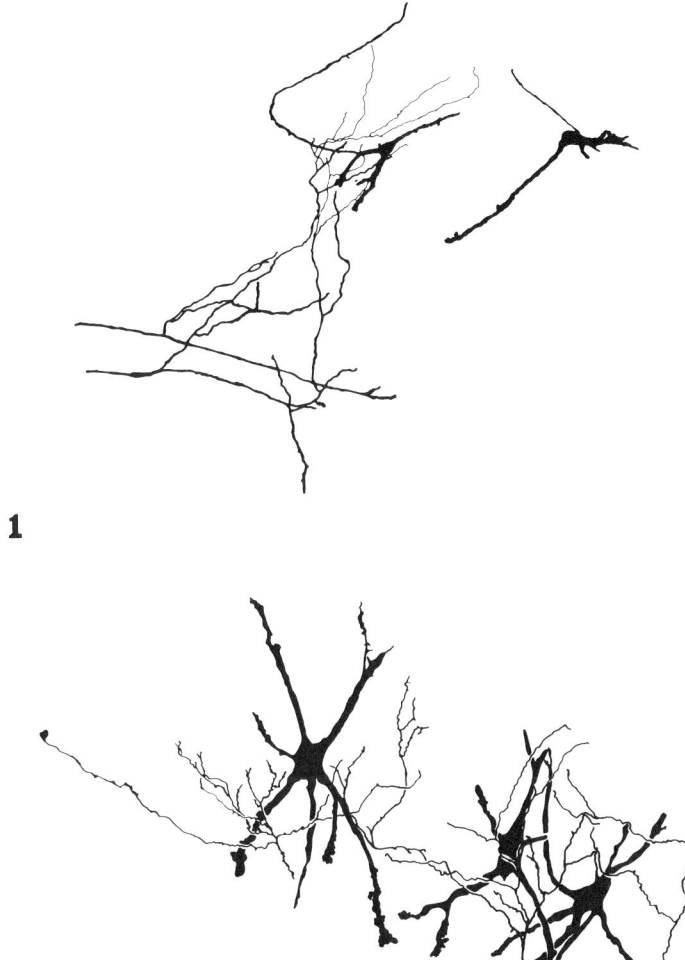

FIGS. 1 AND 2. Camera lucida drawings of, respectively, transverse and horizontal sections from a 5-day-old kitten brain impregnated with the rapid Golgi–Cox procedure. Figure 1 illustrates medial superior olivary nucleus (MSO) principal cells in relation to terminal arbors from collaterals of axons crossing the trapezoid body from the contralateral cochlear nucleus. The midline is to the left. Figure 2 illustrates the candelabra-like rostrocaudal spread of these axons.

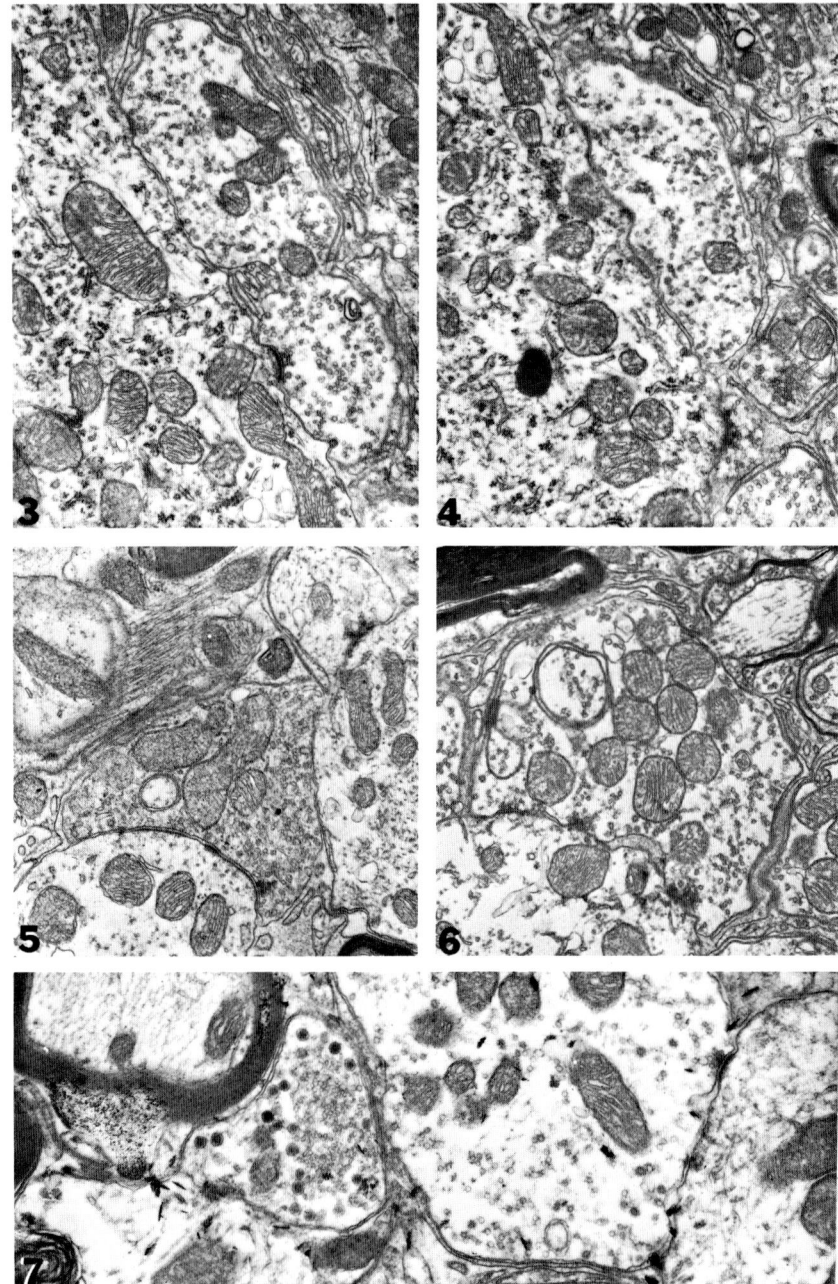

are the ultrastructural substrate for the neurofibrils and boutons seen with reduced silver methods. Mitochondria and small elements of smooth endoplasmic reticulum are present. In many cases the axon giving rise to terminals having all these features could not be observed. The axons that were observed were myelinated. Boutons were frequently separated by an unmyelinated stretch of axon, but myelinated stretches between boutons were observed in only a few instances.

Vesicles in some PI endings appeared more or less pleiomorphic under certain fixation conditions. Even under the most extreme conditions (25% sucrose or 0.5% NaCl) all of the vesicles in some terminals remained spherical. These differences in the physical properties of vesicles in different endings of a class identified by nonvesicular characteristics suggest that a subgroup based on vesicular features may exist that can be obscured with some fixation procedures routinely employed. Endings with pleiomorphic rather than round vesicles but with all the other characteristics of PI endings, including origin from a myelinated axon (Fig. 6), seem to represent a substantial proportion of the total terminal population. In contrast to the flat vesicle endings described below, these endings do not survive massive lesions of the AVCN.

In six cats surviving 2–6 days after sustaining lesions of the AVCN, PI endings demonstrated neurofilamentous hypertrophy and other signs of degeneration before they disappeared. The pattern of ending loss seen in these animals is consistent with that reported by Stotler (1953) and Lindsey (1975) in the cat and Perkins (1973) in the chinchilla. Six days postlesion only a few dendritic profiles were completely denuded of all their PI synaptic connections. Remaining endings included those in various stages of degeneration as well as some that appeared normal. In the longest surviving specimens endings containing small flat

---

FIGS. 3–7. These figures illustrate the different classes of synaptic terminals found in the MSO. Figure 3 shows the curved asymmetric contact region, round synaptic vesicles, and glial ensheathment characteristic of principal input (PI) terminals. A second synaptic region is cut obliquely in the upper left. Other examples of PI terminals are found at the right of Fig. 7 and at the lower right of Fig. 4. Glutaraldehyde (1.25%) and paraformaldehyde (1%) in phosphate buffer, uranyl block stain. ×13,350. Figure 4 shows a terminal found adjacent to that in Fig. 3 that is less well enclosed by glia, has a more regular apposition with the soma, a more symmetric synaptic junction, and which contains pleiomorphic vesicles. This represents the second major group. ×13,350. Figure 5 illustrates the very regular apposition, moderately symmetrical synaptic densities, and the dense packing of small vesicles characteristic of the third major group. Glutaraldehyde (1%) and paraformaldehyde (1%) in phosphate buffer, uranyl block stain. ×13,275. In Fig. 6 a large terminal arising from a myelinated axon has pleiomorphic vesicles but otherwise has all the features characteristic of the PI. It may represent a subclass of the cochlear nucleus (CN) input. From the same material as listed for Figs. 3 and 4. ×12,225. Figure 7 illustrates the single example of a small vesicle ending with large numbers of dense-cored vesicles found in the fiber zone in material prepared with Peracchia's peroxide method. ×9000.

vesicles and some containing larger flat ones appeared normal. Degenerated terminals occurred on dendrites and perikarya and were preferentially distributed on dendrites in the lateral half of the MSO ipsilateral to the lesion and the medial half of the contralateral MSO. In any given region the number of affected endings per dendritic profile ranged from none to all.

The transverse sections of the central cell band and fiber zones cut for electron microscopic observation include profiles of rostrocaudally, dorsoventrally, and obliquely oriented dendrites of rostrocaudally elongated and multipolar cells. Differences in the proportions of affected terminals on any given dendritic profile may be related to the type of cell from which that dendrite arises, or to the orientation of that dendrite. Because there are no diagnostic ultrastructural features for the various MSO cell types, the character of the cell giving rise to the various dendritic profiles could not be established in the material examined. Our observations of variability in the fraction of degenerating terminals on isolated dendritic profiles are consistent with the observations of Lindsey (1975), which were restricted to positively identifiable medial and lateral dendrites of bipolar and multipolar central cells, and to marginal cells.

Thus, information from Golgi, Bodian, and Nissl, together with electron microscopic examination of normal and lesioned material (with special attention to synaptic vesicle shape), suggest the possible existence of additional subpopulations of the major input to the MSO from the AVCN. Chemical techniques for selectively lesioning the specific subpopulations of neurons within a single area such as the AVCN are just beginning to be developed. Such techniques, together with the identification of chemical markers for the axons of each cell type, will be required to fully resolve the details of the axonal relationships with specific neurons.

2. OTHER ULTRASTRUCTURALLY DISTINCT ENDINGS

Terminals of the non-CN input to the MSO are boutons generally less than 2 μm in diameter. These boutons may make more than one synaptic contact with the MSO neuron but have flat contact areas with more symmetrical submembranous densities. These densities are less pronounced than the postsynaptic density in the PI terminals. Depending upon the fixation conditions, the agranular synaptic vesicles may vary in shape from round to flat and appear qualitatively similar to the vesicles in PI endings (Figs. 4, 8–11). These endings apparently correspond to the large flat vesicle endings described by Lindsey (1975) and the intermediate vesicle endings of Perkins (1973).

In some endings the synaptic vesicles are smaller, more numerous, and more densely packed than in either PI or intermediate-sized vesicle endings. These small vesicle endings are more likely to be found adjacent to one another without interposed glial processes and without ICS between pre- and postsynaptic elements (Figs. 5 and 8). Dense-cored vesicles are sometimes found in these endings. These endings correspond to the small flat vesicle endings described by Lindsey (1975) and Perkins (1973). One example of a small ending densely packed with flat vesicles and containing many dense-cored vesicles (Fig. 7) was observed in a fiber zone of the MSO in material treated with the hydrogen peroxide–glutaraldehyde fixative and uranyl block stained. The single example could be a result of the special fixation, could be an anomalous axon, or could represent a numerically small but truly different class of terminals.

We conclude that, in addition to the two possible subgroups of the PI endings (type 1), there is (1) a class of smaller endings (type 2) similar to one of the PI classes but which survives CN lesions, has intermediate-sized vesicles, and more symmetric synaptic membrane densities, and (2) at least one class of small endings (type 3) with symmetric synaptic membrane specializations that contain smaller, more densely packed vesicles than the preceding group and which tend to occur in clusters, may be apposed to one another, and also survive AVCN lesion. Subtle morphologic differences suggest that there may be several types of small vesicle endings. A single example of a possible fourth class was found in the fiber zone, containing small, densely packed vesicles and numerous dense-cored vesicles. Type 2 and 3 endings make up a higher percentage of the synaptic terminals on, and also occupy a higher percentage of the surface of, marginal cells (Schwartz, 1980b).

Ultrastructural analyses have provided a detailed picture of terminal distributions based on one classification scheme. The development of additional chemical markers or selective lesioning agents is required to allow correlation of the ultrastructural data with information already available from Golgi studies of axonal arborization patterns presented below.

3. GOLGI STUDIES OF OTHER INPUTS

Golgi material was systematically searched for axons that might correspond to those that survive CN lesions or that could be associated with the other morphologically distinct terminal classes. We found at least three other extrinsic inputs and one intrinsic input to the MSO that have courses and arborization patterns distinct from that of the principal input. These include two different arborization patterns that have been traced to periolivary cells of origin, one group of axons that traverse the MSO in the mediolateral direction, occasionally giving off a small branch at the margins of the MSO, one group of rostrocaudally oriented axons with a different pattern than any previously described, and one group of axon arbors that probably arises from collaterals of intrinsic MSO axons.

a. Periolivary Inputs. Figure 12 shows a transverse section of a 5-day-old kitten brain impregnated with the Golgi–Cox procedure. The cell marked by the large arrow is apparently located in the dorsomedial periolivary nucleus (DMPO)

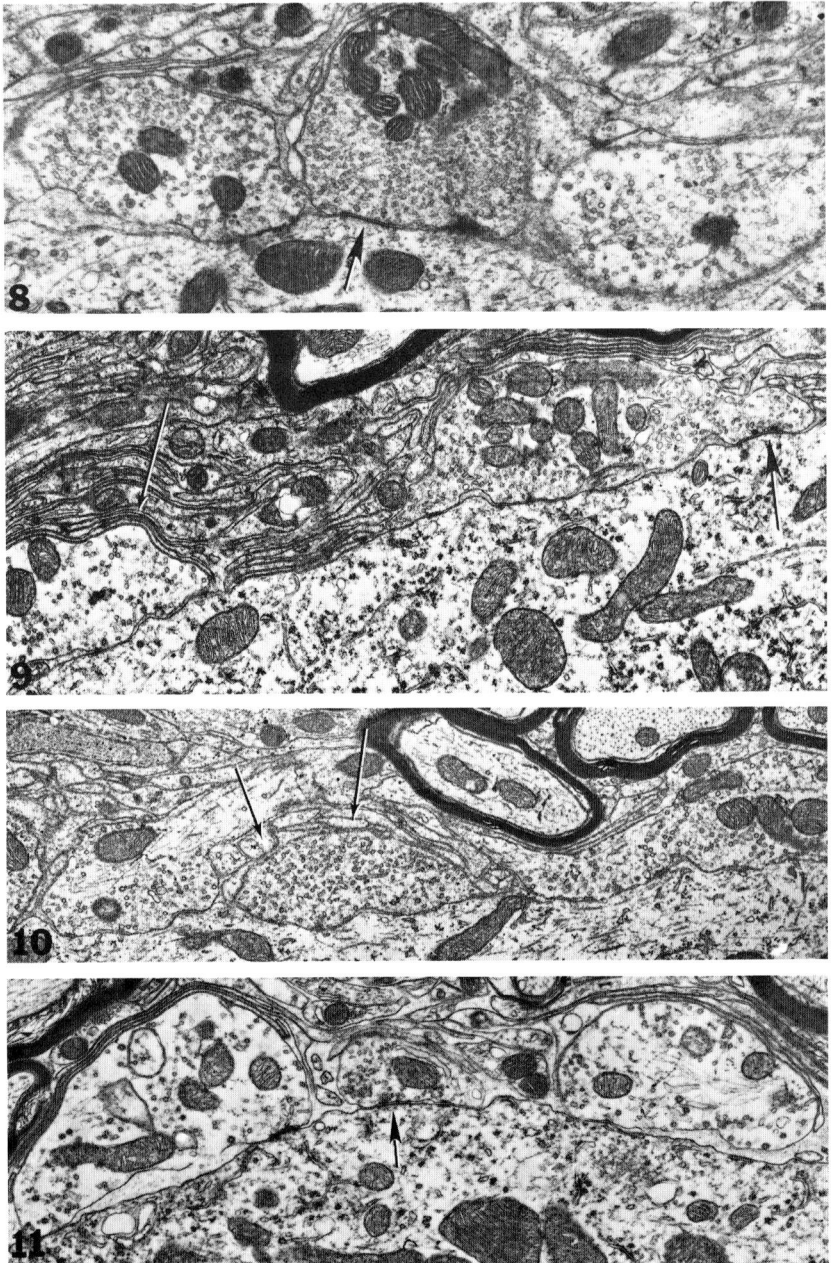

FIGS. 8–11. Multiple synaptic terminal types are shown following various preparative procedures. All three vesicle classes are illustrated in Fig. 8. The round vesicles characteristic of the PI are seen in the terminal at the right. The pleiomorphic vesicles characteristic of the second class of

and is shown in a camera lucida drawing in Fig. 13. Its axon passes over the dorsal pole of the MSO and gives off two collaterals that cross the MSO dorsoventrally, giving rise to branched arbors that can intersect several laminar sheets of rostrocaudally oriented cells, dendrites, and axons.

A brushlike arborization pattern has been observed in various parts of the Golgi–Cox-impregnated MSO, always directed laterally (Fig. 15). In one case such an arbor was traced to its cell of origin close to the medial edge of the ventral portion of the MSO (Fig. 14). Nuclear borders are fuzzy at this point, but it appears to be located in the ventromedial periolivary nucleus (DMPO) (see Morest, 1968, for a complete description of periolivary cell group nomenclature). Axons of elongate cells in the medial nucleus of the trapezoid body (MNTB) have a similar brushlike arborization pattern in the DMPO (Morest, 1968).

b. Presumed Extrinsic Inputs. A class of axons, frequently impregnated with a variety of methods, crosses the MSO from the convex to the concave surface without giving off any branches. These axons are commonly seen in brains impregnated with rapid Golgi methods and have the largest caliber of any axons in those preparations. A few axons in both adult animals and kittens did show small branches near the edges of the MSO. One such axon is illustrated in a photograph from a transverse section of a 5-day-old kitten brain impregnated with the Golgi–Cox procedure (Fig. 12, arrowhead). The origin of these axons is unknown, although they are presumed to arise either in the contralateral AVCN or from the ipsilateral MNTB.

In addition to the arborization patterns identified in transverse sections, a variety is observed in sagittal sections which could be either extrinsic or intrinsic.

Rostrocaudally oriented axons in a sagittal section from a 2-day-old kitten brain are illustrated in Fig. 16. The brain was fixed by immersion in mixed aldehyde fixative and impregnated with the Golgi–Kopsch procedure (Colonnier, 1964). The principal input is not well shown with this procedure. The

---

endings are seen in the terminal at the left. The symmetrical junction (arrow) and small, closely packed vesicles in the middle terminal characterize the third type of ending. Glutaraldehyde (1%) and paraformaldehyde (1%) in phosphate buffer. ×15,392. In Fig. 9 extensive glial lamellae ensheath a PI terminal (small arrow) and one of the second class (large arrow). Paraformaldehyde (1%) and glutaraldehyde (1.25%) in phosphate buffer followed by paraformaldehyde (4%) and glutaraldehyde (5%) in the same buffer, uranyl block stained. ×12,432. In Fig. 10 glial processes (arrows) separate a type 2 terminal containing intermediate-sized, pleiomorphic vesicles (below) from an elongated PI ending that passes over it. Another portion of the elongated PI ending is seen contacting the dendrite at the right. Paraformaldehyde (1%), glutaraldehyde (1%) in phosphate buffer. ×11,618. In Fig. 11 numerous coated vesicles and neurofilaments are present in the PI terminals at the right and left. The small terminal between them (arrow) has pleiomorphic vesicles and represents the second class. Glutaraldehyde (1%) and paraformaldehyde (1%) in phosphate buffer, uranyl block stained. ×11,470.

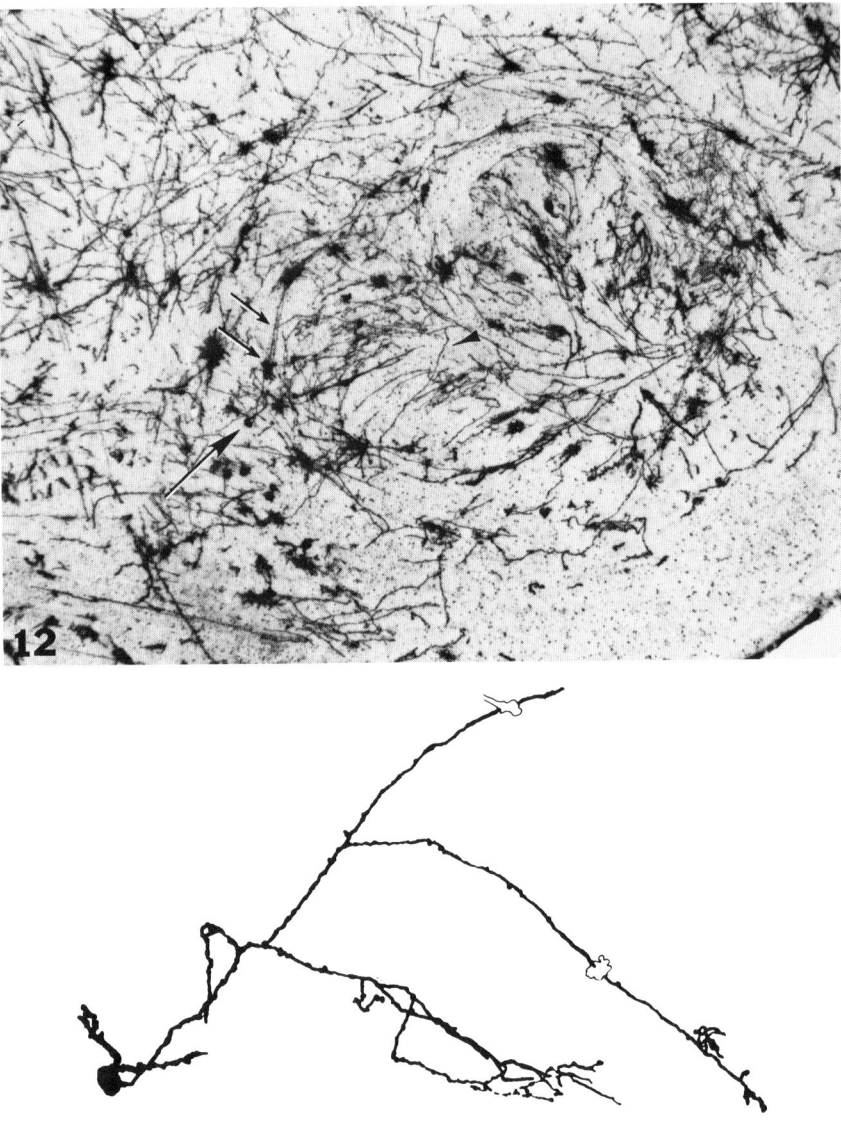

FIGS. 12 AND 13. The large arrow in Fig. 12 identifies a neuron at the edge of the dorsomedial periolivary nucleus (DMPO) in a transverse section through a 5-day-old kitten brain impregnated with the rapid Golgi–Cox method. The axonal arborization pattern of the neuron is shown in a camera lucida drawing in Fig. 13. The small arrows indicate axonal branch points.

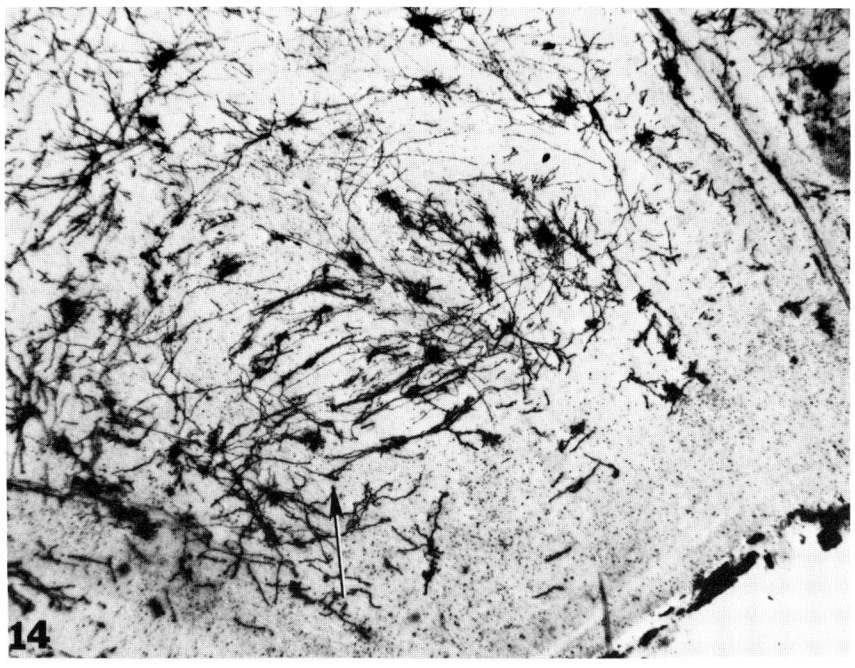

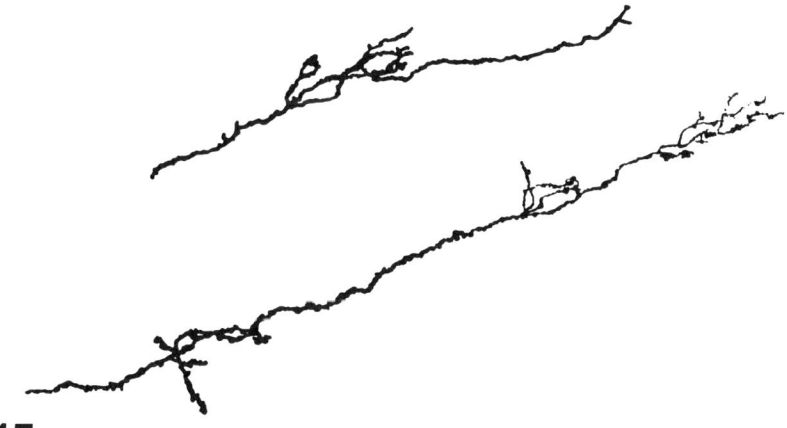

FIGS. 14 AND 15. Illustrating a brush type of axonal arbor from axons originating medial to the MSO. In Fig. 14 a cell in the ventromedial periolivary (VMPO) region (arrow) gives rise to an arbor similar to the two shown in Fig. 15. The arbor is associated with the terminal dendritic branches of an MSO principal cell. The transverse section is from a 5-day-old kitten brain impregnated with the rapid Golgi–Cox method.

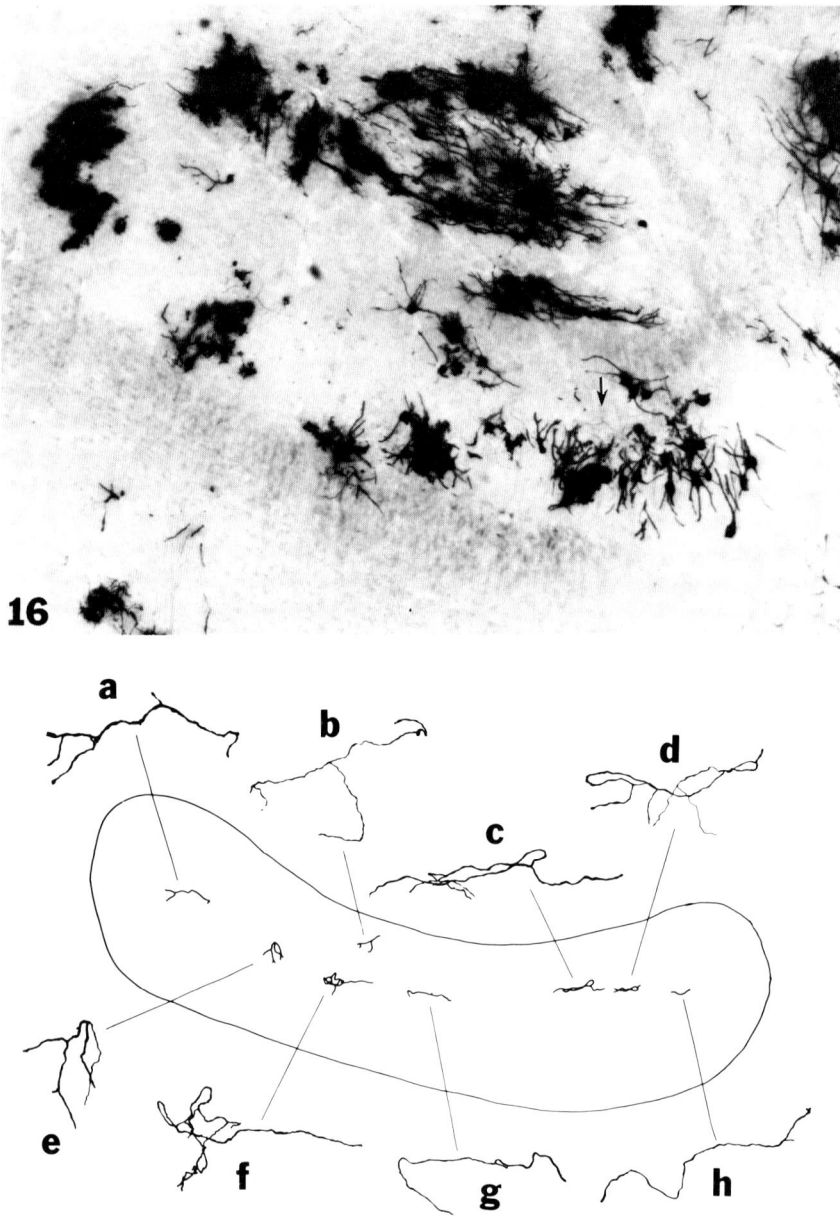

FIGS. 16 AND 17. Illustrating in sagittal sections a variety of axons with a rostrocaudal spread. The camera lucida drawings in Fig. 17 were made from the section shown in Fig. 16 and a section adjacent to it. Arbor (c) in Fig. 17 is shown at the arrow in Fig. 16. It is primarily associated with dendrites. Rostral is to the left.

rostrocaudally running axons near the periphery of the principal cell dendrites exhibit a distinctly different pattern from that of the candelabra-like pattern of the CN input. They are illustrated in camera lucida drawings of the section in Fig. 17 and in an adjacent section.

c. Intrinsic Axons. In seeking evidence of the nature of the terminal arbor of intrinsic collaterals, we have followed over 100 axons impregnated beyond their initial segment. These axons belonged to bipolar and multipolar central cells and marginal cells of young kittens and were followed until they were lost from the 90-μm-thick sections. Most axons were seen in transverse sections. They turned toward the closest edge of the MSO and ran dorsally or ventrally to the edge of the nucleus before being lost among the fibers around the nucleus that LaVilla (1898) observed turning posteriorly (Fig. 18).

Central cell axons were sometimes seen to make a turn at the medial or lateral edge in the vicinity of a marginal cell. Of the more than 100 axons followed, only 4 possible examples of collaterals were found (Fig. 19). One cell (Fig. 19a) at the ventromedial edge of the nucleus could be a marginal cell with a collateral extending into the ventral edge of the cell band. A marginal cell at the lateral edge (Fig. 19b) sends one branch into the cell band and one beyond the lateral border. One principal cell (a somewhat ambiguous case because of the quality of the impregnation) apparently gives off a collateral cluster in the central cell band (Fig. 19c). A similar arborization pattern is observed in a horizontally sectioned cell (Fig. 19d) at the lateral edge of the nucleus. We have also observed several arborizations (Fig. 19e,f) that could not be traced to their cells of origin, but with similar distribution and roughly comparable shape to the two traced to central cell band cells. The failure to impregnate collaterals in any significant numbers cannot be taken as evidence of their relative infrequency. The data indicate that at least some are present and we must continue to look for better examples of the type.

C. Discussion

Golgi studies have confirmed and clarified the horizontally oriented candelabra-like spread of axons of AVCN spherical cells and the interrelationships of branches of these axons with more than one adjacent, horizontally oriented sheet of cells. These studies have also identified four additional Golgi patterns: one of intrinsic collaterals of axons of MSO neurons, two of axons of periolivary neurons, and one belonging to axons of unknown origin. In describing the relationships between MSO neurons, their intrinsic axons, extrinsic axons, and periolivary cells, these studies have established the existence of an anatomical basis for complex processing of auditory information, opening new possibilities to consideration and testing in physiological studies.

114 *Ilsa R. Schwartz*

Golgi studies do not allow a quantitative evaluation of the relative frequency of occurrence of the different classes within the MSO, the relative proportions of each type of ending found on particular neurons, or their relationships to one another, nor do they provide any information about differences in chemical properties. Although three classes of synaptic terminals can be distinguished on the basis of their ultrastructural characteristics, many endings remain difficult to classify. Through lesion studies the type 1 endings have been shown to correspond to the PI from the AVCN, and because of the correspondence between

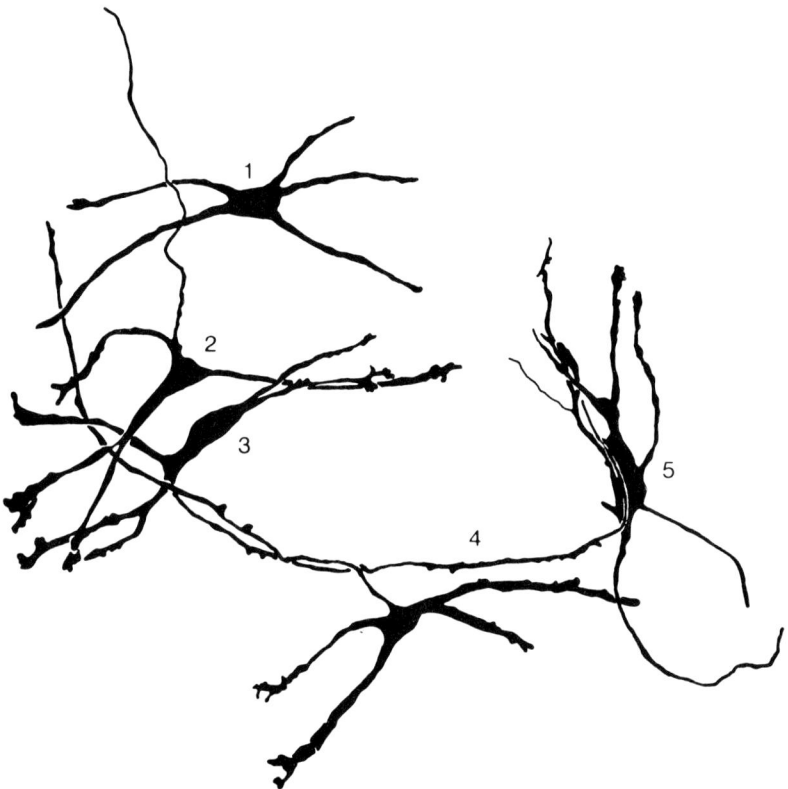

FIG. 18. Illustrating camera lucida drawings of five neurons from a transverse section of a 5-day-old kitten brain impregnated with the rapid Golgi–Cox method of Ramon-Moliner. Cells 1–4 are principal cells, cell 5 is a marginal cell. Axons of principal and marginal cells were best seen in transverse sections. They turned toward the closest edge of the nucleus before being lost among the fibers around the nucleus. As illustrated by cell 5, principal cell axons were sometimes seen to make a turn at the medial or lateral edge in the vicinity of a marginal cell.

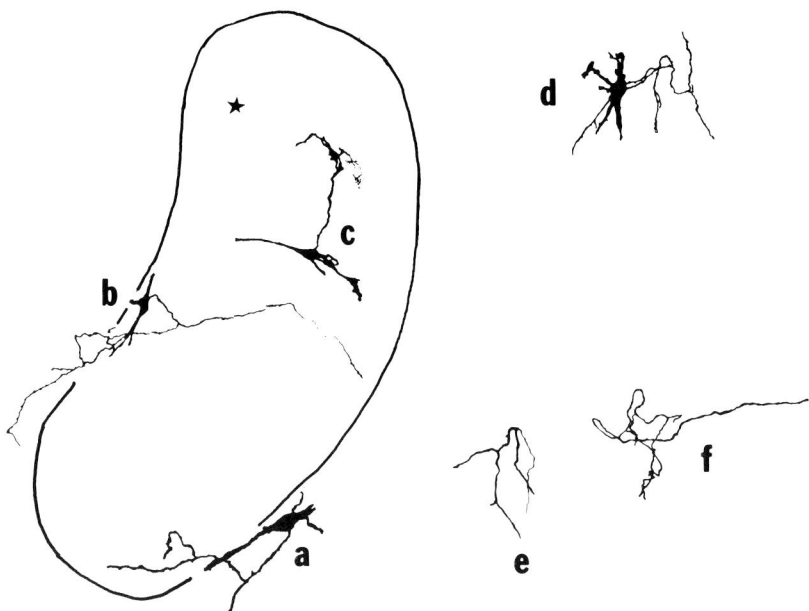

FIG. 19. A composite of cells and axons from a number of animals. One cell (a) at the ventromedial edge of the nucleus could be a marginal cell with a collateral extending into the ventral edge of the cell band. (b) A marginal cell at the lateral edge with one branch into the cell band and one ramifying beyond the lateral border. (c) A central cell whose axon ramifies in a restricted area within the central cell band. (d) A cell from a horizontal section located at the lateral edge of the nucleus (★) [(d) is a principal cell that apparently gives off a collateral cluster in the central cell band and is a somewhat ambiguous case because of the quality of the impregnation]. If (c) and (d) illustrate collateral arbors, cells (e) and (f) from the sagittal sections (Fig. 17) have a similar distribution and roughly comparable shapes.

light microscopic neurofibrillar silver staining methods and the presence of bundles of neurofilaments in these endings, their distribution can be mapped at both the light (Stotler, 1953) and electron microscopic (Lindsey, 1975; Perkins, 1973) levels. Electron microscopy has allowed us to map the distribution and relationships of the ultrastructurally identified classes and gain insights into their functions, although definitive correlations between Golgi arborization patterns and ultrastructural characteristics have not yet been possible for endings other than those of the PI. Because Golgi data indicate that some axons belong to intrinsic and periolivary neurons, lesion studies of these neurons are not possible by conventional methods. Chemical markers that can distinguish between the different synaptic and neural populations will be required to allow selective chemical lesioning or selective terminal marking to map their distribution.

1. Correlations of Axon Arborization Patterns with Synaptic Terminal Types

In accord with studies of previous authors in the chinchilla and the cat (Perkins, 1973; Lindsey, 1975), our examination of the ultrastructural features of synaptic terminals in the MSO reveals three major classes: (1) large, multiple contact synapses with large vesicles, (2) intermediate-sized terminals with more regular appositions and pleiomorphic vesicles of intermediate size, and (3) small boutons with very regular appositions, symmetric junctions, and small, densely packed synaptic vesicles that can be flattened under some fixation conditions. However, our experiments with fixation suggest that some terminals that belong to the first class on the basis of most of their morphologic features vary with regard to the response of their vesicles to hyperosmotic conditions and may represent a subpopulation in the projections from the CN. This is not surprising in light of the several cell types identified in the cat AVCN with Golgi methods (Brawer et al., 1974). Our lesion studies have involved destruction of all the CN cells, i.e., small and large spherical, globular, and multipolar types, and do not allow us to make any distinctions between them with regard to their terminal distribution within the MSO. However, studies with small lesions (Warr, 1982) demonstrate differences in the location and density of projections from each cell type to the superior olivary complex (SOC). Although differences in vesicle morphology (especially in terms of size) are now generally accepted to correlate with differences in cell of origin, as may be the case here, it should be noted that additional factors (e.g., intrinsic chemical differences and functional state, both of which can be affected by fixation conditions) can also contribute to the degree of pleiomorphism or flattening.

Subtle differences in distribution, in vesicle size and shape, and in the number of dense-cored vesicles present suggest that the broad class of small vesicle endings may include terminals of different origins and functional abilities. Neither these terminals nor the intermediate class of terminals of non-CN origin can yet be correlated definitively with any of the axon arborization patterns described in this article. It seems likely that some of the small vesicle endings found distally on principal cell dendrites in the fiber zones correspond to rostrocaudally running axons found in the fiber zones or to the small branches given off by straight axons crossing the MSO from medial to lateral. Both small and intermediate-sized vesicle endings are found on somata and proximal dendrites, with a distribution pattern that could correspond to the arborization patterns of intrinsic axons. Additional information is required to correlate the classes with respect to ultrastructure and arborization pattern.

2. Segregation of Inputs within the MSO

Previous electron microscopic studies of the MSO have revealed ultrastructurally distinct populations of axon terminals in adult animals, but it has been difficult to interpret the significance of differential distributions of these terminals except with regard to the medial–lateral separation of the principal CN input to central and marginal cells. The findings of this article enlarge our understanding of the different inputs received by the MSO and indicate some restrictions in their projections within the nucleus that suggest segregation of different groups of inputs to specific cell types in the MSO. Such a segregated pattern is consistent with previous physiological and anatomical studies of the MSO and with similar observations in nuclear groups at all levels of the auditory system.

3. THE PRINCIPAL INPUT

The PI from the ipsilateral and contralateral AVCN distributes, respectively, to the lateral and medial dendrites of single central cells, and unilaterally to ipsilateral lateral and contralateral medial marginal cells (Stotler, 1953; Lindsey, 1975; Perkins, 1973). The large size and ultrastructural features of the synaptic endings of this input are consistent with a high-security synapse. Synapses with a high probability of firing the postsynaptic cell would be necessary to preserve time and phase information. Large synaptic terminals with all their multiple synaptic sites directed onto a single postsynaptic cell and having an association with ICS are found at each level of the central auditory system [MNTB, Lenn and Reese, 1966; Nakajima, 1971; CN, Kane, 1973; inferior colliculus (IC), Rockel and Jones, 1972]. The bilateral nature of the principal projection to the MSO central cells suggests that these synapses are involved in relaying information about differences in the time of arrival of sound at the two ears. The rostrocaudal spread of the candelabra-like arbor parallels the rostrocaudal spread of multipolar central cells and is large enough to involve several cells in a rostrocaudal sheet. Axons branching at the nuclear margins may contribute to several nearby sheets. The dorsoventral array of sheets of cells and axons in the MSO preserves the tonotopic projection of the cochlea onto the CN. It is not known whether there are any differences in the distributions of these endings to central multipolar and bipolar cells. However, because there is some indication in kittens that terminal dendritic arbors of the two cell types tend to run at right angles to one another (Schwartz, 1977), one possibility is that multipolar cells with a more rostrocaudal spread could be sensitive to a narrower frequency band, whereas bipolars might contribute to coding intensity information that involves recruitment of neurons neighboring those optimally driven by a particular frequency and thus involving more sheets. There are many alternative possibilities that can only be resolved by information about the differential distribution of single axon arbors on the different cell types and by intracellular recordings with marking of the cell to allow its histologic identification.

4. PERIOLIVARY INPUTS

Two periolivary inputs identified in young kittens (preliminary report, Schwartz and Wittebort, 1976) present additional substrates for modulating MSO output to higher levels. The small branches given off by some of these axons have been observed in older animals as well as in young kittens. From their location at the periphery of the MSO fiber zones, they could contact marginal cells or terminal dendritic arbors of bipolar or multipolar cells. Such a distribution is consistent with the ultrastructural observation of a higher percentage of type 2 and type 3 endings present on marginal cells (Schwartz, 1980b).

5. Axons of Unknown Origin

Rostrocaudally running axons ramifying in the MSO fiber zones are observed in both neonatal and adult cats. From their location they probably make contacts primarily on dendrites, or on rostrocaudally elongated cell bodies that have a similar orientation and location. None of these axons has been traced to its cell of origin, which could be either intrinsic or extrinsic.

6. Axons of MSO Neurons

The arborization pattern that we have traced to central cell band cells involves branching within a restricted area within the central band, such as might be associated with one or more somata and proximal dendrites. Although the ultrastructure of the terminals associated with these arbors has yet to be established, several authors have reported groups of flat vesicle endings with a similar distribution (Clark, 1969a,b; Perkins, 1973; Lindsey, 1975). In our experiments with hyperosmotic fixatives, the vesicles in the small endings were much more resistant to flattening than vesicles in endings in the spinal cords of the same cats. Flat vesicles in spinal cord terminals have sometimes been associated with glycine or inhibiting behavior (Bodian, 1966, 1970; Uchizono, 1966; Matus and Dennison, 1971). Thus, more specific information about the chemistry of these endings, or indeed about the other "flat" vesicle endings, is required before we can presume anything about their functional role. One axon arose from a small, rather spherical cell body dorsomedial to the MSO in the region of the DMPO. The DMPO receives collaterals of axons of MNTB principal cells. The peridendritic plexus around these cells is formed in large part by collaterals of the axons from the contralateral AVCN, which form the PI to the medial MSO (Morest, 1968). Morest also illustrated a collateral arbor in the DMPO from one MSO marginal cell. Thus, the axon that courses ventrally through the central cell band from the dorsal pole of the MSO could represent (1) a possible disynaptic pathway from the contralateral AVCN capable of either enhancing or inhibiting the primary response of selected MSO cells, or (2) a feedback loop from MSO marginal cells. With only a single example impregnated in one 5-day-old kitten we can do no more than recognize the possibility of such pathways.

It is even more difficult to reconstruct the route of information arriving in the MSO via broomlike arbors directed laterally at several levels in the MSO. Only one could be traced to a cell of origin ventromedial to the MSO and close to the

MSO boundary in a region that is probably VMPO. The neonatal character of the kitten, with its ill-defined MSO fiber zones, makes it difficult to interpret the location of the arbors within the MSO; although some arbors at least appear to be centrally located, some could be distributing to marginal or peripheral cells on either side. Portions of the multipolar cell and globular cell regions of the VCN apparently project via the ventral trapezoid body to the VNTB and the VMPO (Warr, 1972). Most of the straight axons that cross the MSO presumably arise from the contralateral CN or from the principal cells of the ipsilateral MNTB. Presumably they terminate in the lateral superior olive.

7. New Possibilities for Processing Auditory Information

Since Stotler (1953) demonstrated the projections of the cochlear nuclei onto opposite polar dendrites of individual bipolar cells, the MSO has been thought of as a system capable of analyzing time differences in the arrival of action potentials related to binaurally processed signals (Goldberg and Brown, 1968, 1969). With the identification of four cell types within the MSO (Schwartz, 1977) and the three extrinsic inputs and one intrinsic input described in this article, in addition to the well-known bilateral PI from the CN, we can now recognize a morphological basis for several different pathways that could serve to analyze or code binaural differences in intensity, pitch, or other cues important to localization of sound in space. How, or indeed whether, these pathways operate in processing auditory information remains to be determined.

The need to establish the precise patterns of segregation of different axonal inputs to different cell types within the MSO is clear. New methods that can help to resolve these patterns are discussed in the next section. But the results of application of classical methods described in this section have expanded our ideas about the information-processing capabilities of the MSO and point up the need for physiological investigations of new pathways through the MSO.

III. DIFFERENTIAL AMINO ACID-LABELING STUDIES

A. Rationale

A key to understanding how a synapse functions is identification of its transmitter. Furthermore, synaptic populations are most likely to differ in their neurotransmitters. Thus, markers related to neurotransmitters are most likely to allow us to differentiate among synaptic populations.

This section will describe light and electron microscopic techniques utilized in this laboratory to differentiate and map the distribution of synaptic terminal populations on the basis of their chemical properties, especially those that may assist in identifying their neurotransmitter.

In the auditory system a growing body of data suggests that glutamate and aspartate may be excitatory transmitters between the cells of the eighth nerve and neurons in the CN; whereas glycine (Gly) and γ-aminobutyric acid (GABA) may be involved as inhibitory transmitters in the CN and elsewhere (Klinke, 1981; Daigneault, 1981; Wenthold, 1981; Moore and Caspary, 1983). A correlary of the potential involvement of several amino acid transmitters in the auditory system is that, if they are transmitters, mechanisms should exist for their rapid clearance from the synaptic cleft. One type of mechanism found elsewhere in the CNS is the presence of a high-affinity uptake system for the transmitter or its breakdown product either back into the presynaptic terminal, into the postsynaptic cell, or into glia (Storm-Mathiesen and Iversen, 1977, 1979; Marc and Lam, 1981; Marc *et al.*, 1978). The availability of both radiolabeled amino acids and methods for screening for the presence of high-affinity uptake systems for radiolabeled compounds formed the basis of our strategy for differentiating among auditory synaptic terminal populations. When fresh tissues are incubated in physiological salt solutions containing micromolar quantities of radiolabeled compounds, those structures capable of high-affinity uptake take up significantly more label than other structures. Thus, after fixation the selectively labeled structures can be identified autoradiographically. By incubating adjacent slices of the same auditory areas in media containing different labeled compounds, specific labeling patterns can be detected by light microscopy, and the ultrastructural features and relationships of the labeled structures can be determined by electron microscopy.

B. Methods

The preparative procedures used in slicing, incubation, and autoradiographic preparation and analysis of SOC slices are similar to those detailed in Schwartz (1981). Briefly, anesthetized cats were decapitated or rapidly perfused with saline nitrite (200 ml at room temperature, followed by 500 ml at 0°C). The skull was opened rapidly and the brain stem removed and immersed in a cold, oxygenated salt solution. Blocks containing the SOC were chopped with a Sorval TC2 tissue chopper or hand sliced. Trimmed slices containing the SOC were incubated for 10–20 minutes in oxygenated salt solutions containing micromolar quantities of the amino acid to be studied, rinsed briefly (1–2 minutes), fixed in a mixture of paraformaldehyde and glutaraldehyde in phosphate buffer, osmicated, uranyl block stained, dehydrated, and embedded in Epon–Araldite (see Schwartz, 1982a, for special flat embedding techniques.) Sections (1 μm) were cut for light microscopic autoradiography (LMARG), deplasticized, dipped in Kodak NTB-2 emulsion, and exposed for 1–37 weeks at 4°C. Adjacent sections of the same blocks were cut with diamond knives and processed for electron microscopic autoradiography (EMARG) with the procedures described in Schwartz and Bok (1979). Sections were dipped in Ilford L-4 emulsion and exposed for 2–25 weeks. The animals, varying experimental conditions, and the amino acids tested are given in Table I. The amino acids and variables compared in each animal studied are listed in Table I in Schwartz (1983b).

C. Results

1. Differential Distribution of Labeling Patterns in the MSO and SOC

Although a variety of putative neurotransmitter amino acids and related compounds have been investigated, so far only Gly and GABA provide distinctive synaptic terminal labeling patterns within the MSO that can be related to specific synaptic terminal populations. Occasional terminals are infrequently observed to be labeled after incubations with Glu, Asp, Ala, Pro, and taurine (Tau), but no clear set of distributional or ultrastructural characteristics associated with these terminals has yet emerged. No terminal labeling was observed with Leu, Met, or muscimol (Mus). Details of the GABA and Gly terminal labeling patterns have

TABLE I

Experimental Variables

Amino acid[e]	Specific activity	Number of animals	Other conditions
L-Asp	15.0, 17.3	5	
D-Asp	16.0	2	
Gly	15.0, 53.5	12	a
Glu	20.0, 43.0, 46.15	10	b
GABA	28.2, 34.6, 97.0	9	c
Tau	23.146	5	
Ala	22.9	?	
Gln	33.6	3	d
Mus	9.3	1	
Met	0.2	1	
Pro	102.0	2	
Leu	152.0	1	

[a] Low Na (2), NaCN (1), high K$^+$ rinse (1), cold GABA (2).
[b] +/− amino oxyacetic acid (AOAA) (2), low Na (1).
[c] +/− AOAA (4), low Na (3), NaCN (1), cold Gly (2).
[d] +/− AOAA (1), low Na (1).
[e] Asp, aspartic acid; Glu, glutamic acid; Ala, alanine; Gln, glutamine; Met, methionine; Pro, proline; Leu, leucine.

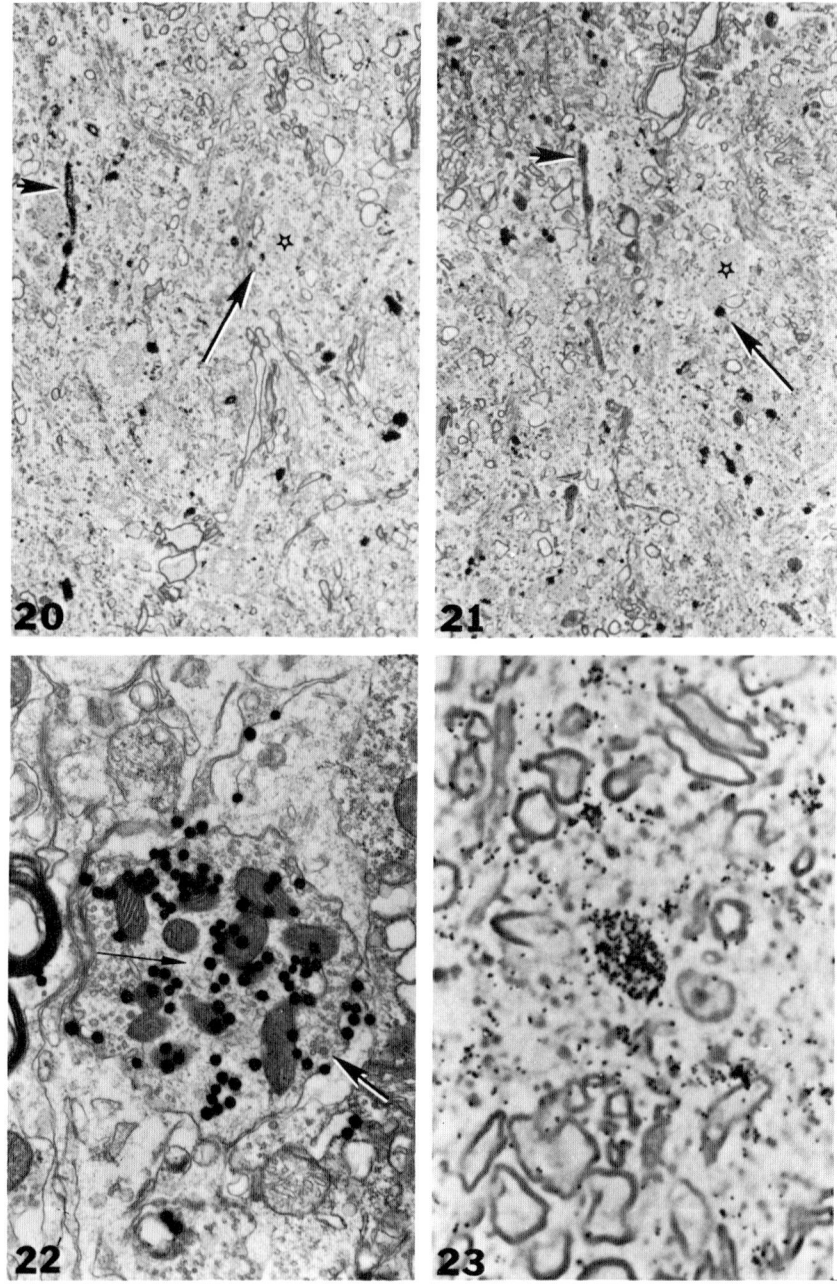

been reported elsewhere (Schwartz, 1982, 1983a,b, 1984b). They may be summarized as follows.

1. Labeled terminals are primarily located perisomatically and are relatively evenly and sparsely distributed through the central cell band (Figs. 20 and 21).
2. Unlike the DCN, no laminar pattern is obvious.
3. In typical sections, central cell band (CCB) cells are apposed to one or two labeled terminals, although some profiles contact none and some may contact as many as four to six.
4. Some marginal cells are apposed to 8 to 10 labeled endings and in general receive more labeled contacts than CCB cells, although some marginal cells receive none or 1 or 2.
5. Gly-labeled endings tend to be larger than GABA-labeled endings.
6. Nonperisomatic labeled endings in the CCB and those found among myelinated axons in the fiber zones tend to be smaller in size.
7. The accumulation of Gly label is not inhibited by the presence of a 100-fold excess of unlabeled GABA. The accumulation is sodium dependent and the accumulated label in synaptic terminals can be depleted by rinsing the slices with solutions containing high potassium ion concentrations.

In contrast to the general absence of terminal labeling, most amino acids tested produced variable degrees of labeling of some neuroglial elements. With both Asp and Glu a few cells, which at the light microscopic level could not be distinguished from small neuronal profiles, were moderately heavily labeled. At the electron microscopic level, no labeled neuronal somata have yet been found, but a few protoplasmic astrocytes with dimensions similar to small neuronal profiles and light-appearing nuclei and cytoplasm were moderately labeled. In all Asp and Glu cases, most neuroglial profiles, both astrocytes and oligodendrocytes, were seen to be unlabeled or much more lightly labeled. With Glu, endothelial cells were moderately heavily labeled and tangential cuts through such cells must be distinguished from the less intensely stained glial elements.

FIGS. 20–23. Figure 20 is a light microscopic autoradiograph of a portion of the MSO central cell band from a slice incubated with GABA. Note the heavily labeled blood vessel (▶) and a small cluster of silver grains (arrow) adjacent to a central cell band neuron (★) (exposure, 90 days). Figure 21 shows a comparable region from an adjacent slice from the same animal incubated with Gly. The blood vessel (▶) is only sparsely labeled. A perisomatically located cluster of silver grains (arrow) is typically larger than those labeled by the GABA incubation (exposure, 122 days). ×86. Figure 22 is an electron microscopic autoradiograph of a typical type 1B ending labeled after incubation of a slice from another cat with Gly in the presence of a 100-fold excess of unlabeled GABA. Note the presence of characteristic neurofilaments (thin arrow) and coated vesicles (large arrow) (exposure, 49 days). ×13,500. Figure 23 is a light microscopic autoradiograph of an MSO slice from another cat, showing an astrocyte labeled after incubation with L-Asp (exposure, 28 days). ×353.

Other amino acids that produced moderately heavy labeling of neuroglia include Gln, Pro, Ala, and Tau. The Pro and Gln patterns were similar to those of Asp and Glu in that a very few cells were significantly more heavily labeled than any others, and they were similarly located in the MSO. Only light labeling of some neuroglial elements occurred with GABA and Gly, although endothelial cells were heavily labeled after GABA incubations. In all cases, glial and blood vessel labeling was markedly less intense than that occurring in terminals and axons. No obvious labeling of glia or endothelial cells occurred with Leu, Met, or Mus. Details of the various amino acid-labeling patterns are reported in Schwartz (1984a).

2. Ultrastructural Correlates of Labeled Ending Populations

Systematic examination of Gly-labeled terminals revealed the presence of a subpopulation found apposed to neuronal perikarya and large dendrites, and consistently characterized by the following ultrastructural features: rounded profiles generally up to 7 µm in diameter, pleiomorphic vesicles, modestly assymetrical junctions, inclusions of coated vesicles and neurofilaments, and a position frequently directly apposed to other synaptic terminals (Fig. 22).

Ultrastructural characteristics associated with GABA-labeled endings show a greater heterogeneity. Labeled endings are usually less than 5 µm in diameter and have relatively symmetrical synaptic appositions, but vesicle size, shape, and density are variable, suggesting that more than a single type of terminal may be labeling. None of the labeled terminals had large round vesicles. Rather, pleiomorphic vesicles and small, densely packed vesicles typical of type 2 and 3 endings were observed.

D. Discussion

1. Anatomical and Chemical Correlations

These studies have successfully identified distinctive chemical properties of at least two different synaptic terminal populations. Although these populations can be distinguished chemically by the fact that they selectively accumulate label during incubations with [^{3}H]Gly or [^{3}H]GABA they can also be differentiated morphologically. A majority of Gly-labeled endings seem to belong to a single subgroup. The ultrastructural characteristics of this subgroup correspond to those of a subpopulation of type 1 endings that were previously distinguished on purely morphological grounds (see Section III,C,1 above). Also, there is good correspondence between the preferential distribution of type 2 and 3 endings on marginal cells (Schwartz, 1980b) and the preferential distribution of Gly- and GABA-labeled terminals on some marginal cells (Schwartz, 1982b). Although lesion studies are required to verify the suspected CN origin of the large Gly-labeled endings and selective lesions will be needed to identify origin from specific cell types in the CN, on the basis of the presently available data (Schwartz, 1983a) we have tentatively identified them as type 1B endings.

By demonstrating a correspondence between a chemical marker and a synaptic terminal population, the label uptake studies allow the distribution patterns of these terminal populations to be easily mapped. Thus, the limitations of the Golgi methods and the ambiguities in morphological classification schemes are overcome, and the ability to distinguish these radiolabeled populations at the light microscopic level allows us to map the distribution throughout the entire extent of a large nucleus.

2. IMPLICATIONS FOR TRANSMITTER IDENTIFICATION

Although chemical markers provide a powerful anatomical tool, we must be careful not to assume too much about the physiology of the structures marked. In order to prove that a substance is a neurotransmitter it must satisfy a number of criteria. Among the most generally accepted of these are the following: (1) the exogenously applied putative transmitter substance must have the same action as the naturally released transmitter; (2) pharmacological agents that inhibit or enhance the effects of the natural transmitter should have the same action on the effects of the presumptive transmitter; (3) the putative transmitter must be available presynaptically—either by transport, uptake, or synthesis; and (4) the putative transmitter must be rapidly removed from the synaptic cleft—either by uptake or inactivation.

Although the first two criteria are the most important, they are also the most difficult to prove for small neural elements in complex neuropils, where direct recording from the postsynaptic cell or recovery of the released transmitter may not be possible. Because of the difficulty of proving that putative transmitters satisfy all the primary criteria, a number of indirect types of evidence are frequently adduced. Such evidence includes (1) histochemical demonstrations of the presence of relevant synthetic enzymes presynaptically and of degradative enzymes in the cleft, (2) autoradiographic demonstrations of binding of related ligands (presumably postsynaptically), and (3) biochemical evidence of decreased concentration of the putative transmitter following lesion-induced loss of the presynaptic terminals. Studies of synaptosomes and slices have shown that in situations where many other kinds of evidence have implicated a substance as the neurotransmitter, its uptake is sodium dependent and its stimulated release is calcium dependent (Cotman *et al.*, 1981; Vargas *et al.*, 1977).

Although no single piece of data is conclusive, it now appears that a good case can be made to support the hypothesis that Gly is a transmitter between some neurons in the CN or contralateral MNTB and some neurons in the lateral superior olivary nucleus (LSO) and MSO. There is good evidence that the identity of action criterion has been met for LSO neurons (Moore et al., 1981) and preliminary studies suggest that some MSO neurons show similar properties (Moore and Caspary, 1983). Zarbin et al. (1981) have reported strychnine-binding sites in frozen sections of the LSO, and their results appear consistent with the relative density of labeled sites, seen after our Gly incubations of fresh brain slices. Our studies have demonstrated an efficient mechanism for accumulating label after Gly incubations in a specific population of synaptic terminals in both the MSO and LSO. The morphological characteristics of these terminals are consistent with the features known to characterize endings of CN projections. The label uptake is sodium dependent and stimulated release of label occurs in the presence of calcium. Although the number of such terminals in the MSO is small and they are sparsely distributed, some neurons are contacted by a larger number of labeled terminals. Lesion studies of the multipolar cell region of the PVCN (Warr, 1982) have shown a sparse collateral projection to the LSO and MSO of the major projection to the IC via the lateral lemniscus. Clearly, further lesion studies of the CN will be required to confirm this suspected origin of the Gly-labeled terminals. Although biochemical analyses must be performed to confirm that the ^{3}H label is still on Gly, analyses of slice preparations similar to ours indicate that 85% of the [^{3}H]Gly remains in that form (Storm-Mathisen and Iversen, 1979).

Gly may not be the only transmitter at these endings, but the preceding data provide strong support for the idea that it is a transmitter of at least one group of axons to the LSO and MSO.

3. LIMITATIONS

Autoradiographic comparisons of uptake and concentration of label derived from probe concentrations (in the micromolar range) provide a useful way to screen individual elements in complex neuropils for differing chemical properties. As discussed in the preceding section, simply demonstrating localization of label is not enough to prove a transmitter role, although it is certainly helpful in identifying likely candidates that can then be analyzed more extensively physiologically and pharmacologically. For the present, the methodologies described in this article must be viewed as a powerful anatomical tool with physiological implications. Their use has allowed us to identify and characterize previously unrecognized populations of synaptic terminals on the basis of their chemical properties as well as their morphological ones.

We anticipate that identification of chemical markers for additional populations will allow the integration of information from Golgi, Bodian, and a variety of other light microscopic methodologies with ultrastructural analyses and experimental manipulations of the sorts described above to finally solve the problem of fully describing the environment of individual neurons in the auditory system.

ACKNOWLEDGMENTS

This work was supported by USPHS Research Grants NS 09823, 09996, and 14503. The excellent technical assistance of Elizabeth Osborne, Susan Mirolli, Susan Sharp, Mary Gustin, M. Rita Watson, and Gary Fink is gratefully acknowledged.

A portion of the work in Section II was performed by Andrea Zaranz Wittebort and was submitted by her to the Medical Sciences Program, Indiana University, Bloomington, Indiana in partial fulfillment of the requirements of the M.S. degree.

Preliminary reports of portions of this work have appeared (Schwartz and Wittebort, 1976; Schwartz, 1981, 1982b).

REFERENCES

Bodian, D. (1966). Synaptic types on spinal motoneurons: An electron microscopic study. *Bull. J. Hopkins Hosp.* **119,** 16–45.

Bodian, D. (1970). An electron microscopic characterization of classes of synaptic vesicles by means of controlled aldehyde fixation. *J. Cell Biol.* **44,** 115–124.

Brawer, J. R., Morest, D. K., and Kane, E. C. (1974). The neuronal architecture of the cochlear nucleus of the cat. *J. Comp. Neurol.* **155,** 251–300.

Clark, G. M. (1969a). The ultrastructure of nerve endings in the medial superior olive of the cat. *Brain Res.* **14,** 293–305.

Clark, G. M. (1969b). Vesicle shape versus type of synapse in the nerve endings of the cat medial superior olive. *Brain Res.* **15,** 548–551.

Colonnier, M. (1964). The tangential organization of the visual cortex. *J. Anat.* **98,** 327–344.

Cotman, C. W., Foster, A., and Lanthorn, T. (1981). An overview of glutamate as a neurotransmitter. *In* "Glutamate as a Neurotransmitter" (G. DiChiara and G. L. Gessa, Eds.), pp. 1–27. Raven, New York.

Daigneault, E. A. (1981). Pharmacology of the cochlear efferents. *In* "Pharmacology of Hearing: Experimental and Clinical Bases" (R. D. Brown and E. A. Daigneault, Eds.), pp. 137–151. Wiley, New York.

Goldberg, J. M., and Brown, P. B. (1968). Functional organization of the dog superior olivary complex: An anatomical and electrophysiological study. *J. Neurophysiol.* **31,** 635–636.

Goldberg, J. M., and Brown, P. B. (1969). Response of binaural neurons of dog superior olivary complex to dichotic tonal stimuli; some physiological mechanisms of sound localization. *J. Neurophysiol.* **32,** 613–636.

Guinan, J. J., Jr., Norris, B. E., and Guinan, S. E. (1972). Single auditory units in the superior olivary complex. II. Locations of unit categories and tonotopic organization. *Int. J. Neurosci.* **4,** 147–166.

Guth, P. S., and Melamed, B. (1982). Neurotransmission in the auditory system: A primer for physiologists. *Annu. Rev. Pharmacol. Toxicol.* **22,** 383–412.

Harrison, J. M., and Irving, R. (1965). The anterior ventral cochlear nucleus. *J. Comp. Neurol.* **124,** 15–42.

Kane, E. (1973). Octopus cells in the cochlear nucleus of the cat: Heterotypic synapses upon homeotypic neurons. *Int. J. Neurosci.* **5,** 251–279.

Karnovsky, M. J. (1967). The ultrastructural basis of capillary permeability studied with peroxidase as a tracer. *J. Cell Biol.* **35,** 213–236.

Klinke, R. (1981). Neurotransmitters in the cochlea and cochlear nucleus. *Acta Otolaryng.* **91,** 541–554.

LaVilla, I. (1898). Algunos detalles concernientes a la oliva superior y focos acusticos. *Rev. Trimestr. Micrograf.* **3,** 75–83.
Lenn, N. J., and Reese, T. S. (1966). The fine structure of nerve endings in the nucleus of the trapezoid body and the ventral cochlear nucleus. *Am. J. Anat.* **118,** 375–390.
Lindsey, B. G. (1975). Fine structure and distribution of axon terminals from the cochlear nucleus on neurons in the medial superior olivary nucleus of the cat. *J. Comp. Neurol.* **160,** 81–104.
Marc, R. E., and Lam, D. M. K. (1981). Glycinergic pathways in the goldfish retina. *J. Neurosci.* **1,** 152–165.
Marc, R. E., Stell, W. K., Bok, D., and Lam, D. M. K. (1978). GABA-ergic pathways in the goldfish retina. *J. Comp. Neurol.* **182,** 221–245.
Matus, A. I., and Dennison, M. E. (1971). Autoradiographic localization of flat vesicle synapses in spinal cord. *Brain Res.* **32,** 195–197.
Moore, M., and Caspary, D. M. (1983). Strychnine blocks binaural inhibition in lateral superior olivary neurons. *J. Neurosci.* **3,** 237–242.
Moore, M., Caspary, D. M., and Havey, D. C. (1981). Iontophoretic application of putative inhibitory neurotransmitters into binaural units in the superior olive. *Soc. Neurosci. Abstr.* **7,** 389.
Morest, D. K. (1968). The collateral system of the medial nucleus of the trapezoid body of the cat, its neuronal architecture and relation to the olivo-cochlear bundle. *Brain Res.* **9,** 288–311.
Morest, D. K. (1973). Auditory neurons of the brain stem. *Adv. Oto-Rhino-Laryngol.* **20,** 337–356.
Nakajima, Y. (1971). Fine structure of the medial nucleus of the trapezoid body of the cat with special reference to two types of synaptic endings. *J. Cell Biol.* **50,** 121–134.
Peracchia, C., and Mittler, B. S. (1972). Fixation by means of glutaraldehyde-hydrogen peroxide reaction products. *J. Cell Biol.* **53,** 234–238.
Perkins, R. E. (1973). An electron microscopic study of synaptic organization in the medial superior olive of normal and experimental chinchilla. *J. Comp. Neurol.* **148,** 387–416.
Ramón y Cajal, S. (1909). "Histologie du Systeme Nerveux de L'Homme et des Vertebres," Vol. I. Consejo Superior de Investigaciones Cientificas, Madrid, 1972 reprint.
Ramon-Moliner, E. (1970). The Golgi–Cox technique. *In* "Contemporary Research Methods in Neuroanatomy" (W. J. H. Nauta and S. V. O. Ebbesson, Eds.). Springer-Verlag, Berlin and New York.
Rockel, A. J., and Jones, E. G. (1972). Observations on the fine structure of the central nucleus of the inferior colliculus of the cat. *J. Comp. Neurol.* **147,** 61–92.
Scheibel, M. E., and Scheibel, A. B. (1974). Neuropil organization in the superior olive of the cat. *Exp. Neurol.* **43,** 339–348.
Schwartz, I. R. (1972). Axonal endings in the cat medial superior olive: Coated vesicles and intercellular substance. *Brain Res.* **46,** 187–202.
Schwartz, I. R. (1977). Dendritic arrangements in the cat medial superior olive. *Neuroscience* **2,** 81–101.
Schwartz, I. R. (1979). Differential distribution of glutamic acid, aspartic acid and glycine uptake in the cochlear nucleus. *Soc. Neurosci. Abstr.* **5,** 30.
Schwartz, I. R. (1980a). Localization of label from (H3)GABA in parallel fibers in the outer molecular layer in the cat dorsal cochlear nucleus. *Soc. Neurosci. Abstr.* **6,** 43.
Schwartz, I. R. (1980b). The differential distribution of synaptic terminals on marginal and central cells in the cat medial superior olivary nucleus. *Am. J. Anat.* **159,** 25–31.
Schwartz, I. R. (1981). The differential distribution of label following uptake of H^3-amino acids in the dorsal cochlear nucleus of the cat: An autoradiographic study. *J. Exp. Neurol.* **73,** 601–617.

Schwartz, I. R. (1982a). A simple method for osmicating and flat embedding large tissue sections for light and electron microscopy. *Stain Tech.* **57,** 52–54.

Schwartz, I. R. (1982b). Differential tritiated amino acid labeling of synaptic terminals in the cat medial superior olivary nucleus. *Assoc. Res. Otolaryng. Abstr. Midwinter Meet.*

Schwartz, I. R. (1983a). H3 labeling following glycine incubations identifies a distinctive population of synaptic terminals in the cat medial superior olivary nucleus. *Assoc. Res. Otolaryng. Abstr. Midwinter Meet.*

Schwartz, I. R. (1983b). Differential uptake of H3-amino acids in the cat cochlear nucleus. *Am. J. Otol.* **4,** 300–304.

Schwartz, I. R. (1984a). Amino acid labeling patterns in fresh brain slices of the cat superior olivary complex. In preparation.

Schwartz, I. R. (1984b). Uptake of glycine by endings in the cat medial superior olive. In preparation.

Schwartz, I. R., and Bok, D. (1979). Electron microscopic localization of ^{125}I-α-bungarotoxin binding sites in the outer plexiform layer of the goldfish retina. *J. Neurocytol.* **8,** 53–66.

Schwartz, I. R., and Wittebort, A. Z. (1976). Axon terminals in the cat medial superior olivary nucleus. *Anat. Rec.* **184,** 525.

Sotelo, C., and Palay, S. L. (1968). The fine structure of the lateral vestibular nucleus in the rat. I. Neurons and neuroglial cells. *J. Cell Biol.* **36,** 151–179.

Storm-Mathisen, J., and Iversen, L. L. (1977). Glutamic acid and excitatory nerve endings. Reduction of glutamic acid uptake after axotomy. *Brain Res.* **120,** 379–386.

Storm-Mathisen, J., and Iversen, L. L. (1979). Uptake of (^{3}H)glutamic acid in excitatory nerve endings: Light and electron microscopic observations in the hippocampal formation of the rat. *Neuroscience* **4,** 1237–1253.

Stotler, W. A. (1953). An experimental study of the cells and connections of the superior olivary complex of the cat. *J. Comp. Neurol.* **98,** 401–431.

Uchizono, K. (1966). Excitatory and inhibitory synapses in the cat spinal cord. *Jpn. J. Physiol.* **16,** 570–575.

Vargas, O., DeLorenzo, M. D. C., Saldate, M. C., and Orrego, S. (1977). Potassium-induced release of (^{3}H)GABA and of (^{3}H)noradrenaline from normal and reserpinized rat brain cortex slices. Differences in calcium-dependency and insensitivity to potassium ions. *J. Neurochem.* **28,** 165–170.

Warr, W. B. (1966). Fiber degeneration following lesions in the postero-ventral cochlear nucleus of the cat. *Exp. Neurol.* **14,** 453–474.

Warr, W. B. (1969). Fiber degeneration following lesions in the postero-ventral cochlear nucleus of the cat. *Exp. Neurol.* **23,** 140–155.

Warr, W. B. (1972). Fiber degeneration following lesions in the multipolar and globular cell areas in the ventral cochlear nucleus of the cat. *Brain Res.* **40,** 247–270.

Warr, W. B. (1982). Parallel ascending pathways from the cochlear nucleus: Neuroanatomical evidence of functional specialization. *Contrib. Sensory Physiol.* **7,** 1–38.

Wenthold, R. J. (1981). Glutamate and aspartate as neurotransmitters for the auditory nerve. In "Glutamate as a Neurotransmitter" (G. DiChiara and G. L. Gessa, Eds.), pp. 69–78. Raven, New York.

Wittebort, A. Z. (1976). Axon terminals in the medial superior olivary nucleus of the cat: A Golgi study. Master's Thesis, Indiana University.

Zarbin, M. A., Wamsley, J. K., and Kuhar, M. J. (1981). Glycine receptor: Light microscopic autoradiographic localization with ^{3}H-strychnine. *J. Neurosci.* **1,** 532–547.

Auditory Temporal Integration at Threshold: Theories and Some Implications of Current Research

DANIEL ALGOM AND HARVEY BABKOFF

DEPARTMENT OF PSYCHOLOGY
BAR-ILAN UNIVERSITY
RAMAT GAN, ISRAEL

I.	Introduction	131
II.	Major Empirical Findings	132
	A. Graphic Presentations	133
	B. Review of Empirical Findings	137
III.	Theories of Auditory Temporal Summation	140
	A. Statistical Probability Formulations	141
	B. Other Nonsummation Interpretations	143
	C. Hyperbolic Models of Integration	143
	D. Exponential Models of Integration	145
	E. Short Time Constants versus Long Time Constants	149
IV.	Some Implications of Current Research	151
	A. Integration and Resolution	151
	B. Recent Models of Temporal Integration	154
V.	Conclusions	156
	References	157

I. INTRODUCTION

Psychophysical studies of auditory temporal integration have demonstrated a reciprocal relation between stimulus intensity and duration necessary to obtain a constant response. The phenomenon has been studied extensively at threshold and somewhat less at suprathreshold levels of stimulation. Although there is general agreement with regard to the fundamental empirical findings involved in the time–intensity relation, there is no such consensus with regard to a theoretical formulation. Various theoretical interpretations have appeared in the literature over the last 40 years. These theoretical formulations have been mainly independent developments by different authors rather than representative of an organic development of a dynamic field of interest. The interpretations that have been offered differ in terms of the coverage of data as well as in their level of mathematical sophistication. This situation makes it difficult to assess the "state of the art" reliably, as well as to incorporate new experimental findings into an accepted body of relevant knowledge. The purpose of this article is to attempt to review the data and the various hypotheses that have been advanced to explain temporal summation in audition over the past 40 years. To elucidate the discussion, examples from other sensory modalities will occasionally be given. Following this, we shall attempt to discuss the implications of some recent findings for the different theoretical frameworks presented for auditory temporal integration.

II. MAJOR EMPIRICAL FINDINGS

The most frequent stimulus parameters considered in the context of auditory temporal integration are frequency and bandwidth of stimuli, the effects of masking, the mode of stimulation, the phasic characteristics of the stimuli, and the level of stimulation. The interactions among these dimensions are quite complex. Several authors posit that there probably are more instances of nonlinear temporal summation in the auditory system than in other sensory modalities (Bekesy, 1960; Goldstein, 1967).

At threshold, the ear integrates the acoustic energy of a sinusoid signal linearly up to about 250 msec; that is, in this range a 10-fold increase in duration decreases the signal intensity necessary for threshold by 10 dB. For durations longer than around 250 msec, the change in threshold is slight and the integration process may be considered complete at around 2 seconds (see, for example, Garner and Miller, 1948; Watson and Gengel, 1969). Among the most frequent indices used to describe such data are either the critical duration[1] (i.e., the

---

[1]The term critical duration has been used by most investigators as describing that value of stimulus duration at which there is an intersection of the lines of zero slope ($I \times t = C$) and unit slope ($I = C$). Where there is a period of partial integration, critical duration usually describes that stimulus duration at which the first deviation from complete integration occurs. It is clear that the use of these terms is permissible only in those cases where integration results are described by a linear approximation of data (in which case the intersection of lines may be observed). However, the use of these terms in conjunction with nonlinear models of integration is unintelligible and, thus, totally unacceptable. Most nonlinear models of temporal summation share in common the view that one curve might provide a better description of data than several straight lines. Most of such models that have been

longest duration producing reciprocity) or the time constant of the function relating intensity to duration for a given psychophysical response.

A. Graphic Presentations

There are several ways of plotting the results of the reciprocity studies. The ways of displaying data discussed in this section refer to graphic displays in which both stimulus parameters, intensity and duration, are plotted in the same units, e.g., logarithmically. There are other types of data displays that present the intensity and duration parameters plotted in different units, or which use second-order transforms. Such data displays are based on certain theoretical considerations that will be discussed below. We chose the following means of graphic display (Fig. 1) as illustrative of a more empirical (closer to the raw data) format of data presentation.

In Fig. 1A a response measure (response probability or detection level such as d') is plotted on the ordinate with stimulus intensity (usually log I) plotted on the abscissa. The parameter is stimulus duration. Each of the parallel straight lines represents a psychometric function for stimuli of different durations ($t_{i+1} > t_i$). The longer the stimuli (moving to the left), the less the intensity needed to preserve a constant response (e.g., detection level). The parallelism of the lines, as well as their relatively constant distances from each other, show that different constant combinations of intensities and durations result in constant detectability. This example of perfect reciprocity breaks down at the longer durations as, e.g., $t = t_5$. The psychometric function at the longer duration (t_5) almost overlaps with the function at a shorter duration (t_4), indicating that in this range increasing

---

suggested (e.g., Plomp and Bouman, 1959) proposed some version of the negative exponential curve as the proper form of the temporal integration function. The time constant of such a function is one of its mathematical properties, defining its rate of decline. When the model is applied to integration data, this time constant may serve as a summary figure to describe the rate of integration of stimulation over time. Therefore, these two summary indices—critical duration and the time constant of integration—should not be used interchangeably; reporting data in terms of one of them implies an underlying model of integration which is incompatible with that of the other. In spite of this mathematical state of affairs, one can still benefit from a practical relationship that does seem to hold between critical duration and the time constant of integration. The value of the time constant seems to set a conservative lower limit on the value of the corresponding critical duration if a linear model is to be applied to the same data. This is so because that segment of the exponential curve that lies in the time region below the value of the constant may be treated as linear for all practical purposes (hence it may be concluded that the respective durations are shorter than the hypothetical critical duration). Thus, if a time constant τ is estimated in an experiment by the application of an exponential model to fit data, the probability is great that the critical duration will assume a value of at least τ if a linear approximation is attempted to the same data. This practical relationship is of great importance when making comparisons across studies, the data of which are reported in terms of different theoretical models.

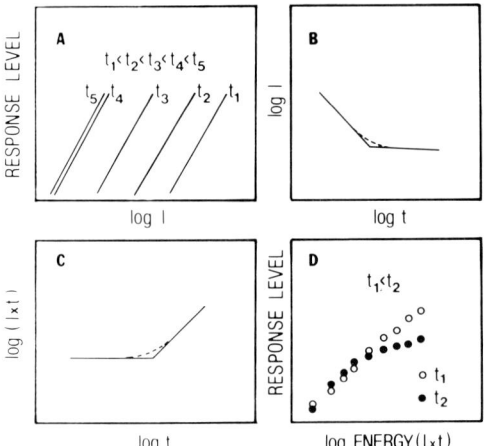

FIG. 1. Some traditional ways of illustrating stimulus reciprocity results, showing the range over which time and intensity are reciprocally related. I, Intensity; t, duration.

duration does not allow a further reduction in stimulus intensity. By convention, a straight line is drawn across the psychometric functions at the 50% detection level (usually defined as threshold). The resulting ordinate and abscissa values serve as the estimates of the $I \times t$ trading function, an example of which is shown in the next two panels. In Fig. 1B, at short durations, the points describing threshold intensity fall along a straight line as a function of stimulus duration with a slope of -1 when both parameters are plotted in log units, indicating that the $I \times t$ (energy) product is constant for a constant (e.g., threshold) response. Such data accord with Bloch's Law ($I \times t = C$). At longer durations, the points tend to fall on the line of zero slope, indicating that a further lengthening of stimulus duration ceases to have any effect on the behavioral response ($I = C$). This is the region of no integration. Although the transition from complete to no integration may be fairly abrupt under special conditions (e.g., Hartline, 1934; Graham and Margaria, 1935), a more gradual change is evident in most studies. In the latter case, the period lasting from the first deviation from complete integration—the critical duration—up to the duration above which there is no integration has been termed "partial integration" (e.g., Pieron, 1952). In Fig. 1C, the same characteristics may be seen somewhat differently. This plot describes the $I \times t$ product for threshold as a function of stimulus duration. At short durations, the points fall along a straight line of zero slope, indicating that the $I \times t$ product at threshold is constant—a result achieved by a corresponding decrease in intensity with each increase in duration. At longer durations, the points fall on a line of unit slope, indicating that intensity alone determines the constant response ($I = C$). In Fig. 1D, a response measure is plotted on the ordinate with energy plotted on the abscissa. The symbols represent stimuli of different durations at varying energy levels. The energy of these stimuli is manipulated by varying their intensity and duration in order to produce differently configured, equal-energy stimulus pairs at a number of energy levels. The functions, thus produced, overlap at durations shorter than the critical duration—meaning equal level of detectability of equal-energy stimuli, irrelevant of their time–intensity construction. Beyond that duration, the function for the longer (less intense) stimuli shows poorer performance.

Some illustrative data, generated by different organisms and different modalities, will be shown to emphasize the different ways of looking at stimulus integration.

Computer-averaged electroretinographic (ERG) data from an anesthetized, dark-adapted adult cat (Babkoff, 1975a,b) were generated by light stimuli (Sylvania F14712-CWX fluorescent tube driven by 500-V dc pulses) of three different durations and recorded by platinum chloride wick electrodes. The number of ERGs averaged for a given stimulus condition depended upon the noise level of the recording and ranged from 10 to 20.

The three panels of Fig. 2 illustrate three different ways of presenting the data.

The left and middle panels show plots of the response variables as functions of

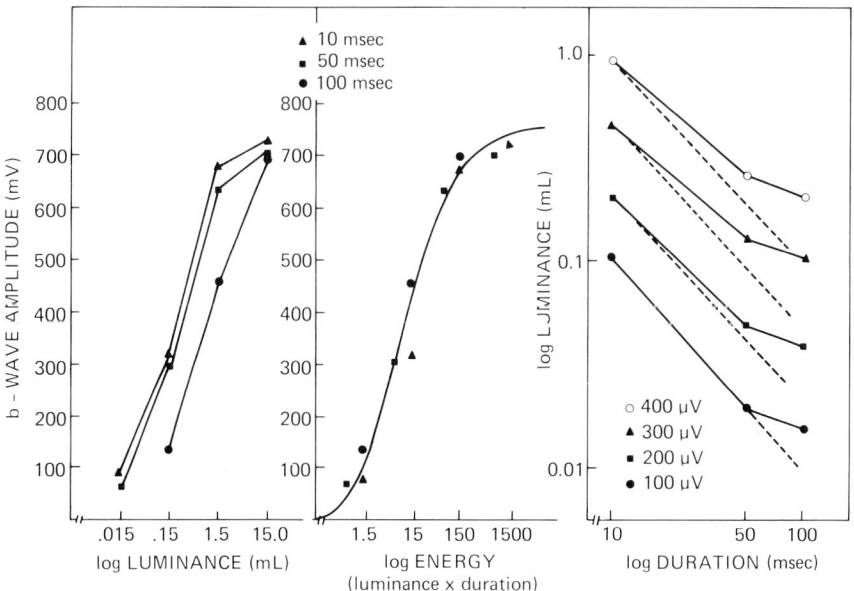

FIG. 2. Temporal summation in the adult cat electroretinographic (ERG) data. Three different illustrations; see text for explanation.

the stimulus variables. In the left panel, ERG b-wave amplitude, measured from the baseline to the peak of the positive-going wave, is plotted in microvolts (μV) on the ordinate as a function of stimulus luminance in log millilambert (mL) on the abscissa. Stimulus duration is the parameter. Data plotted this way emphasize the direct effect of the independent variables (luminance and duration) on the dependent variable. Integration is not emphasized and the exact interaction of stimulus luminance and duration is not clear from this figure.

The middle panel shows ERG b-wave amplitude plotted on the ordinate as a function of log stimulus energy (luminance × duration) on the abscissa. A single function is drawn. Integration can be ascertained by noting the extent to which all of the data fall on the same function regardless of the different luminances and durations. The effect of stimulus energy (luminance × duration) as the "adequate stimulus" (Boring, 1942) is emphasized by the goodness of fit of the data to the single function drawn in this figure. Note that the single curve provides a slightly better fit for the b-wave data generated by the 10- and 50-msec duration stimuli than for the data generated by the 100-msec duration stimulus.

The right panel differs from the left and middle panels in that it relates the values of the two stimulus parameters necessary to generate a fixed response level. Log luminance is plotted on the ordinate as a function of log duration on the abscissa. Data are shown for four different levels of ERG b-wave amplitude, 100, 200, 300, and 400 μV. For each datum set, a theoretical curve (broken line) is drawn that indicates total integration ($I \times t = C$). The extent of integration can be ascertained by noting the goodness of fit of the data points to the theoretical functions. Note that for all of the four response levels, the data for the 100-msec duration stimulus fall above the theoretical function, indicating relatively more luminance necessary than predicted by total integration. Critical duration seems to lie between 50 and 100 msec for the lower amplitude ERG b-waves. Furthermore, although for the 100-μV level data for both 10- and 50-msec durations fall on the theoretical line, the data for the 200, 300, and 400-μV levels show a different pattern. At these response levels, only data for the 10-msec duration fall on the theoretical line. The data for both the 50- and 100-msec durations fall above the theoretical line, indicating that critical duration lies between 10 and 50 msec for higher amplitude ERG b-wave levels (Schevelev and Hicks, 1971; Wasserman and Kong, 1979; Wicke et al., 1964).

Temporal summation in audition for the human listener is illustrated in Fig. 3. Psychometric functions for several subjects were generated for 988-Hz tones of 16- and 64-msec duration (Algom and Babkoff, 1978). Detection levels in standard scores (z scores) are plotted on the ordinate as a function of *total* stimulus energy on the abscissa (see Fig. 1D). Data are plotted separately for the two stimulus durations for two subjects. Note that for these subjects a single line can be drawn through the data points representing the two stimulus durations when

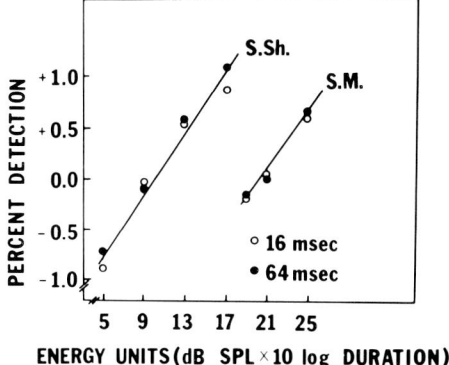

FIG. 3. Sample psychometric functions are plotted for two subjects. Detection levels in z scores are plotted on the ordinate as a function of total stimulus energy in decibels, i.e., 10 × log intensity (dB SPL) × duration on the abscissa. (After Algom and Babkoff, 1978, Fig. 1.)

plotted on the total stimulus energy axis, thus illustrating complete reciprocity or total integration of the 16- and 64-msec 988-Hz tones.

In summary, there are four characteristics of temporal integration that may be observed in the graphic data displays of most studies: (1) complete integration or intensity–duration reciprocity, (2) a critical duration, (3) partial integration, and (4) no integration.

B. Review of Empirical Findings

Most acoustic integration data may be described in terms of Garner's well-known general equation, $I \times t^a = C$, where the exponent a is the slope of the line relating log I to log t. Perfect trading relationships (i.e., where $a = 1$) are found only with threshold tonal stimuli. For broad-band noise stimuli, however, only partial integration has been found even at threshold. Most studies report values of a at around 0.7, which means a 7 dB change in threshold for a 10-fold change in duration for noise stimuli (Babkoff and Algom, 1976; Garner, 1947; Miller, 1948; Penner, 1978). In contrast, the value of a changes sharply when the same stimuli are presented at suprathreshold levels. The exponent a may then assume values exceeding 1.0, with 1.25 as a representative figure (McFadden, 1975; Small et al., 1962; Stevens and Hall, 1966). It seems curious, as some researchers have noted, that for the same noise spectrum, the exponent a should assume values both greater and smaller than 1.0, depending on overall stimulus level. This alteration in the slope of the integration curve implies that subjective loudness grows less rapidly as a function of duration than as a function of sound pressure at threshold (partial integration), but that the opposite phenomenon occurs at suprathreshold levels (see also Békésy, 1960).

Since the study reported by Garner (1947) of the effect of critical bands on integration, many studies have shown that integration is constant and most efficient whenever the bandwidth of the signal does not exceed the critical bandwidth (the size of which is frequency dependent). In that range, the slope of integration is about -3 dB per doubling of duration. When successive doublings of signal bandwidth cause power to fall outside the critical bandwidth, performance decreases. At these short durations the integration function becomes steeper, with a slope of -4.5 dB per doubling of duration (Green et al., 1957; Olsen and Carhart, 1966; Sheeley and Bilger, 1964). It is now accepted that only the power concentrated in a narrow frequency band is integrated without loss (see Zwislocki, 1960). It has further been shown that a listener is able to detect only one critical band at a time (Greenberg and Larkin, 1968).

The role of frequency in auditory temporal integration has become an important subject of discussion (Olsen and Carhart, 1966; Watson and Gengel, 1969; Zwislocki, 1960). Although there is a trend across studies for the critical duration (or the time constant) of integration to decrease with increasing frequency (Zwicker and Wright, 1963; Wright, 1968), the role of frequency analysis in temporal summation still remains unresolved to some extent. In particular, the spread of energy, especially at low frequencies, makes the detection of very brief tones a complex problem. Mainly for this reason, Miller (1948) introduced the method of testing temporal integration with noise bursts. Noise, unlike tones, does not change materially in spectrum as the duration is shortened. Of course, with such stimuli perfect integration was never demonstrated.

Temporal summation has also been shown to hold for trains of auditory stimuli (e.g., Garner, 1947; Plomp, 1961; Pollack, 1973). In general, using such a mode of stimulation, different studies demonstrated temporal summation of energy to hold irrespective of the manner in which the energy is packaged, i.e., repetition rate, duration of the periodically repeated pulses, number of pulses, etc. Two-pulse measures of temporal summation may be considered as special cases of such stimulation (e.g., Irwin and Zwislocki, 1971; Zwislocki, 1960).

A stimulus parameter, which is of special importance in temporal summation studies in audition, is that of the form of the stimulus envelope. The dilemma confronting the experimenter in such studies has been discussed by Dallos and Olsen (1964). One must ensure that all stimuli have a definite pitch quality and that they do not contain an appreciable amount of energy at frequencies other than those of the fundamental tone. These requirements may be met by several means of specifying the duration; for example, by including the rise and fall times in the signal duration, by designating the duration between the half-energy points on the stimulus envelopes, or by correcting the gross duration for the rise–fall times, etc. (Olsen and Carhart, 1966).

Most studies of auditory temporal summation have employed monaural conditions of stimulation. Recent investigations nevertheless indicate that summation over time is identical for both monaurally and binaurally presented stimuli (Babkoff and Algom, 1976; Schenkel, 1967). An illustration of such data is shown in Fig. 4.

Two parallel functions for conditions of binaural and monaural stimulus presentation are shown. Threshold, in decibels, is plotted on the ordinate as a function of noise burst duration, on the logarithmic abscissa for the two modes of stimulation separately. The average slope for both conditions is approximately 6 dB/decade, and the intercept difference between the integration functions is about 3 dB.

In summary, the influence of different stimulus conditions on auditory temporal summation has proven to be complex. Interaction among variables seems to be the rule rather than the exception. Examples include the interaction between the level and the bandwidth of stimuli, as well as that between the level and the effect of the number of stimuli in a train. Given these results to date, one might expect to discover even more complex interactions in future experimentation. In view of this situation, it would seem inappropriate to designate any given value as the critical duration or the time constant of integration in the auditory system. Moreover, the results of most studies of auditory temporal integration indicate a quite gradual transition from complete to no integration in the threshold–duration functions rather than an abrupt transition. This fact, combined with the fairly broad range of partial summation observed in the threshold–duration functions, explains the relatively rare use of the critical duration as a summary statistic in audition as compared to its wide use in vision.

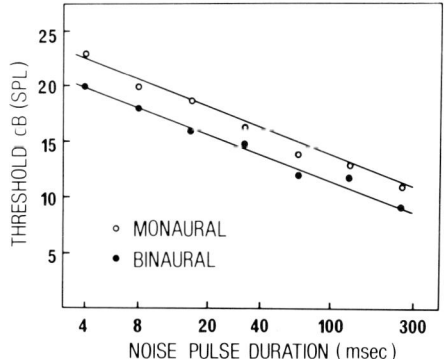

FIG. 4. Threshold in decibels (SPL) is plotted on the ordinate as a function of noise burst duration on the logarithmic abscissa. The two curves represent data for the different stimulation modes, monaural (upper curve) and binaural (lower curve). (After Babkoff and Algom, 1976, Fig. 1.)

From a methodological point of view, a variety of methods have been employed with relatively little attention to their effects on the form of the integration function. The procedures used are varied and range from Békésy audiometry, through the methods of adjustment, constant stimulus, to forced choice methodology, including a forced choice modification of the method of limits. The common experimental approach is to determine the duration and intensity of the signal necessary for the subject to report he heard the stimulus or to report he heard a stimulus at a constant loudness level. Thus, especially for threshold studies, the procedure involves measuring the signal intensity necessary to obtain a constant detection level at each of a number of stimulus durations. For suprathreshold investigations, magnitude estimation has become a popular method of studying integration.

What is common to all of these procedures is the measurement of a constant response as a function of alternative stimulus configurations. Little consideration has been given to the question whether these constant psychophysical responses also imply constant or equivalent nondiscriminable psychological responses. This issue has been raised more frequently in the recent literature (Algom and Babkoff, 1978; Zacks, 1970).

Apart from stimulus and procedural variables, the specific response measures used have been shown to be of importance in determining the characteristics of integration even for threshold-level stimuli. For example, although the stimuli presented and the procedure used may be identical, the estimate of the critical duration differs if the measurement is reaction time or response frequency. In vision, the estimated critical duration for threshold measured by reaction time is shorter than the estimate obtained with a psychophysical measure (e.g., Bruder, 1971).

To conclude, empirical studies over the past 40 years indicate a rather complex influence of stimulus conditions, procedural variables, and response measures on temporal integration. The possible confounding of the effects emerging from these different classes of variables must be taken into account in the evaluation of any estimate of temporal summation, as well as in comparisons across studies.

III. THEORIES OF AUDITORY TEMPORAL SUMMATION

The different theoretical explanations of auditory temporal summation that have appeared during the last 40 years have been concerned mainly with the following issues: the basic nature of the underlying mechanism (probabilistic or deterministic), the locus of integration (peripheral or central), the type of energy integrated (acoustic or neural), the effect of the power spectrum (the extent to which the critical band imposes limits on integration and whether there is a frequency effect), and the effects of the temporal pattern of stimuli (tones versus periodical pulses). Almost all of the possible alternatives have been suggested by different theorists. Several classifications of these theoretical interpretations are possible. We propose the following classification of theoretical constructs: those theories that posit the existence of true integration (acoustic or neural) somewhere in the auditory system as the basis for the observed temporal integration, versus those theories that posit mechanisms other than true integration. We shall first review those theories that do not assume an underlying acoustic or neural integrator.

A. Statistical Probability Formulations

The probability summation hypothesis is the major rival formulation to the assumption of an actual power integration that takes place somewhere in the auditory system. In fact, probability hypotheses have been advanced in almost every case of improved performance due to various intra- and intermodality interactions, the most outstanding cases in this respect being those of binocular or binaural summation. Most probability summation predictions are based on the classic probability theorem for independent observations. Thus, the probability summation hypothesis posits that the decrease in the threshold as a function of an increase in stimulus number is due to an increase in the probability of reporting one of a series of independent events as the number of these events increases. While the most straighforward application of this hypothesis is to the analysis of multiple (including two)-pulse data, it can also be applied to experiments employing single pulses. In this case, the hypothesis assumes that the decrease in threshold occurs as a result of the independent probability summation of detections due to an increasing number of segments of the single pulse as its duration increases. In most of its direct applications in predicting temporal integration data, the hypothesis has underestimated the actual amount of integration that was measured (see, for example, Babkoff *et al.*, 1975; Westendorf *et al.*, 1972; Zwislocki, 1960). However, one may not exclude the possibility that probability summation takes place in addition to neural summation or the possibility that some modified probabilistic model can predict the data (Dember, 1960; Eriksen, 1966).

More elaborate probability formulations, benefiting from known statistical probability density distributions, have also been tested. Crozier (1940) proposed a statistical theory for threshold and suprathreshold visual phenomena that may also be applied to the corresponding auditory phenomena. The statistical nature of the theory is derived from its assumption that the basis for sensory discrimination lies in the comparison of the statistical effects of two stimuli (in the case of threshold, one of these stimuli is taken to equal zero). The theory assumes that the sensory effects produced by stimuli are normally distributed when plotted against log intensity. Thus, the normal probability integral expresses the sensory effect as a function of log I. It is further assumed that the probability of excitation depends upon the amount of the sensory effect available and that the reciprocal of the excitatory stimulus intensity measures this capacity. Given these assumptions, the theory is able to explain many kinds of visual data by rather direct extensions (Brown and Mueller, 1965). In the case of temporal integration, it is assumed that the normal distribution of the neuronal thresholds is reflected when sensitivity ($1/I$) is plotted as a function of duration—the resultant curve being the normal probability integral.

Crozier's theory was tested empirically for auditory stimulation (e.g., Garner and Miller, 1948; Plomp and Bouman, 1959) and its predictions were found to be in good quantitative agreement with experimental results. Nevertheless, the theory was regarded with certain reservations due to its assumptions and its allowance for more constants to be determined directly from data than from other theoretical formulations.

Another probabilistic approach to the study of the characteristics of auditory integration is associated with the "theory of signal detectability." The question that arises from a signal-to-noise ratio standpoint relates to the identification of the noise in the situation. More generally stated, the thrust of the experimentation is directed toward understanding why it is difficult to detect the time–intensity-defined signal and how the characteristics of detection can be explained. The concept of critical bands was employed in this context to answer the above questions. The optimum procedure for detecting a signal of known duration is to adjust the receiver bandwidth to approximately the reciprocal of the signal duration (Green *et al.*, 1957). The effects of mismatching the receiver bandwidth and the reciprocal of signal duration are known (approximately a 3 dB signal-to-noise ratio loss per octave mismatch when both signal energy and noise level are held constant) and may be understood in terms of several characteristics of the output of the filter. One may assume either a variable or a fixed bandwidth on the part of the receiver. Whereas this and other models using the filter analogy suffer from some serious difficulties, one may think of other models that might provide more favorable comparisons between predictions and data.

It seems that the major impact of "signal detection" studies upon the conceptualization of the time–intensity relationship was a methodological one. It encouraged the use of forced-choice procedures, the use of somewhat more sensitive response measures, and allowed for more flexibility in the experimental designs (see, for example, Green *et al.*, 1957).

To summarize, the probabilistic approach (that is, the assumption of improved performance because of multiple opportunities to detect) may be considered as the converse of the complete summation hypothesis to the extent that it assumes the absence of any physical or physiological summation.

B. Other Nonsummation Interpretations

From time to time, attempts have been made to explain acoustic temporal summation by means of other, somewhat more simple neural phenomena. Thus, according to Miller (1948), the ear is more of a delaying device than an integration device. He assumes that different neural elements have different latencies, especially at higher centers. Loudness is correlated with the instantaneous level of neural activity in these centers. The level of activity is a function of time due to the different latencies of the neural elements in these higher centers, rather than an expression of acoustic summation; "perception of noise is the integral of the distribution of transmission times of the various pathways from the cochlea to the higher center, and not the integral of sound intensity" (Miller, 1948). Miller was also able to predict other auditory phenomena by using this theory, as well as by determining a value of the neural pathway transmission time.

A somewhat similar explanation, involving the assumption of a short temporal integration as part of a neural process, was advanced by Gersuni (1965) and Watson and Gengel (1969). Gersuni also postulated that the more sensitive receptors had much longer time constants (100 msec) than the less sensitive receptors (10 msec). The differential arrival times thus produced could explain the observed, quite long integration data. The assumption of a wide range of receptor thresholds, implicit in Gersuni's hypothesis, requires a stronger empirical base than is presently available. According to an alternative formulation, brief and more intense inputs give rise to a neural process of spatial summation due to the synchronization of impulses, whereas longer and weaker stimuli give rise to synaptic transmission by temporal summation of asynchronous impulses. If such processes are executed in successively higher neural stages, the total effect might account for quite large time constants of integration (Watson and Gengel, 1969).

Although the final theoretical framework for temporal summation data has not been formulated, most authors prefer the hypothesis of an authentic power integration in the auditory system. In this context, the probabilistic formulations may at least serve as useful null hypotheses. In the following section we attempt to review some of the theories that assume actual power summation.

C. Hyperbolic Models of Integration

Some authors, especially in earlier studies, assumed that an actual process of integration of acoustic power was taking place somewhere in the auditory system. This was a very useful working hypothesis because the auditory system does appear to act as a linear energy integrator, at least at threshold. If we denote the stimulus power by I and the stimulus duration by t, we obtain the equation for an energy integrator:

$$It = k \tag{1}$$

This perfect power integration does not hold for very short or long durations of pure tone stimuli and would not predict results at low frequencies. Recognizing this, Garner and Miller (1947) introduced a modification of the model that has been called the "diverted input hypothesis."

$$t(I - I_\infty) = k \tag{2}$$

This hypothesis maintains that a certain portion, I_∞, of the stimulus intensity is not an effective stimulus for the ear. All stimulus energy above this value is integrated linearly with time. I_∞ in this equation is the value of intensity necessary for the detection of an extremely long signal (i.e., from 1–2 seconds long).

A more general equation that might also encompass the phenomenon of partial summation (for noise bursts and long tones) has also been advanced by Garner.

$$t^n(I - I_\infty) = k \tag{3}$$

This function approaches a hyperbola as n approaches unity. Hughes (1946) presented a similar means of symbolizing the integration process that might also lend itself to a somewhat different interpretation. It seems obvious that the integration process implied at least a momentary storage of energy by a device of finite capacity. Thus, a time constant, τ, of this momentary energy storage system might be used as the unit of measurement, and any monotonic, negatively accelerated function may be selected as the predicted form of the integration. Hughes chose the following hyperbolic version:

$$I_t/I_\infty = 1 + (\tau/t) \tag{4}$$

or

$$I_t = I_\infty(1 + \tau/t) \tag{5}$$

Equation (4) can also be written

$$(I - I_\infty)t = I_\infty \tau = k \tag{6}$$

yielding Garner and Miller's corresponding equation. Although explanations have been suggested for this equation, no adequate suggestion has been advanced as to why the diverted input hypothesis should approximate the empirical data. Nor has it been explained why some intensity should not be an effective stimulus for the ear (Green et al., 1957).

Other researchers, working mainly in the field of vision, tended to posit an authentic summation process with a time constant whose value could be estimated from the experimental data without going into any further quantitative considerations. However, they stressed the implication that our senses receive the physical input in discrete time units within which it is not possible to discriminate between stimuli when the discrimination is based upon duration alone (Boynton, 1961). Hartline (1934) argued that the critical duration reflected the time needed by the nervous system to produce a given response (which may or may not be the one recorded by the experimenter). Other authors (i.e., Stroud, 1955; White, 1963) explicitly interpreted the critical duration as the limit on our ability to perceive and process stimulus durations under given experimental conditions. Such a limitation on neural resolving power was considered to be offset by the obvious adaptive value of integration with low-energy stimuli. Implicit in all of these hypotheses is the assumption that over some temporal range, equal-energy stimuli are equally detectable because such stimuli produce essentially identical neural responses (see Zacks, 1970; see also Zwislocki, 1960, 1969).

In summary these formulations all yield graphic data displays in which both stimulus parameters, I and t, are plotted in the same units (e.g., either linear or logarithmic; see Section II,A).

D. Exponential Models of Integration

Plomp and Bouman (1959) formulated a theory of temporal integration similar to that of Hughes, the main difference being their assumption of a negative exponential curve as describing the form of the integration. They argued that with stimulus onset, an intermediary effect arises with negative acceleration in the auditory system, but reaches a limit depending upon the stimulus intensity (I). The stimulus is perceived when this effect reaches some critical value (s_0). Thus, the following relationship holds between s and I:

$$s = kI_t(1 - e^{-t/\tau}) \qquad (7)$$

yielding an integration function in the form of

$$I_t = I_\infty / (1 - e^{-t/\tau}) \qquad (8)$$

The similarity of this equation to that of Hughes [Eq. (5)] is obvious. The main difference is that Plomp and Bouman's equation represents a circuit that discharges after a threshold is reached. Thus, according to this theory, the summation process at threshold can be explained with only one time constant. In addition, the theory may be extended to explain summation phenomena with periodic tone pulses (Plomp, 1961). When the data do not approach asymptote (a line of zero slope) over the durations employed in a given study (as is frequently the case, but not as is required by the model), the following modifications may be introduced (Morgan *et al.*, 1977),

$$\text{SPL} = A + [I/(1 - e^{-t/B})] + Ct \qquad (9)$$

where SPL is the sound pressure level required for threshold and A, B, and C are the parameters of the best fitting function. A is a scale factor, B is analogous to a time constant, and C is the slope (slightly negative) of the line at which the data approach asymptote.

The model of Plomp and Bouman is one of the most popular used in the literature when trying to fit experimental data and in fixing the time constant of integration. Its appeal may partially be accounted for by its relative simplicity.

Another model that is usually used to describe the summation data involves an integrator or a running average device. These interpretations have postulated that the ear performs a running average on the sound in accordance with the convolution integral. In other words, at time t, the subject does not perceive the instantaneous intensity of the stimulus, but instead perceives a weighted average of the components of the stimuli that have occurred in the recent past (Penner, 1978). The corresponding convolution integral may be written as follows:

$$y(t) = \int_0^\infty \chi(t-\tau)h(\tau)d\tau \tag{10}$$

where $y(t)$ is a quantity directly related to the effect of the sound [i.e., the subject's percept at time (t)], $h(t)$ is a weighting function, and $\chi(t)$ is the intensity of the incoming stimulus. The various versions of the running average model differ from each other in their specification of both the weighting and the stimulus functions.

An early version of this type of model was developed by Munson (1947). His basic assumption posited that each pulse on arrival at a higher neural center mediated a small elemental contribution to the magnitude of the sensation experienced. He further assumed that the effectiveness of the element diminishes as time elapses after its advent. The corresponding equation is

$$\Delta N = k\Delta n F(t_1 - t) \tag{11}$$

where N is the magnitude of a sensation t_1 seconds after the onset of a stimulus, and ΔN is the magnitude of the contribution mediated by the arrival of n pulses during the interval $t \pm \Delta t/2$. k is a constant related to the units of measurement of N, and $F(t_1 - t)$ is a dissipation function that describes the diminution in effectiveness of the quantal distribution after it emerges at time t. Equation (11) may be converted to a differential equation, with a subsequent integration yielding

$$N = k \int_{t=0}^{t-t_1} r(t)F(t_1 - t)dt \tag{12}$$

where r is the rate at which nerve pulses are incident upon the higher neural centers. Equation (11) may be considered as Munson's fundamental formula, whereas Eq. (12) serves as the computational one.

The stimulus function $r(t)$ is determined after the adaptation phenomena shown by the pulsing rate of a single nerve fiber to steady stimulation. Shortly after the stimulus onset the rate is very high, but it soon drops to one-fourth of the initial rate and thereafter continues to decrease very slowly. The following equation is proposed by Munson:

$$r(t) = \tfrac{1}{2}\exp-(60t) + \tfrac{1}{2}\exp[-(0.75t)^{0.15}] \tag{13}$$

where the first term reflects the rapid initial descent and the second term, the slow secondary decrease.

The general form of the weighting function $F(t_1-t)$ was already implied by the fundamental formula [Eq. (11)]. Munson finally specified it to be a decaying exponential function:

$$F = e^{-c(t_1-t)} \tag{14}$$

What this weighting function means is that the ear's integration favors the relatively recent portions of the sound.

Thus, by so specifying the functions of Eq. (12), we arrive at the convolution integral. While the stimulus function $r(t)$ involves an initial large-rise effect that quickly settles down to a slower steady level, the weighting function $F(t_1-t)$ favors the recent portion of the sound. This may be stated in terms of the fundamental formula: although an old pulse is less effective than a recent one $[F(t_1-t)]$, there are much fewer recent pulses $[r(t)]$.

Zwislocki (1960, 1969) developed a very similar theory, in which he tried to supply a physiological base to the proposed forms of the functions. His stimulus function is very similar to that of Munson,

$$r(t) = \epsilon_b e^{-\beta t} + \epsilon_c e^{-\gamma t} + \epsilon_\infty \tag{15}$$

where β and γ are time constants, and ϵ_b, ϵ_c, and ϵ_∞ are other constants. This function, which represents the peripheral neural effect of the stimulus, involves (in physiological terms) the combined effect of the decay of single-unit activity with a process of neural group equilibration. Zwislocki's weighting function is identical to that of Munson,

$$F(t_1-t) = e^{-\alpha(t_1-t)} \tag{16}$$

Substituting the above stimulus and weighting function in Eq. (10) gives the following solution of the convolution integral:

$$y(t) = [\epsilon_b/(\beta-\alpha)](e^{-\alpha t} - e^{-\beta t}) + [\epsilon_c/(\gamma-\alpha)](e^{-\alpha t} - e^{-\gamma t}) + (\epsilon_\infty/\alpha)(1 - e^{-\alpha t}) \tag{17}$$

where the values of the constants are to be determined from the data.

A special feature of Zwislocki's theory lies in his assumption that each sinusoid cycle (or pulse in a train) produces a neural change that decays exponentially. Using sufficiently high frequencies, only the envelope of these neural spikes is of importance. At threshold, a direct proportionality may be assumed to hold between stimulus intensity and neural excitation [i.e., the stimulus function written in Eq. (15) does not hold for the threshold of audibility] and, thus, the basic theory at threshold involves only one time constant—that of the exponential decay. The theory as posited in the form of Eqs. (15), (16), and (17) holds at suprathreshold levels of stimulation.

The basic difference between Zwislocki's and Plomp and Bouman's theories for integration at the threshold lies in the former's assumption of a neural response to each of the sinusoids contained in a tone burst. The advantage of making this assumption and performing the corresponding computations is the direct applicability of the theory to practically any auditory stimulus pattern. Apart from this difference, both theories share in common the idea that a single time constant may explain integration phenomena at the threshold for various temporal patterns of pulses.

At the suprathreshold level, Zwislocki attaches great importance to the form of the stimulus function [Eq. (15)], which reflects the temporal decay of neural activity. He argues that this temporal process can counteract the effects of the nonlinear stimulus transformation taking place in the auditory system ($\epsilon = I^n$, where ϵ is the magnitude of neural excitation). Because these opposite temporal processes are taking place either prior to or at the input to an integrator, psychoacoustic data show the characteristics of a linear temporal integrator. Thus, the theory does assume the existence of a linear temporal integrator with a time constant of 200 msec within the auditory nervous system. The apparent anomaly aroused by the known compression of the neural response to stimulus intensity preceding integration is offset by another temporal process—the decay of neural activity. Near the threshold, both the nonlinearity and the temporal decay disappear, and the psychoacoustic function directly reveals the characteristics of the integrator.

In essence, then, Zwislocki argues that the observed temporal integration of acoustic stimuli reflects the operation of an underlying integrator device, albeit not an auditory one. He suggests that a neural integrator operates somewhere in the nervous system both for threshold and suprathreshold stimuli, with some complexities evident at the suprathreshold level. In this basic sense, the theory is the simplest one possible because it assumes an underlying integration process for an observed integration process. Its great success is in fitting together the various auditory and neural facts and in showing them to be compatible with the above assumption.

Although both Zwislocki and Munson proposed fairly complicated forms for their stimulus and weighting functions, it was, in fact, shown that most available psychoacoustic data can be predicted by a very simple form of the running average hypothesis. In this form (Robinson, 1974), both the stimulus and the weighting functions are rectangular. A rectangular weighting function

$$h(t) = \begin{cases} k & \text{for } 0 \leq t \leq t_m \\ 0 & \text{otherwise} \end{cases} \quad (t_m \text{ is the critical duration}) \tag{18}$$

acts like a window in time so that the ear integrates all the sound perceived through the window. Using this weighting function, the integral may be written in a very simple way (Penner, 1978),

$$y(t) = k \int_{t-t_m}^{t} \chi(\tau) d\tau \tag{19}$$

meaning that the percept at time (t) is the simple sum of all input stimulation for the t_m msec preceding t. However, this is just the "classical" formulation of the temporal integration phenomenon. This was achieved with a rectangular integrator because it is easy to see that such a function gives rise to a maximum value of the percept just as the stimulus ends.

Both versions of the running average models (i.e., those of Munson and Zwislocki, and of Robinson) account reasonably well for most experimental findings on temporal summation in hearing. However, there are a few experimental findings that favor Zwislocki's theory (Irwin and Kemp, 1976).

It seems that several authors share the traditional view that temporally integrated responses are incapable of discrimination on the basis of differences in duration. Temporal summation seems to set a limit upon temporal resolution. Zwislocki, for example, partly bases his decision regarding the possible location of the temporal summation mechanism upon such considerations. Thus, he argues for a high neural locus because "otherwise it would be difficult to explain the amazing auditory sensitivity to dichotic time differences" (1960) or "A peripheral summation with a time constant of the order of 200 msec would make the auditory system insensitive to small dichotic time differences" (1969).

E. Short Time Constants versus Long Time Constants

Recently, several studies have reported finding very short time constants in auditory resolution (Green, 1971, 1973; Patterson and Green, 1970), which Ronken (1970) and Penner (1978) have attempted to explain in view of the data in the acoustic integration literature implying much longer time constants. The models of Ronken and Penner, for example, suggest that stimuli approximately 20 msec apart are treated as separate inputs. This result is, of course, in sharp contrast with the traditional view of time–intensity data, which posits that stimulus power is accumulated for about 100–200 msec. A possible solution to this discrepancy is proposed by Penner. First, she proposes a more general statement of the running average hypothesis (even for threshold) in which the weighting function may also depend on the driving function of stimulus intensity.

$$y(t) = \int_0^\infty f[\chi(t-\tau)]h[\tau,\chi(t)]d\tau \tag{20}$$

In a usual application, however, she proposes that $h(t)$ is independent of $\chi(t)$, as was assumed in previous models. The major departure from the previous form lies in the assumption of a nonlinear function of stimulus intensity driving the integrator. Penner proposes a power law or a compression function of stimulus intensity to drive the integrator,

$$f[\chi(t-\tau)] = \chi[(t-\tau)]^p \quad p < 1 \tag{21}$$

thus arriving at the following model:

$$y(t) = \int_0^\infty \chi^p(t-\tau)h(\tau)d\tau \tag{22}$$

For this model a weighting function may be specified that could generate the classical time–intensity data. One of the possibilities is

$$h(t) = \begin{bmatrix} s_0 apt^{ap-1} & \text{for } t \geq 1 \\ s_0 & \text{for } t < 1 \end{bmatrix} \tag{23}$$

where s_0 is a constant (reflecting the instantaneous value of the driving function at time t) and a is the slope of the function relating log I to log t. It can be seen that by choosing an appropriate value for p, the exponent of t (time constant) may be made small even when a is close to 1 (or rather to -1). Thus, the time–intensity trade data (a in the vicinity of 1) can be predicted by an integrator having a small time constant as long as a compression factor is assumed. Equation (23) may be rewritten so as to show that the weighting function has the form of an exponential function of log t.

The problem tackled by Penner is the same one treated by Zwislocki's (1969) analysis of suprathreshold summation. Both authors try to show how linear (or close to linear) integration is produced in audition in spite of an inherently nonlinear stimulus transformation also typical of the system. Zwislocki and Munson propose a stimulus transformation function at the input of the integrator to describe neural transformations of physical stimulation. This hypothesized process counteracts the ever-present stimulus compression effect, which again occurs at a stage preceding integration. The mutual neutralization of these processes allows for the effect of the linear integrator to show itself in experimental data. Penner, in contrast, places the compression process at the integrator itself; it is the driving function of the integrator. Thus, prior to the integrator, the input is directly proportional to stimulus intensity (Penner's stimulus function). The effect of the compression is tempered by an appropriate weighting function of the integration. The weighting function, which is related to log t by an exponential equation, accomplishes this by producing a rescaling of the temporal dimension so that shorter durations become relatively more important. Thus, both duration and intensity are transformed by a power function. This is just what is needed to counteract the effects of the nonlinear compression, but at the same time it yields an integrator with a very short time constant.

Thus, Zwislocki and others who suggest the existence of a linear integrator assume that the time constant of its weighting function reflects the time constant obtained in the experimental results. Penner, on the other hand, who suggests a nonlinear integrator driven by a power function, is able to show that quite long time–intensity trades are producible with an integrator having a short time constant. "Thus the existence of time-intensity trade data does not necessarily imply that there is a long-term integrator in the auditory system" (Penner, 1978). The model proposed by Penner is able to reconcile the apparently contradictory results regarding the length of time constants (brief versus long).

Although Penner's formulation is an interesting mathematical possibility, it is more difficult to explain it in physiological terms. The main difficulty lies in the (implicit) assumption of direct proportionality between the input to the integrator and stimulus intensity. If the common assumption that the power law transformations occur at peripheral loci, perhaps even at the receptor levels, is correct, then the most likely location for Penner's integrator is at the periphery of the auditory system or very close to it. However, in that case the integrator should directly summate incoming acoustic energy, a possibility that must be regarded with some reservation due to the highly damped sound transmission system of the ear.

IV. SOME IMPLICATIONS OF CURRENT RESEARCH

A. Integration and Resolution

The puzzle of duration–intensity reciprocity is still unresolved nearly a century after its first formulation by Bloch in the visual modality. The problem in audition is similar to that in vision (e.g., Kahneman, 1979), the crux of the matter being the reliable demonstration of the viability of a simple linear law in spite of a complex and mainly nonlinear auditory system. The experimental findings accumulated in the literature, as well as their logical consequences stated as theoretical propositions, constitute a detailed set of constraints for a really comprehensive theoretical framework to be developed that can fit all of the temporal summation data. At present there is no conclusive evidence to allow one to decide among the various theoretical alternatives that have been offered. A comprehensive theoretical framework must await more detailed experimentation.

For the theorist, what are the constraints that do appear well founded from previous research and theoretical formulations?

An early view of temporal summation relates the notion of critical duration to a response measure (see Wasserman and Kong, 1979). Hartline's (1934) tautology may have played a role in preparing for this approach. According to Hartline, the critical duration is an index that reflects the time needed to process a neural response in order to determine a proper motor response. The germ of an "absolute timing of mental activities" (Wasserman and Kong, 1979) may also have been contained in this hypothesis as well as the more problematic implication regarding integration as a peripheral process determining the critical duration. Such a concept, has, of course, difficulties in reconciling the possibility that temporal integration and temporal resolution may occur within the same temporal range.

The assumed incompatibility of resolution and integration is reflected in Zwislocki's (1960, 1969) argument for a more central mechanism for temporal summation, because "otherwise it would be difficult to explain the amazing auditory sensitivity to dichotic time differences." Researchers in the field of simultaneity perception or perceptual numerosity have considered the critical duration as a valid index of the so-called "perceptual moment" (Stroud, 1955; White, 1963). Temporal integration of incoming information seemed to imply a "loss of order." This led some researchers to interpret the critical duration as a limit on our ability to perceive and process stimulus durations under given experimental conditions (Murch, 1973, p. 106). Thus, Boynton (1961, p. 753) concludes his discussion of temporal factors in vision with "A common unifying principle apparently consistent with the data is the idea of temporal quantization of visual input by the higher visual nervous system, so that the input is 'packaged' into discrete time frames within which a purely temporal discrimination is not possible."

This assumed psychophysiological equivalence of temporally integrated stimuli yielding a given response may have stemmed partly from studies demonstrating the practical interchangeability of different configurations of equal-energy stimuli for a variety of psychophysical tasks (masking, binaural and binocular summation, etc.). For example, Westendorf *et al.* (1972) showed that binocular summation occurred equally well for a condition in which the flashes to each eye were of equal energy, but different in terms of their luminance and duration parameters as well as for a condition in which the flashes were equal in duration and luminance. However, these are but additional instances of isosensitivity functions saying nothing about the questions of the psychological and/or physiological equivalence of the integrated responses (see Pollack, 1973).

Recent results, however, indicate that a clear and explicit distinction must be drawn between temporal integration and temporal resolution with the *same* set of stimuli presented within the *same* range of time. Neither of these processes should be taken as imposing limits on the other; rather, they should be considered as a demonstration of independent operations of the auditory system reflected by different response classes, although sharing a common time domain. The fact that subjects are able to *discriminate* between the stimuli giving rise to their temporally integrated *constant* responses (Zacks, 1970; Algom and Babkoff, 1978; Algom et al., 1980) is of major importance in this respect. Thus, the argument is made here that temporal summation shows little about the organism's time-resolving power. Equal sensation or isosensitivity functions—of which the time–intensity trade-off is a member—may reflect the specific demands of the experimental tasks rather than the lack of ability to process individually the component physical dimensions.

We (Algom and Babkoff, 1978; Algom et al., 1980) tested the ability of subjects to discriminate between pairs of equal-energy, equally detectable pure tones. These threshold-level stimuli were shown to be within critical duration and yielded intensity–duration reciprocity for a detection response. The results indicated that equal-energy, equally detectable tones of different intensities and durations were discriminable from one another although the durations did not exceed the limits of complete reciprocity when the response measure was detection.

The discrimination level was found to increase as a function of the overall energy level and, consequently, as a function of the detection level. However, when we plotted the discrimination level against the detection level, both on normal coordinates, it was invariably found that the discrimination level increased at a faster rate than did the detection level as a function of the same parameter, energy (the functions always followed a straight line in such coordinates). The slopes ranged from 1.41 to 1.77, regardless of the frequency of tones (ranging in frequency from 0.5 to almost 8 kHz). An example of such a function is shown in Fig. 5.

How should one interpret these results? Our own linking hypothesis (Brindley, 1960) states that these recurring findings about greater-than-unity discrimination–detection slopes are indicative of two separate—if not totally independent—neural processes. Note that because both the ordinate and abscissa scales are in z scores, the slopes reflect the relations of the two standard deviations of the best fitting cumulative normal equations of discrimination and detection. A slope ranging from 1.4 to 1.7 implies that the variance of the discrimination distribution is smaller than that of the detection distribution. One probable explanation for this difference may be stated in terms of the number of independent, relevant sources of information available to the subject in a sensory task. In particular, as the number of such sources for a decision increases, the variability of the subject's responses should decrease proportionally. In a detection task, the only relevant basis for a decision is the presence (or absence) of the stimulus, regardless of its duration or intensity. In a discrimination task, the decision that a difference exists between two equal-energy stimuli may be based on any number of available cues, such as stimulus duration or intensity, each of which can serve

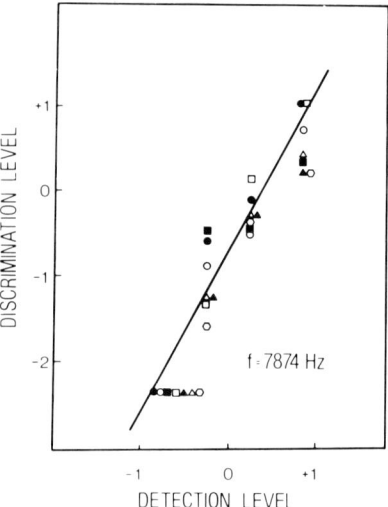

FIG. 5. Discrimination level in z scores is plotted on the ordinate as a function of detection level (also in z scores) on the abscissa for four pairs of equal-energy, equal-detection-level stimuli. Data are plotted for each subject; a single linear function is drawn through the data based on the median slope. The frequency of the tone is 7874 Hz. (After Algom et al., 1980.)

as a basis for the discrimination response. Therefore, at higher energy levels, the differences in intensity and duration between the members of the equal-energy pairs can become more discriminable. In a broader sense our results stress the task-dependent nature of auditory temporal summation in humans, as well as the implication that even within the range of reciprocity, the sensory system might retain the cues associated with each of the parameters, intensity and duration.

In view of these results, the hypothesis (e.g., Campbell and Counter, 1968) that the two processes, temporal resolution and temporal summation, are incompatible is no longer self-evident. Neither is the explanation of temporal summation in terms of stimulus persistence as opposed to stimulus temporal resolution (e.g., Penner, 1978). If summation of stimuli over time means their temporal quantization into "discrete time frames within which a purely temporal discrimination is not possible" (Boynton, 1961) our results would not have been possible; neither would the results of several other studies of auditory temporal acuity (e.g., Patterson and Green, 1970; Efron, 1973).

B. Recent Models of Temporal Integration

In light of the above findings some modifications seem desired in a more empirically based account of temporal integration.

Most behavioral studies of temporal integration have not been directly concerned with the question of the "real" psychological equivalence of the psychophysically determined constant responses. Emphasis was placed on the extent to which a constant response (e.g., constant detectability) could be preserved despite the alternative ways of packaging stimulus energy over time. Whether these constant responses also imply an underlying physiological equivalence or a psychophysical nondiscriminability of the responses was not systematically studied.

A possible way of viewing recent temporal acuity and temporal integration data allows for the possibility that stimulus integration begins as a peripheral sensory event. However, only those aspects of the neural code to equal-energy stimuli that determine their detectability result in equivalent neural events; other aspects of the neural code of these stimuli, such as those that determine their discriminability from each other, may result in different neural events (Bruder, 1971; Zacks, 1970). Kong and Wasserman (1978) suggest the possibility of different CNS neurons being used for different perceptual tasks, so that "detection and discrimination are mediated by central neurons with different integration times."

Wasserman and Kong (1979) have extended the argument and introduced a hypothesis according to which all physiological and behavioral summation characteristics subsequent to the receptor are determined by two major factors, the receptor output and the way the information is processed by the recipient. In fact, receptors supply various kinds of output and these can be analyzed and processed in several ways, either by recoding into a single output regardless of the amount or way the energy is presented (no integration), or by structuring the output as neural "events" (specific features occurring at a particular time) or as a neural "process" (stressing those properties that are related to the entire sensory signal). In the latter two cases, summation is found; however, the extent and specific characteristics of the intensity–duration function may differ extensively depending upon which of the procedures are used to analyze the receptor output.

With respect to behavioral measures, Wasserman and Kong (1979) hypothesized that the behavioral critical duration is an expression of the particular way in which the CNS analyzes a given peripheral sensory signal. Critical duration covaries with changes in the analysis of the same peripheral signal. The nervous system is capable of recomposing the available signals from the periphery in accordance with task requirements. When the task is changed, the processing operations are changed. Critical duration is thus considered to be task dependent.

The Wasserman–Kong model needs modifications, however, if it is to be successfully applied to audition (see Feth, 1979). In particular, the role of the primary receptor in determining the dynamics of temporal integration (i.e., supersummation) should be reconsidered. Babkoff (1979) provided evidence that indicates that it seems highly unlikely that receptor nonlinearity is a necessary or sufficient explanation for supersummation. The same conclusion can also be drawn from Zwislocki's (1969) analysis of suprathreshold temporal integration.

The issue of the locus of temporal summation, although relevant to this discussion, will not be elaborated further. Such a discussion clearly requires a much fuller treatment than is possible within this article. Of all the alternatives reviewed in this article, only the probability summation hypothesis and Penner's (1978) theory are compatible with a peripheral explanation. Zwislocki (1960, 1969) argued for a central (although not necessarily cortical) mechanism mainly because of the lack of long latencies and the slow building of neural activity in the periphery. The issue is, of course, intimately linked with the question of the type of energy integrated. Only the "diverted input hypothesis" and Penner's formulation are compatible with the parsimonious but empirically questionable assumption of a direct integration of acoustic energy. In particular, Penner's (1978) model does not require the long latencies at the periphery. Penner's model is also the only integrator formulation in the literature that seems compatible with the discrimination and integration data without introducing major modifications. This is achieved by assuming that a nonlinear integrator with a brief time constant operates even at threshold. As noted, Penner's main suggestion allowing for such a reconciliation of the different results demands the presence of a dynamic rescaling of the temporal dimension of the stimulus.

V. CONCLUSIONS

The major findings reviewed in the empirical section of this article illustrate the emphasis of most of the earlier studies on the influence of a variety of stimulus variables on the characteristics of temporal integration (some of which are still unresolved). Recent investigations, by comparison, have tended to include the importance of the response class as well. It seems generally accepted now that the various measures arbitrarily selected by experimenters may not be equally meaningful to the study of integration (Bruder and Kietzman, 1973; Kong and Wasserman, 1978; Leshowitz and Wightman, 1972). Different measures are probably related to different underlying neural processes. However, none of these should be taken as "discounting" or "filtering out" temporal information in any way (see, for example, the "recoding" option, Wasserman and Kong, 1979). We agree with Marks (1979) in viewing temporal integration as an (adaptive) operation of the sensory system in the time domain that can bring the organism to the point where an invariant response is possible.

The situation suggested by the results of recent investigations calls for the design of experiments aimed at a systematic mapping of the relations among different integration and acuity measures utilizing a variety of behavioral tasks, all within a *common* framework. Such an effort may yield a better understanding of the underlying neural dynamics producing the different behavioral–temporal measures. In addition, research programs of this kind should be performed in parallel in different modalities—in vision and audition, for example. Differences, to be sure, are to be expected. It is, however, the discovery of differences as well as invariances within and across modalities that may serve to prepare an overall theoretical framework to explain stimulus integration in sensory systems.

REFERENCES

Algom, D., and Babkoff, H. (1978). Discrimination of equal-energy, equally detectable auditory stimuli. *Psychol. Res.* **40**, 149–157.

Algom, D., Babkoff, H., and Ben-Uriah, Y. (1980). Temporal integration and discrimination of equally detectable, equal-energy stimuli: The effect of frequency. *Psychol. Res.* **42**, 305–318.

Babkoff, H. (1975a). The effect of light-deprivation on the adult electroretinogram. *Vision Res.* **15**, 870–872.

Babkoff, H. (1975b). The effect of light deprivation of the B-wave input-output function, *Ann. Ophthalmol.* **7**, 1335–1338.

Babkoff, H. (1979). Deviations from intensity-duration reciprocity as possible indicators of pathology. *Behav. Brain Sci.* **2**, 255–257.

Babkoff, H., and Algom (Gombosh), D. (1976). Monaural and binaural temporal integration of noise bursts. *Psychol. Res.* **39**, 137–145.

Babkoff, H., and Sutton, S. (1971). Monaural temporal interaction. *J. Acoust. Soc. Am.* **50**, 459–465.

Babkoff, H., Brandeis, R., and Bergman, Y. (1975). Partial integration of single electrocutaneous pulses. *Percept. Psychophys.* **17**, 285–292.

Bekesy, G. (1960). "Experiments in Hearing." McGraw-Hill, New York.

Boring, E. G. (1942). "Sensation and Perception in the History of Experimental Psychology." Appleton, New York.

Boynton, R. M. (1961). Some temporal factors in vision. *In* "Sensory Communication" (W. A. Rosenblith, Ed.), pp. 739–756. M.I.T. Press, Cambridge, Massachusetts.

Brindley, G. S. (1960). "Physiology of the Retina and the Visual Pathway." Arnold, London.

Brown, J. L., and Mueller, C. G. (1965). Brightness discrimination and brightness contrast. *In* "Vision and Visual Perception" (C. H. Graham, Ed.), pp. 208–250. Wiley, New York.

Bruder, G. E. (1971). The temporal integration of luminous energy for response frequency, response latency, and signal detectability. Unpublished doctoral dissertation, City University of New York.

Bruder, G. E., and Kietzman, M. L. (1973). Visual temporal integration for threshold signal detectability and reaction time measures. *Percept. Psychophys.* **13**, 293–300.

Campbell, R. A., and Counter, S. A. (1968). Temporal integration and periodicity pitch. *J. Acoust. Soc. Am.* **45**, 691–693.

Crozier, W. J. (1940). The theory of the visual threshold. I. Time and intensity. *Proc. Nat. Acad. Sci. U.S.A.* **26**, 54–60.

Dallos, P. J., and Olsen, W. O. (1964). Integration of energy at threshold with gradual rise-fall tone pips. *J. Acoust. Soc. Am.* **36**, 743–751.

Dember, W. N. (1960). "Psychology of perception." Holt, New York.

Efron, R. (1973). Conservation of temporal information by perceptual systems. *Percept. Psychophys.* **14**, 518–530.

Eriksen, C. W. (1966). Temporal luminance summation effects in backward and forward masking. *Percept. Psychophys.* **1**, 87–92.
Feth, L. L. (1979). Temporal summation in the auditory system. *Behav. Brain Sci.* **2**, 260–261.
Garner, W. R. (1947). The effect of frequency spectrum on temporal integration in the ear. *J. Acoust. Soc. Am.* **19**, 808–815.
Garner, W. R., and Miller, G. A. (1948). The masked threshold of pure tones as a function of duration. *J. Exp. Psychol.* **37**, 293–303.
Gersuni, G. V. (1965). Organization of afferent flow and the processes of external discrimination. *Neuropsychologia* **3**, 45–109.
Goldstein, J. L. (1967). Auditory nonlinearity. *J. Acoust. Soc. Am.* **41**, 676–689.
Graham, C. H., and Margaria, R. (1935). Area and the intensity-time relation in the peripheral retina. *Amer. J. Physiol.* **113**, 299–305.
Green, D. M. (1971). Temporal auditory acuity. *Psychol. Rev.* **78**, 540–551.
Green, D. M. (1973). Temporal acuity as a function of frequency. *J. Acoust. Soc. Am.* **54**, 373–379.
Green, D. M., Birdsall, T. G., and Tanner, W. P. (1957). Signal detection as a function of signal intensity and duration. *J. Acoust. Soc. Am.* **29**, 523–531.
Greenberg, G. Z., and Larkin, W. D. (1968). Frequency-response characteristic of auditory observers detecting signals of a single frequency in noise: The probe-signal method. *J. Acoust. Soc. Am.* **44**, 1513–1523.
Hartline, H. K. (1934). Intensity and duration in the excitation of single photoreceptor units. *Cell. Comp. Physiol.* **5**, 229–247.
Hughes, J. W. (1946). The threshold of audition for short periods of stimulation. *Proc. R. Soc. London Ser. B* **133**, 486–490.
Irwin, R. J., and Kemp, S. (1976). Temporal summation and decay in hearing. *J. Acoust. Soc. Am.* **59**, 920–925.
Irwin, R. J., and Zwislocki, J. J. (1971). Loudness effects in pairs of tone bursts. *Percept. Psychophys.* **10**, 189–192.
Kahneman, D. (1979). Mechanisms that produce critical durations. *Behav. Brain Sci.* **2**, 265–266.
Kong, K. L., and Wasserman, G. S. (1978). Changing response measures alters temporal summation in the receptor and spike potentials of the *Limulus* lateral eye. *Sensory Processes* **2**, 21–31.
Leshowitz, B., and Wightman, F. L. (1972). On the importance of considering the signal's frequency spectrum: Some comments on MacMillan's "Detection and recognition of increments and decrements in auditory intensity" experiment. *Percept. Psychophys.* **12**, 209–210.
Marks, L. E. (1979). Invariance, richness, recoding. *Behav. Brain Sci.* **2**, 272.
McFadden, D. (1975). Duration-intensity reciprocity for equal loudness. *J. Acoust. Soc. Am.* **57**, 702–704.
Miller, G. A. (1948). The perception of short bursts of noise. *J. Acoust. Soc. Am.* **20**, 160–170.
Morgan, D. E., Gilman, S., and Dirks, D. B. (1977). Temporal integration at the "threshold" of the acoustic reflex. *J. Acoust. Soc. Am.* **62**, 170–176.
Munson, W. A. (1947). The growth of auditory sensation. *J. Acoust. Soc. Am.* **19**, 584–591.
Murch, G. M. (1973). "Visual and Auditory Perception." Bobb-Merill, New York.
Olsen, W. O., and Carhart, R. (1966). Integration of acoustic power at threshold by normal hearers. *J. Acoust. Soc. Am.* **40**, 591–599.
Patterson, J. H., and Green, D. M. (1970). Discrimination of transient signals having identical energy spectra. *J. Acoust. Soc. Am.* **48**, 536–553.
Penner, M. J. (1975). Persistence and integration: Two consequences of a sliding integrator. *Percept. Psychophys.* **18**, 114–120.
Penner, M. J. (1978). A power law transformation resulting in a class of short-term integrators that produce time-intensity trades for noise bursts. *J. Acoust. Soc. Am.* **63**, 195–201.

Pieron, H. (1952). "The sensations: Their functions, processes and mechanisms." Yale Univ. Press, New Haven, Connecticut.

Plomp, R. (1961). Hearing threshold for periodic tone pulses. *J. Acoust. Soc. Am.* **33,** 1561–1569.

Plomp, R., and Bouman, M. A. (1959). Relation between hearing threshold and duration for tone pulses. *J. Acoust. Soc. Am.* **31,** 749–758.

Pollack, I. (1973). Time-intensity equivalence relations for auditory pulse trains. *J. Exp. Psychol.* **100,** 239–245.

Robinson, C. E. (1974). Simple form of the auditory running-average hypothesis: Application to the temporal summation of loudness and to the delayed perception of the offset of brief stimuli. *J. Acoust. Soc. Am.* **55,** 645–648.

Ronken, D. (1970). Monaural detection of a phase difference between clicks. *J. Acoust. Soc. Am.* **47,** 1091–1099.

Schenkel, K. D., von. (1967). Die beidohrigen Mithorschwellen von Impulsen. *Acoustica* **18,** 38–46.

Schevelev, I. A., and Hicks, L. H. (1971). Characteristics of temporal summation at different levels in the visual system of the cat. *In* "Sensory Processes at the Neuronal and Behavioral Levels" (G. V. Gersuni, Ed.), pp. 57–68. Academic Press, New York.

Sheeley, E. C., and Bilger, R. C. (1964). Temporal integration as a function of frequency. *J. Acoust. Soc. Am.* **36,** 1850–1857.

Small, A. M., Brandt, J. F., and Cox, P. G. (1962). Loudness as a function of signal duration. *J. Acoust. Soc. Am.* **34,** 513–514.

Stevens, J. C., and Hall, J. W. (1966). Brightness and loudness as functions of stimulus duration. *Percept. Psychophys.* **1,** 319–329.

Stroud, J. M. (1955). The fine structure of psychological time. *In* "Information Theory in Psychology" (H. Quastler, Ed.), pp. 174–207. Free Press, New York.

Wasserman, G. S., and Kong, K. L. (1979). Absolute timing of mental activities. *Behav. Brain Sci.* **2,** 243–255.

Watson, C. S., and Gengel, R. W. (1969). Signal duration and signal frequency in relation to auditory sensitivity. *J. Acoust. Soc. Am.* **46,** 989–997.

Westendorf, D. H., Blake, R. R., and Fox, R. (1972). Binocular summation of equal-energy flashes of unequal duration. *Percept. Psychophys.* **12,** 445–447.

White, C. T. (1963). Temporal numerosity and the psychological unit of duration. *Psychol. Monogr.* **77,** 1–37.

Wicke, J. D., Donchin, E., and Lindsley, D. B. (1964). Visual evoked potentials as a function of flash luminance and duration. *Science* **164,** 83–85.

Wright, H. N. (1968). Clinical measurement of temporal auditory summation. *J. Speech Hear. Res.* **11,** 109–127.

Zacks, J. L. (1970). Temporal summation phenomena at threshold: Their relation to visual mechanism. *Science* **170,** 197–199.

Zwicker, E., and Wright, H. N. (1963). Temporal summation for tones in narrow-band noise. *J. Acoust. Soc. Am.* **35,** 691–699.

Zwislocki, J. J. (1960). Theory of temporal auditory summation. *J. Acoust. Soc. Am.* **32,** 1046–1060.

Zwislocki, J. J. (1969). Temporal summation of loudness: An analysis. *J. Acoust. Soc. Am.* **46,** 431–441.

The Specialized Auditory System of Kangaroo Rats

DOUGLAS B. WEBSTER* AND MOLLY WEBSTER**

*,**DEPARTMENT OF OTORHINOLARYNGOLOGY
AND *DEPARTMENT OF ANATOMY
KRESGE HEARING RESEARCH LABORATORY OF THE SOUTH
LOUISIANA STATE UNIVERSITY MEDICAL CENTER
NEW ORLEANS, LOUISIANA

I.	Introduction	161
II.	The Middle Ears	165
	A. Kangaroo Rat Middle Ear Anatomy	165
	B. Kangaroo Rat Tympanic Membrane	167
	C. Kangaroo Rat Auditory Ossicles and Intraaural Muscles	168
	D. Mammalian Middle Ear Function	169
	E. Kangaroo Rat Middle Ear Function	170
	F. Adaptive Value of Kangaroo Rat Low-Frequency Hearing	172
	G. Evolution of the Kangaroo Rat Middle Ear	177
III.	The Cochlea	183
	A. Must the Cochlea Match the Middle Ear?	183
	B. Structure of the Kangaroo Rat Cochlea	183
	C. Development of the Kangaroo Rat Cochlea	186
	D. Cochleae of Other Heteromyid Rodents	187
IV.	The Central Auditory System	189
	A. Theoretical	189
	B. Kangaroo Rat Central Auditory Pathway	189
	C. Central Auditory System of Other Heteromyids	190
V.	Summary	192
	References	194

I. INTRODUCTION

A few living rodent species possess extraordinarily large middle ears—so large that they distort the shape of the skull by extending superiorly to the dorsal surface, posteriorly past the foramen magnum, and anteriorly into the orbit (Fig. 1); so large that in some species the combined volumes of right and left middle ears exceed that of the cranial cavity. Such hypertrophied middle ears have evolved independently at least four times in rodent phylogeny and are found

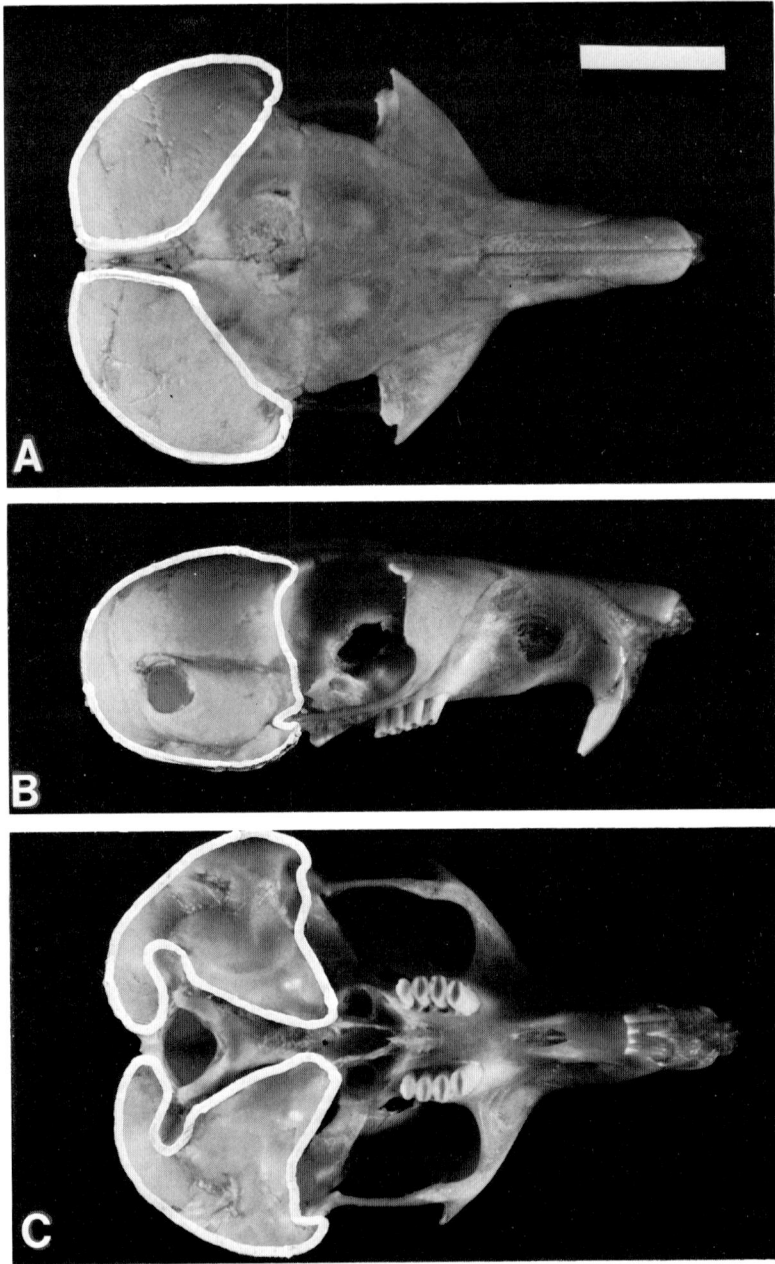

FIG. 1. Dorsal (A), lateral (B), and ventral (C) views of the skull of a banner-tailed kangaroo rat (*Dipodomys spectabilis*). The white lines outline the enlarged middle ears. Bar equals 1 cm.

today in representatives of four separate rodent families: kangaroo rats and kangaroo mice, of the family Heteromyidae; gerbils, of the family Cricetidae; jerboas, of the family Dipodidae; and springhaas of the family Pedetidae (Howell, 1932). Furthermore, these rodents share two other important features: they exhibit a tendency for bipedal, saltatory locomotion, and they live in arid to semiarid habitats characterized by sparse, discontinuous vegetation.

Why these correlations in four diverse groups? Or to put it in biological terms, *what selective pressure(s)* favored evolution of greatly enlarged middle ears and saltatory locomotion in desert environments? Our initial goal, some 20 years ago, was to answer that question.

We began our studies on two species of the genus *Dipodomys*—the kangaroo rats. This genus is native to the western United States and northern Mexico; some of its 28 species inhabit chaparral, but most live in deserts, including some of the most arid regions of North America. As an adaptation to these desert environments, they have evolved specialized water balance systems that enable them to survive without free water by using metabolic water, a byproduct of carbohydrate and lipid metabolism (Schmidt-Nielsen and Schmidt-Nielsen, 1951). However, these same specializations limit their ability to control body temperature when exposed to heat, and therefore these animals are nocturnal, spending the daylight hours in underground burrows that maintain the lower temperature and higher relative humidity they require. At night, when the temperature falls, they come to the surface to forage for the seeds that supply their carbohydrate- and lipid-rich diet.

Merriam's kangaroo rat (*Dipodomys merriami*) (Fig. 2), one of the smallest species (about 40 g adult weight), is found ubiquitously in the southwestern American and northern Mexican deserts, where it lives in relatively small, simple burrows (Fig. 3). The banner-tailed kangaroo rat (*Dipodomys spectabilis*) (Fig. 4), one of the largest (about 130 g adult weight), is restricted to flat, semiarid regions of Arizona and New Mexico. Its elaborate burrows are constructed in prominent mounds containing two or three levels of interconnecting tunnels and large "rooms" for food storage, located above the level of the surrounding terrain and frequent flash floods of the desert rainy season (Fig. 5).

For more than 20 years we studied the anatomy and functioning of the middle and inner ear in these two species and how it compares to the "normal" mammalian situation; we examined their hearing ability and found it, like their anatomy, highly specialized; and we studied the animals in their environment and the interactions of their hearing (and other senses) in "real life" situations. Finally, we applied what we had learned to the evolution of the entire family Heteromyidae, which consists of 5 genera exhibiting considerable auditory diversity; we eventually studied 27 species of these 5 genera. Most of this work has been previously published in research reports; this article is an attempt to pull it together into a coherent, connected story that shows that, properly understood,

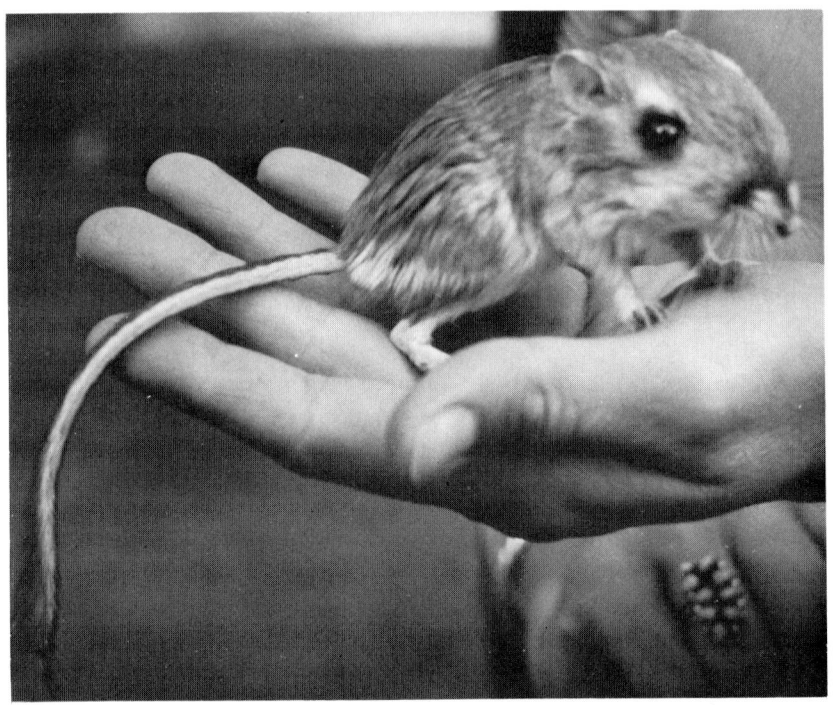

FIG. 2. Merriam's kangaroo rat; note the prominent eyes and broad head.

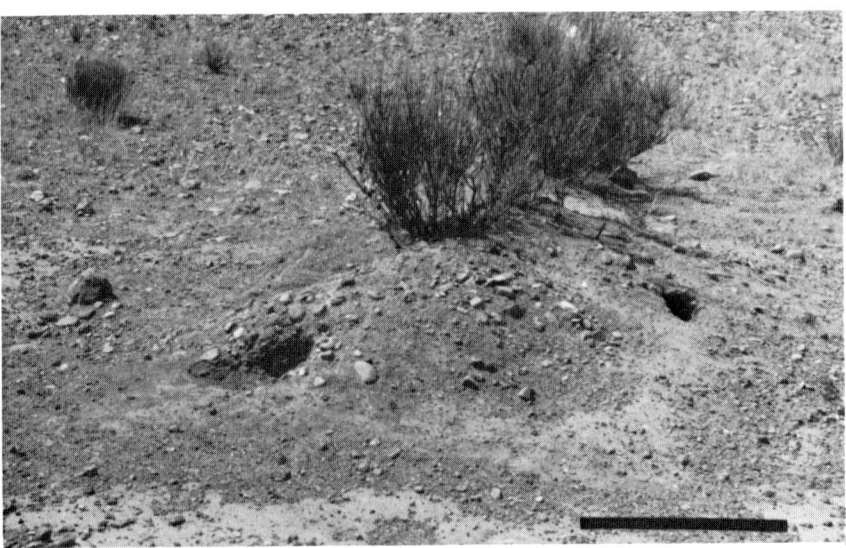

FIG. 3. Typical mound of a Merriam's kangaroo rat. Note the two openings to the simple burrow system. Bar equals 0.5 m.

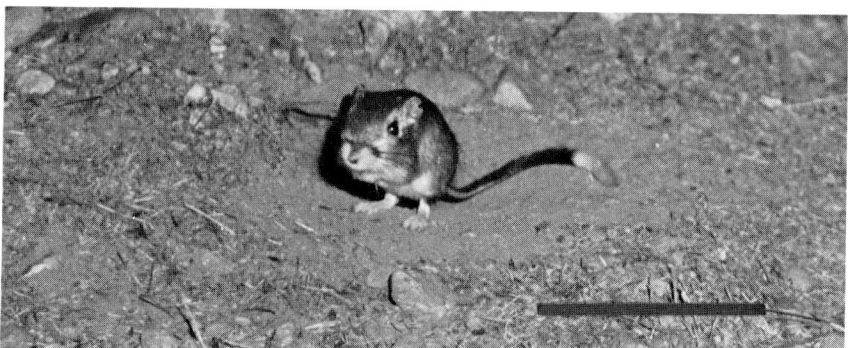

FIG. 4. Banner-tailed kangaroo rat at its mound. Note the bipedal stance and long tail. Bar equals 10 cm.

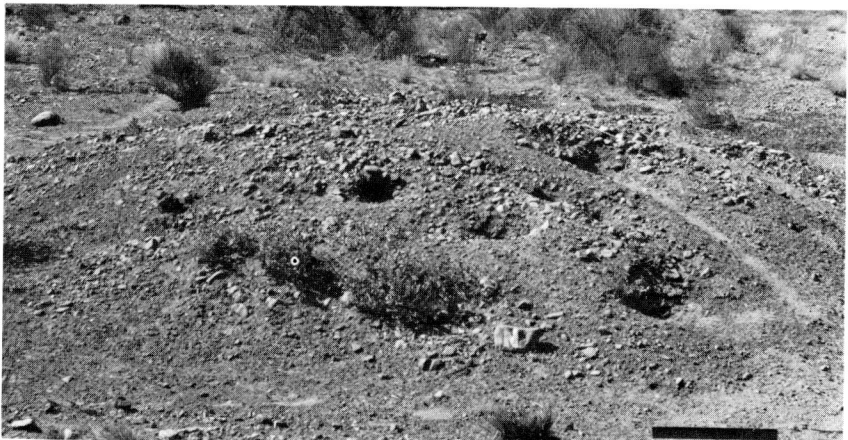

FIG. 5. Elaborate, elevated mound of a banner-tailed kangaroo rat. Note the several burrow openings and trails used by the kangaroo rat. Bar equals 1.0 m.

the question "why?" is meaningful in biology, and can lead one on a fascinating journey.

II. THE MIDDLE EARS

A. Kangaroo Rat Middle Ear Anatomy

The greatly enlarged temporal bone of the kangaroo rat is composed of the fused periotic, ectotympanic, and styloid elements; as in all rodents, the squamosal is a separate bone rather than a part of the complex. The volume of each middle ear is 0.47 cm^3 in Merriam's kangaroo rat, and 1.00 cm^3 in the bannertailed kangaroo rat; relative to body size, the volumes are approximately equal in the two species (Webster, 1961).

The middle ear cavity is composed of three interconnecting portions (Fig. 6): the ventral hypotympanum (18% of the total volume) communicates posteriorly with the antrum (33%) and dorsally with the epitympanum (49%) (Webster, 1961). The epitympanum and antrum, separated by a thin lamina of bone, extend laterally well past the level of the tympanic membrane. In addition to this peripheral expansion the cavity is made even larger, because during the first 4 weeks after birth all "excess" bone is eroded away on the walls adjoining the brain and inner ear. During this time, thick, trabeculated bone is continually laid down on the outer walls of the middle ear cavity, while previously formed bone is continually removed by osteoclastic activity. At 4 weeks this intense osteoblastic and osteoclastic activity comes to an end, and the ultrathin laminar bone of the adult remains (Webster, 1975).

In most areas, laminar bone less than 0.1 mm thick forms the outer margins of

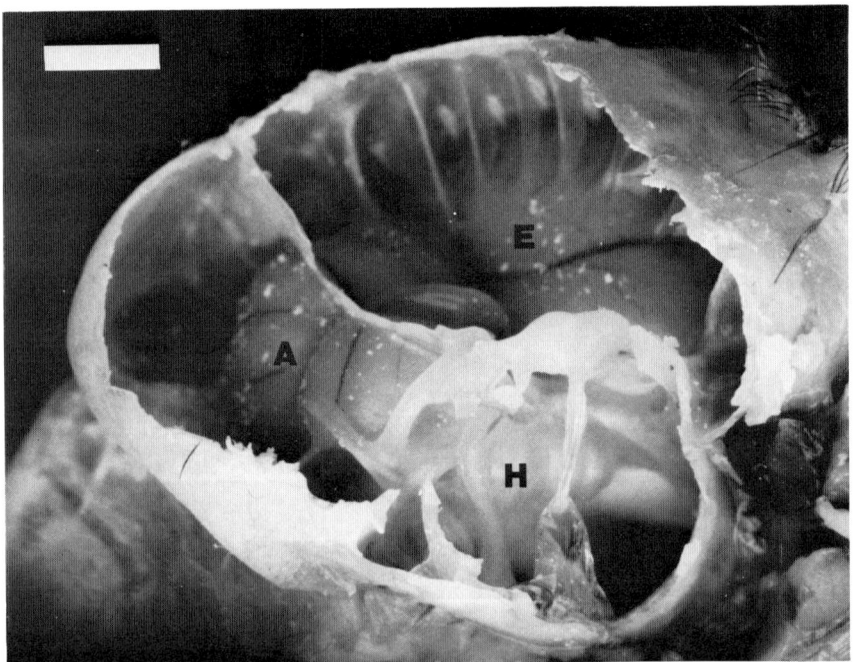

FIG. 6. Ventrolateral view of a dissection of the middle ear of *Dipodomys merriami*. A, Antrum; E, epitympanum; H, hypotympanum. Bar equals 2.0 mm.

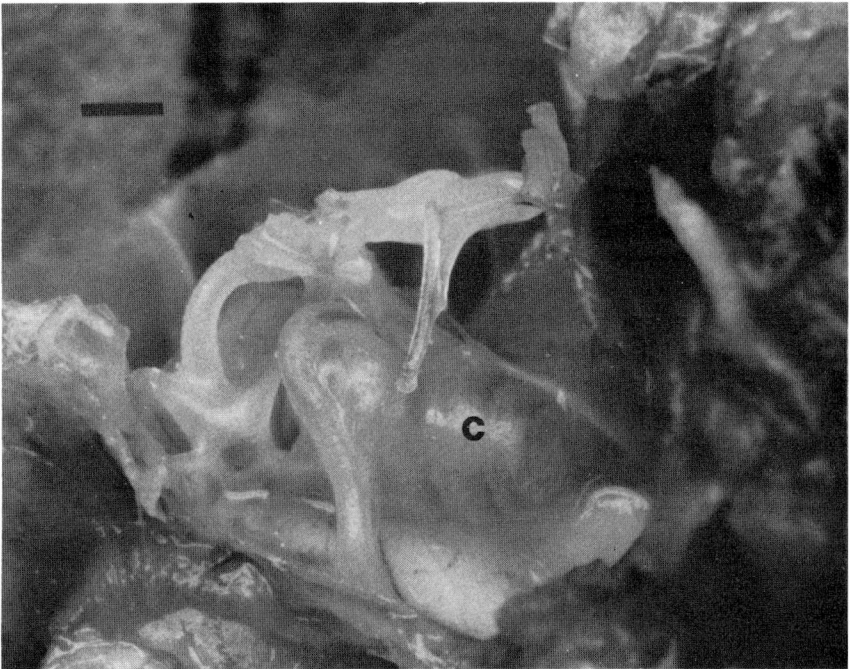

FIG. 7. Ventral view of a dissection of the hypotympanum of *Dipodomys merriami*, showing the prominent cochlea (C) bulging into it. Bar equals 1.0 mm.

the middle ear cavity. The hypotympanum is expanded past the area of the cochlea, so that in effect the cochlea bulges into the cavity (Fig. 7), where it is covered by bone so thin that the spiral ligament can be seen through its translucent walls; medially the hypotympanum is extended nearly to the pharynx, making the eustachian tube little more than a foramen. In the antrum, both the horizontal and posterior semicircular canals, again covered by extremely thin bone, are clearly outlined (Fig. 8); the anterior semicircular canal is similarly outlined in the epitympanum (Webster, 1961).

B. Kangaroo Rat Tympanic Membrane

The tympanic membrane is large for such a small animal, having a diameter of 5.2 mm in Merriam's kangaroo rat and 6.3 mm in the banner-tailed kangaroo rat, as compared to 3.1 mm in the golden hamster (Oaks, 1967). Otherwise, it is quite normal: shaped like a flat cone, composed of a large pars tensa and a very small, superiorly located pars flaccida, with an outer layer of thin stratified

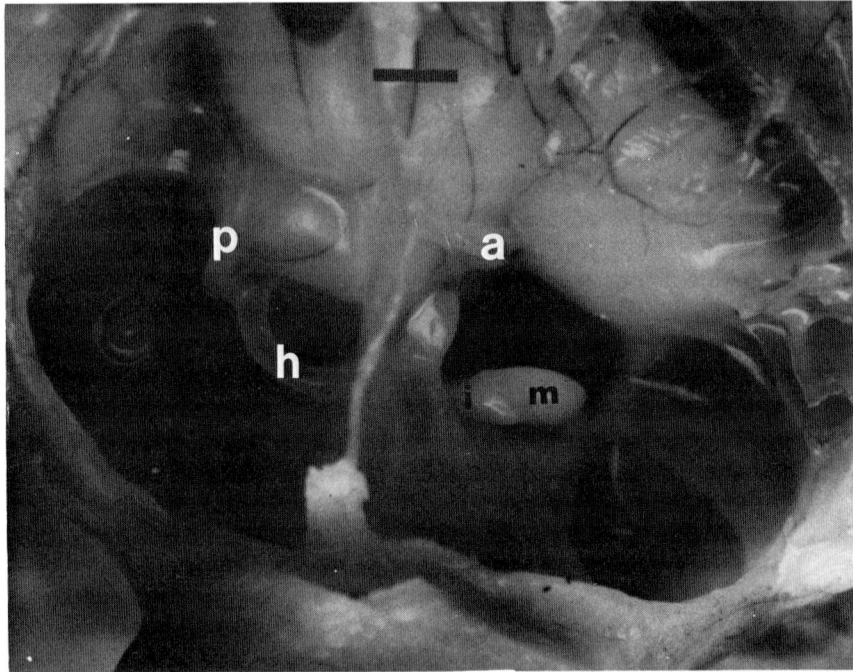

FIG. 8. Dorsal view of a dissection of the middle ear of *Dipodomys merriami*, showing the posterior (p) and horizontal (h) semicircular canals bulging into the antrum and the anterior (a) semicircular canal bulging into the epitympanum. m, Head of malleus; i, body of incus. Bar equals 2.0 mm.

squamous epithelium, a middle layer of radial and circular fibers, and an inner layer of simple squamous epithelium.

C. Kangaroo Rat Auditory Ossicles and Intraaural Muscles

The auditory ossicles are delicately suspended in the middle ear cavity. The malleus has a very short neck, a tenuous anterior process, and a large head; its manubrium, embedded in the fibrous layer of the tympanic membrane, is unusually slender. The incus and the malleus join in a complex double saddle-shaped synovial articulation that allows no relative motion between them. The long process of the incus parallels the manubrium but is less than one-third of its length—a much greater difference than in most mammals. The lenticular process of the incus articulates with the head of the stapes in an amphiplanar joint. The footplate of the stapes is extremely thin and of a bullate shape that bulges into the vestibule of the inner ear; the collagenous fibers of the annular ligament, which hold it in place, are unusually fine (Webster, 1961).

There are only two suspensory ligaments for the ossicular chain: the anterior ligament of the malleus, which is attached to its anterior process, and the posterior ligament of the incus, which is attached to its short process. An imaginary line drawn through these two ligaments passes through the center of gravity of the tympano-ossicular system and defines the axis of rotation during auditory stimulation (Webster, 1961).

Both the tensor tympani and stapedius muscles are very delicate; the former inserts upon the manubrium of the malleus and the latter onto the neck of the stapes (Webster, 1961).

D. Mammalian Middle Ear Function

Several outstanding physiologists (e.g., Zwislocki, 1965; Møller, 1972; Dallos, 1973) have thoroughly analyzed the function of the mammalian middle ear; here we present only enough of an overview to allow comparison of the kangaroo rat with more "standard" experimental animals.

The middle ear acts as an impedance-matching transformer. The more closely the impedance of the fluid-filled cochlea matches that of air, the more acoustic energy can be transferred from the air to the cochlea. Because acoustic impedance is directly proportional to pressure and inversely proportional to particle velocity, anything that either increases pressure at the cochlea or decreases particle velocity at the cochlea will increase the *apparent* impedance of the airborne sound and bring it closer to the impedance of the fluids of the cochlea.

The mammalian tympano-ossicular system does both. The acoustic force impinging upon the relatively large tympanic membrane is transferred to the relatively small footplate of the stapes, thereby increasing the pressure (force per unit area) as a function of the difference in their sizes; because only about two-thirds of the tympanic membrane acts to move the ossicles, the amount of pressure increase at the stapes is the ratio of two-thirds the tympanic membrane area to the stapes footplate. Pressure is also increased as a result of the lever system of the ossicles; because the manubrium of the malleus is longer than the long process of the incus, pressure is increased at the stapes as a ratio of these lever arms. Moreover, because of this difference in lever arm lengths, the particle velocity at the stapes is also decreased as a ratio of the lever arms.

Thus, it is the tympano-ossicular system that does the impedance matching. If there were no tympano-ossicular system, less than 1% of the airborne acoustic energy would be transmitted to the cochlea. However, in humans, for instance, the tympano-ossicular system *theoretically* allows about 75% of the airborne energy to reach the cochlea.

In reality, however, the efficiency of the tympano-ossicular system is reduced by *resistance,* primarily due to friction caused particularly by the ossicular ligaments and tendons and by the enclosed middle ear air space.

In addition to its resistive (frictional) characteristics, the tympano-ossicular system is also affected by *reactive* characteristics, which make it, like any mechanical system, frequency dependent; that is, it will transmit acoustic energy most efficiently at its natural frequency, which is determined by its mass and stiffness. The greater the mass, the lower the natural frequency; the greater the stiffness, the higher the natural frequency. It follows, therefore, that large mammals tend to hear most acutely at relatively low frequencies and small mammals at relatively high frequencies; in fact, most small mammals are essentially deaf below 1 kHz, with their most sensitive hearing far above that. As extreme examples, the auditory frequency range of Indian elephants is from 0.017 to 10.0 kHz (Heffner and Heffner, 1982), whereas that of little brown bats is from 10.0 to 110.0 kHz (Dalland, 1965).

Mammals whose sensitive hearing covers a wide range of frequencies are found to have adaptations which, by one means or another, minimize the *resistive* components of their tympano-ossicular systems. The interactions of these two middle ear characteristics—resistance and reactance—determine almost entirely the frequency range of mammalian hearing.

The easiest way to quantify and describe the effect of these characteristics is by recording cochlear microphonic (CM) potentials, which are AC receptor potentials produced by the cochlear hair cells. The frequency of the CM mimics that of the stimulating sound, and, within physiological limits, the amplitude of the CM is proportional to the intensity of that sound. These potentials are most readily recorded from an active electrode placed on the round window membrane. Because this electrode is closest to the basal portion of the cochlea, it is preferentially sensitive to basal hair cells. Thus, the CM sensitivity curve does not necessarily reflect perceptual (behavioral) auditory thresholds over the entire range, but is an accurate reflection of middle ear mechanics (Dallos, 1973).

E. Kangaroo Rat Middle Ear Function

We measured the sound intensity necessary to obtain a 1-μV CM in kangaroo rats in the frequency range from 0.05 to 100 kHz (Webster and Strother, 1972; Webster and Webster, 1980). The greatest sensitivity was between 0.1 and 16.0 kHz, where it took less than 20 dB SPL to elicit the 1-μV response. The CM remained quite sensitive through 25 kHz, but above that became rapidly less sensitive. Surprisingly, in spite of the bias for basal (high-frequency) hair cells in the CM sensitivity curve, in this case the behaviorally determined audiogram almost perfectly mirrored the microphonic sensitivity curve (Fig. 9) exhibiting the same low-frequency sensitivity (Webster and Webster, 1972; Heffner and Masterton, 1980).

In other small mammals with good sensitivity below 1 kHz, such as gerbils, chinchillas, and guinea pigs, the absolute volume of the middle ear cavity is as

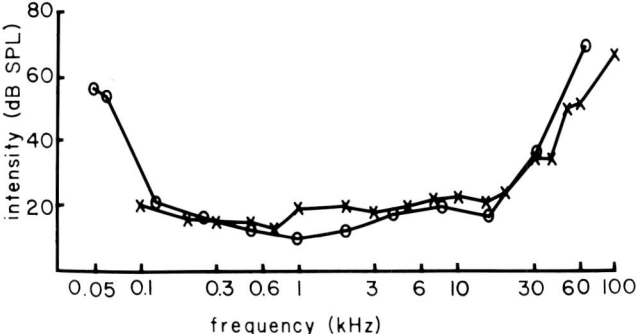

FIG. 9. Behavioral auditory thresholds (○————○) and 1-μV cochlear microphonic thresholds (×————×) of *Dipodomys merriami*.

great, or nearly as great, as that of kangaroo rats. To test the hypothesis that their enlarged middle ears facilitate the low-frequency sensitivity of kangaroo rats, the antrum and epitympanum were filled with clay, using great caution to avoid touching any portion of the tympano-ossicular system, and CM sensitivity or behavioral auditory thresholds were determined (Webster, 1962; Webster and Webster, 1972). Both CM measurements and behavioral tests showed that sensitivity was reduced by more than 10 dB in the frequency range from 0.125 to 2.0 kHz (Fig. 10). Postmortem measurement of the middle ear cavities showed that the procedure had reduced middle ear volume by over 50%. We concluded that enlarged middle ear volume does indeed facilitate low-frequency sensitivity.

How? Lower frequencies have longer wavelengths, which require greater amplitudes of excursion for the tympanic membrane and other moving parts. The larger the enclosed air space of the middle ear, and/or the larger the diameter of the tympanic membrane, the more easily these larger excursions can occur.

Actually, several other characteristics of the kangaroo rat middle ear are responsible for the broad frequency range of best hearing (0.1–16.0 kHz). The middle ear has a small mass reactance, due to the small absolute mass of tympanic membrane and ossicles. It also has a small stiffness reactance, due to the loss of supernumerary suspensory ligaments on the ossicular chain, which not only causes them to be delicately suspended in the middle ear space, but also causes the axis of rotation to pass through their center of gravity. The enlarged middle ear cavity, as well as the loss of ligaments and the small mass, also greatly reduce friction (the resistive components). The unusually large difference in lever arm lengths, together with the enlargement of the tympanic membrane caused by the hypertrophy of the entire cavity, improves the areal and lever ratios so that, theoretically, better than 90% of the acoustic energy, at appropriate frequencies, may be transmitted to the cochlea (Webster and Webster, 1975a).

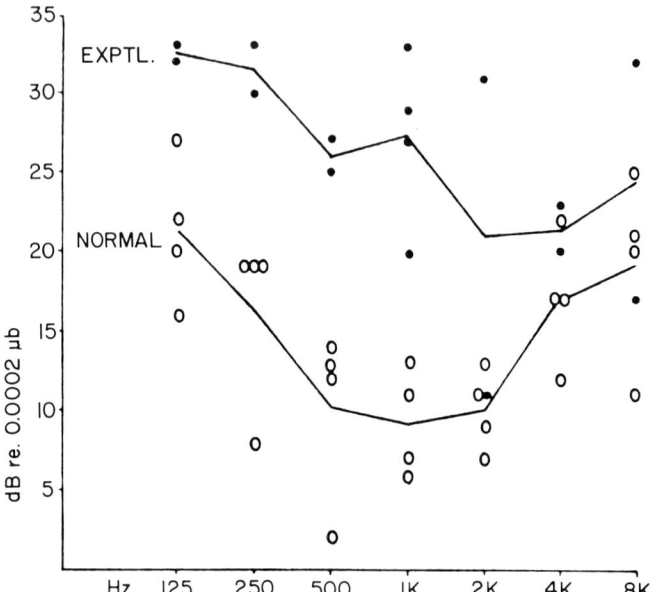

FIG. 10. Behavioral auditory thresholds of normal *Dipodomys merriami* (open circles) and with experimentally reduced middle ear volumes (closed circles). (From Webster and Webster, 1972, with permission.)

Thus, we knew *what* the middle ear specializations of the kangaroo rat do, but we still needed to know *why*. The adaptive value of this low-frequency sensitivity could only be understood in reference to the environmental pressures these species experience.

F. Adaptive Value of Kangaroo Rat Low-Frequency Hearing

Speech and language are so important to humans that we tend to assume that the adaptive value of hearing in other species also involves intraspecific communication. Earlier authors, in fact (Legouix et al., 1954; Legouix and Wisner, 1955), hypothesized that the enlarged middle ears of gerbils enabled them to hear one another's cries over the distances separating their burrows, and were therefore ultimately important in reproduction. However, mammals with enlarged middle ears, including gerbils, are not very vocal; furthermore, analyses of the few sounds they do produce have shown that the predominant frequencies of their calls lie above their most sensitive hearing range!

What, then, could be the adaptive value of unusually good low-frequency hearing in small, relatively nonsocial mammals? Predator detection seemed a reasonable next choice. Specifically, for the seed-eating kangaroo rat, inhabiting an area with little natural cover in which it must forage at night and over fair distances, there could be potent adaptive value to any feature that made it possible to auditorily detect a potential predator. And in that case, perhaps the bipedal, saltatory locomotion associated with enlarged middle ears in all four families could have to do with predator avoidance. We learned that the major predators of kangaroo rats are snakes and owls. We set out, therefore, in search of kangaroo rats, snakes, and owls to test our hypothesis.

Working at night, without artificial light, we placed recently live-trapped kangaroo rats with captive barn owls or sidewinder rattlesnakes in large outdoor enclosures and observed their behavior (Webster, 1962). In the experiments with barn owls, the kangaroo rat foraged quadrupedally while the owl observed from a perch about 8 ft above. When the kangaroo rat stopped moving the owl swiftly flew from the perch, but at what appeared to be the very instant of the strike the kangaroo rat leaped, almost vertically, thus avoiding the strike, and then leaped again in a more lateral direction. Occasionally the owl pursued the kangaroo rat for a short distance, always unsuccessfully; usually it simply flew back to the perch. The sequence was repeated a few minutes later. Neither owl nor kangaroo rat seemed to adapt or modify this general behavior even over 2 hours of observation; of course, because both were in an enclosed area, neither could leave the scene, which might well have been the normal behavior in the open.

Other investigators have demonstrated that owls have acute hearing and extremely good auditory localization; in fact, they successfully hunt mice in total darkness, using only auditory clues (Payne and Drury, 1958; Konishi, 1973). It is also known that their wing feathers are modified so that their flight is almost soundless. Our tape recordings contained no detectable sound until a fraction of a second before the strike, when they "braked" their flight. This braking created a low-intensity, low-frequency sound, the spectrum of which had the greatest energy below 1.2 kHz.

When kangaroo rats with bilaterally reduced middle ear volumes were placed in the enclosure, the same behavioral sequence occurred, except that the experimentally impaired kangaroo rat did not leap to avoid the strike and was caught by the owl (Webster, 1962).

The experiments with sidewinder rattlesnakes had similar results. After a variable period of exploration, the sidewinder coiled itself in the sand of the enclosure. The kangaroo rat was introduced into the cage, explored it, foraged on the seeds we had placed therein, and eventually approached the motionless sidewinder. The kangaroo rat then assumed a bipedal stance oriented toward the snake (Fig. 11) and made short hops toward and away from it (Fig. 12). If the snake struck, the kangaroo rat avoided it with an unusually large, apparently simultaneous, reverse leap. Soon afterward the kangaroo rat began foraging again, the snake resumed its coiled position, and the sequence was repeated (Webster, 1962).

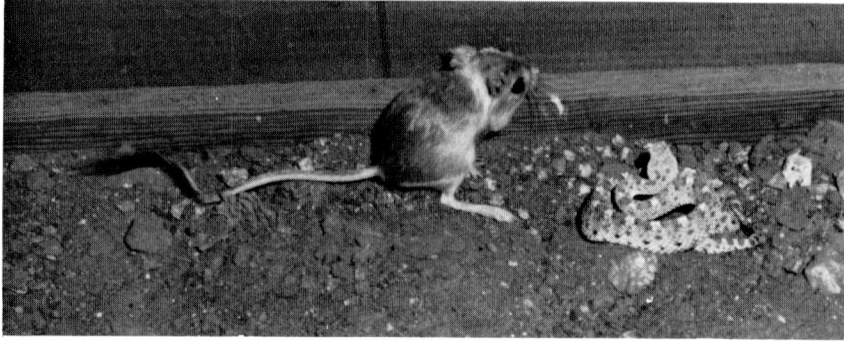

FIG. 11. A *Dipodomys merriami* in a bipedal stance next to a coiled sidewinder rattlesnake in an outdoor enclosure.

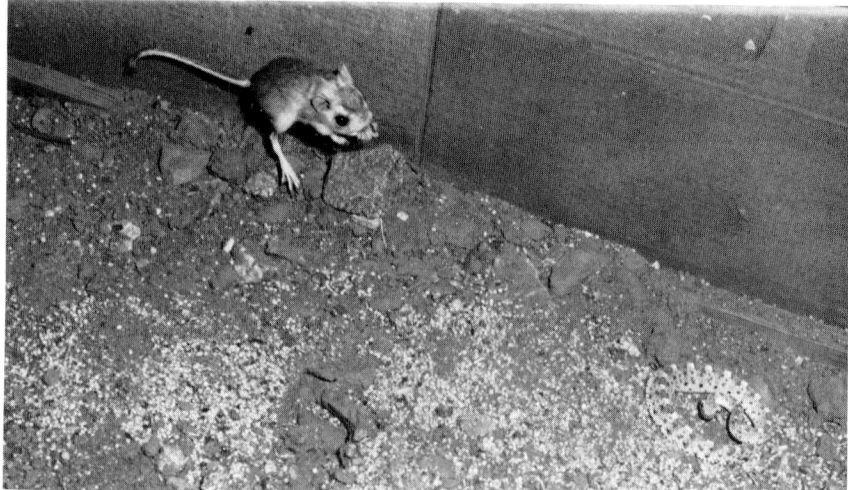

FIG. 12. The same *Dipodomys merriami* as in Fig. 11, making a backward leap away from the sidewinder rattlesnake.

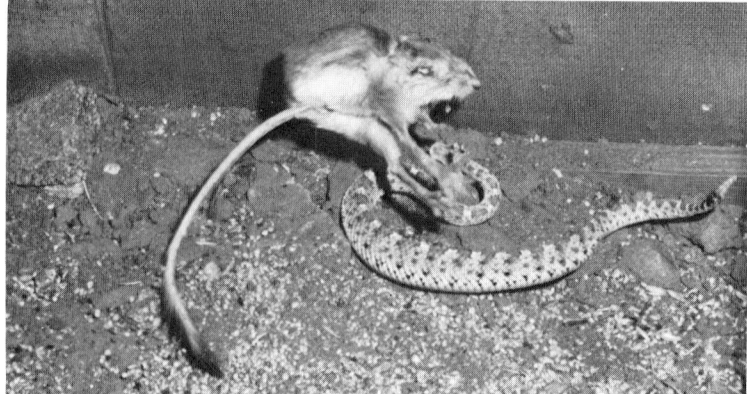

FIG. 13. A blinded *Dipodomys merriami*, with reduced middle ear volumes, being struck and killed by a sidewinder rattlesnake. (From Webster and Webster, 1971, with permission.)

Other investigators have shown that rattlesnakes use infrared receptors called pit organs to detect the presence of small mammals, and can catch mice in total darkness (Bullock and Diecke, 1956; Noble and Schmidt, 1937). Our tape recordings contained a brief low-intensity sound, the main energy of which was at frequencies below 2.0 kHz, just at the initiation of the snake's strike.

As was true in the experiments with the owls, kangaroo rats with bilaterally reduced middle ear volumes exhibited the same basic behavior but did not make the last-second escape leap and were therefore struck and killed (Webster, 1962). It seemed clear that the specialized hearing of the kangaroo rat enabled it to avoid these two common predators.

In what we thought was the experiment to confirm the kangaroo rat's dependence on hearing, to the exclusion of other senses, for predator detection–avoidance, we placed sidewinders with kangaroo rats whose middle ears were experimentally reduced and with kangaroo rats, similarly impaired, who were also blinded. This time the outdoor enclosure was dimly illuminated by a 60-W bulb. The animals whose middle ear volumes were reduced avoided predation as well as did normal animals; those who were also blinded (Fig. 13) did not (Webster and Webster, 1971). We realized that the situation was more complicated than we had expected: vision was also important, despite the nocturnal habits of the animals and our previous results, which seemed to have indicated that these animals relied on hearing alone.

That being so, could olfaction or the vibrissae also play a role in predator detection–avoidance? To test this idea, kangaroo rats with eyes, vibrissae, or olfactory bulbs removed were placed in an outdoor enclosure with a sidewinder. The blind and the vibrissae-less kangaroo rats behaved like normal kangaroo rats, first foraging, then orienting toward the snake, then making short, hesitant hops, and finally making a large reverse leap to avoid the strike. The anosmatic kangaroo rats, however, behaved quite differently, never assuming the alert orientation stance nor making the short, hesitant hops, and, in fact, appearing to be unaware of any potential danger (Webster, 1973). Indeed, when an anosmatic kangaroo rat was placed with a captive sidewinder that displayed no striking behavior (which is not unusual for some captive rattlesnakes), the kangaroo rat nudged at the coils of the snake and eventually even climbed and "rested" upon them.

We wondered about the role of these senses in other life activities, and therefore tested the ability of both normal and sensorily impaired kangaroo rats to run a complex maze. The maze was chosen as a kind of laboratory model of the animal's environment: the often complex tunnels of burrows, the paths through the desert along which they forage and return. The animals were trained in the maze and their performance charted. When they had reached criterion, various specific sensory losses were introduced, one at a time, by bilateral removal of eyes, cochleae, vibrissae, or olfactory bulbs, and by combinations of these surgeries (Webster and Webster, 1975c).

Removing vibrissae, cochleae, or olfactory bulbs, either alone or in combinations, had no effect on the time the animals took to run the maze, on the number of errors (wrong turns), or on the number of collisions with the walls. Removing the eyes alone resulted in a dramatic increase in both time and errors, but not in collisions. As other senses were lost, performance was further degraded; however, collisions occurred only when both the eyes and the vibrissae were gone. Kangaroo rats with all four sensory losses (eyes, vibrissae, cochleae, and olfactory bulbs) could complete the maze, but each trial required about 2 minutes with an average of 13 errors and 3 collisions (Fig. 14), as compared to the normal

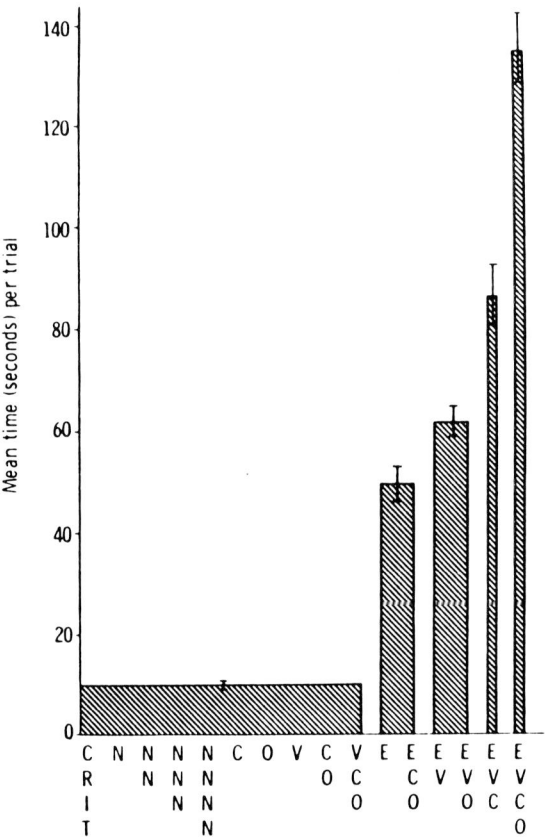

FIG. 14. Means and standard errors of the time required for kangaroo rats (*Dipodomys merriami*) to complete a complex maze under varied sensory deprivation. CRIT, Criterion runs; N through NNNN, normal animal following 1 to 4 control periods; C, bilateral cochlear removal; O, bilateral olfactory bulb removal; V, bilateral vibrissae removal; E, bilateral eye removal. (From Webster and Webster, 1975c, with permission.)

performance of 10 seconds per trial with no errors or collisions (Webster and Webster, 1975c).

This series of results suggested several things. When there is sufficient light, kangaroo rats can use vision to avoid predation, even if their hearing is impaired. Vision is also of prime importance in running a maze; audition is of no importance. Kangaroo rats are alerted to a snake's presence by olfaction and then can avoid a predatory strike either by using hearing alone, or, if hearing is impaired and sufficient light is available, by using vision instead.

While these experiments answered specific questions and were well controlled, they were not able to tell us what really happens in nature. To overcome these problems we also designed a "natural selection experiment." We livetrapped 27 Merriam's kangaroo rats in a 190 × 365 m area of unfenced desert (Webster and Webster, 1971). Nine of the animals were normal controls, nine were operated controls, with Plasticine weights placed subcutaneously above but not within the middle ear cavities, and nine had Plasticine within the middle ears, thus bilaterally reducing their volumes. All animals were coded with ear notches and, within 24 hours of capture, were released in exactly the spot where they had been trapped. The area was retrapped every fourth night for the next month, and captured animals were identified and then released; we had a 79% success rate in retrapping our experimental animals. At the end of the month we retrapped the area on four successive nights in order to identify the animals that were still in the population. Thus, we determined that only 22% of the animals with reduced middle ears were still present, as compared to 67% of the normal animals and 67% of the operated controls. Of the 13 animals that disappeared from the population in that month, 12 did so during the dark phase of the moon (Fig. 15).

Taken together, these experiments strongly indicate that kangaroo rats can use *either* vision or audition to avoid predation. It is easy to understand that nocturnal animals could experience selective pressures strong enough to account for middle ear hypertrophy and other adaptations to improve sensitivity in critical frequency ranges.

G. Evolution of the Kangaroo Rat Middle Ear

The fossil record for the family Heteromyidae, based primarily on teeth and mandibles, is fairly complete (Reeder, 1957; Shotwell, 1957; Wood, 1935); the earliest fossils are from the Oligocene in Colorado, then a semitropical area, and the family evolved as the Rocky Mountains were forming and the climate was becoming more arid. Today there are four genera in addition to the kangaroo rats (*Dipodomys*), which together exhibit considerable diversity of both structure and habitat. Spiny pocket mice (*Heteromys* and *Liomys*) are ratlike in appearance and live in tropical forests and savannah areas in Mexico, Central America, and

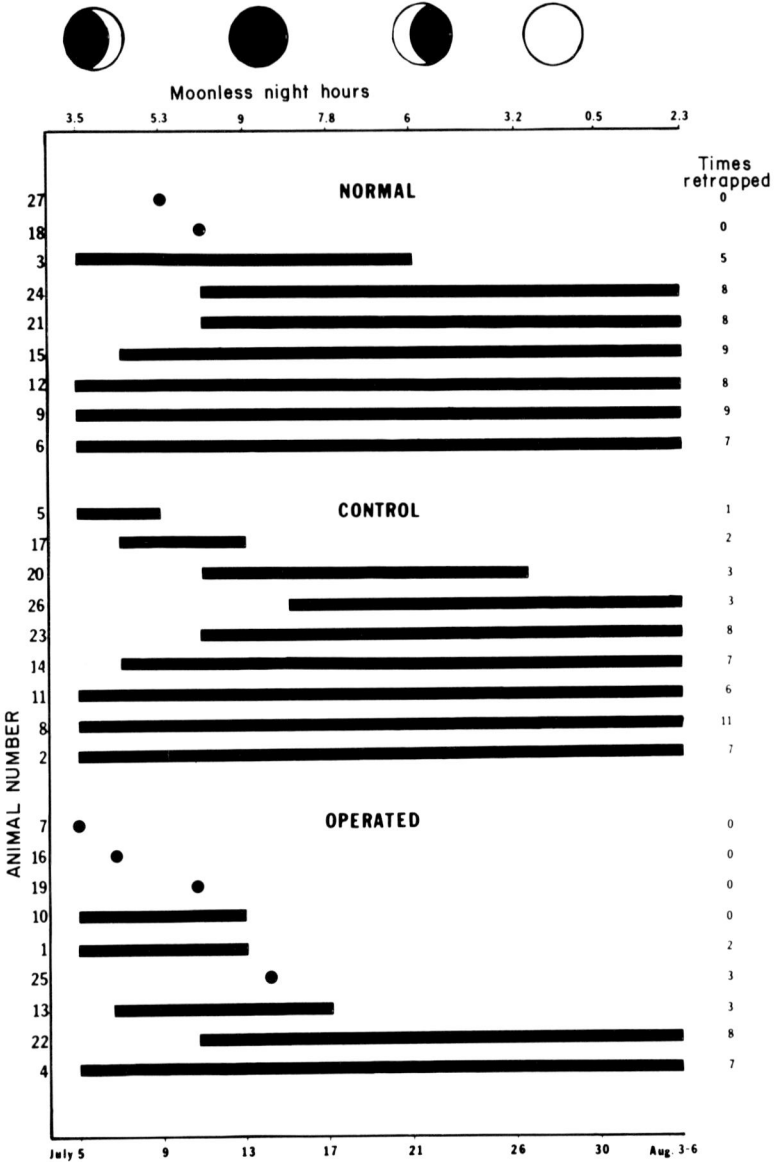

FIG. 15. Retrapping records of each of the 27 marked kangaroo rats, plotted against retrapping dates (lower abscissa) and approximate night hours without moonlight (upper abscissa); phases of the moon from the last quarter through full are diagrammed at top. Dots instead of bars indicate release date of an animal never retrapped. (From Webster and Webster, 1971, with permission.)

northern South America; the fossil record indicates that they are quite similar to the ancestral heteromyids living in similar semitropical environments. Pocket mice (*Perognathus*), more mouselike, live in chaparral and desert regions of Mexico and western North America; the fossil record shows that they are similar to at least some of the fossil heteromyids living in semiarid environments. Kangaroo mice (*Microdipodops*) are very small, primarily bipedal rodents living in high, arid desert regions of the western United States. Apparently the ancestral subpopulation that led to the spiny pocket mice migrated as the climate changed, retaining both their aboriginal ecological niche and much of their structure. The rest remained basically in the same geographical area and, as it became more arid, evolved to fit the new climate; their descendants, the present-day pocket mice, kangaroo rats, and kangaroo mice, exhibit not only highly modified auditory systems, but also bipedal, saltatory locomotion and a water balance system that eliminates the need for free dietary water.

Although no group of living species or genera, no matter how much it appears to form a "sequence," can replicate a phylogenetic sequence (Hodos and Campbell, 1969), we decided to infer the evolution of heteromyid auditory systems from the living genera. This we justify because of the lack of paleontological data on the auditory system, which means that this is the best we can do; and because of the demonstrated similarities in both habitat and other structures between living species and those in the evolutionary past. Underlying this decision is the premise that the auditory system of kangaroo rats, as well as other systems such as locomotion and water balance, are finely tuned to the animals' environment and evolved in response to the selective pressures of that environment. The spiny pocket mice (both *Heteromys* and *Liomys*) have the least modified middle ears of the family. The cavities are small (0.03 cm^3 or 1/22 the volume of the comparably sized kangaroo rat). The antrum is the largest portion and its walls are of thick trabeculated bone containing air cells; the epitympanum and hypotympanum have smooth bony walls and are very small (Fig. 16). The ossicles, however, are also much smaller in spiny pocket mice than in kangaroo rats. The anterior process of the malleus is fused to the ectotympanic element, rather than being suspended by a fine ligament as in kangaroo rats. All these features suggest a low-mass, high-stiffness middle ear, which would not transmit low frequencies efficiently. However, spiny pocket mice also have a few unusual middle ear characteristics, seemingly unrelated to any selective pressures. They lack both a stapedius muscle and a stapedial artery, which are present in most rodents, including kangaroo rats. In addition, the annular ligament of the stapes is much finer than in *Dipodomys*, consisting of fine, connective tissue fibers on both the vestibule and middle ear sides of the oval window, with a synovial space between them (Webster and Webster, 1975a,b).

Although *Perognathus* averages less than half the body size of *Heteromys* and *Liomys*, middle ear volume is about twice that of spiny pocket mice (but still

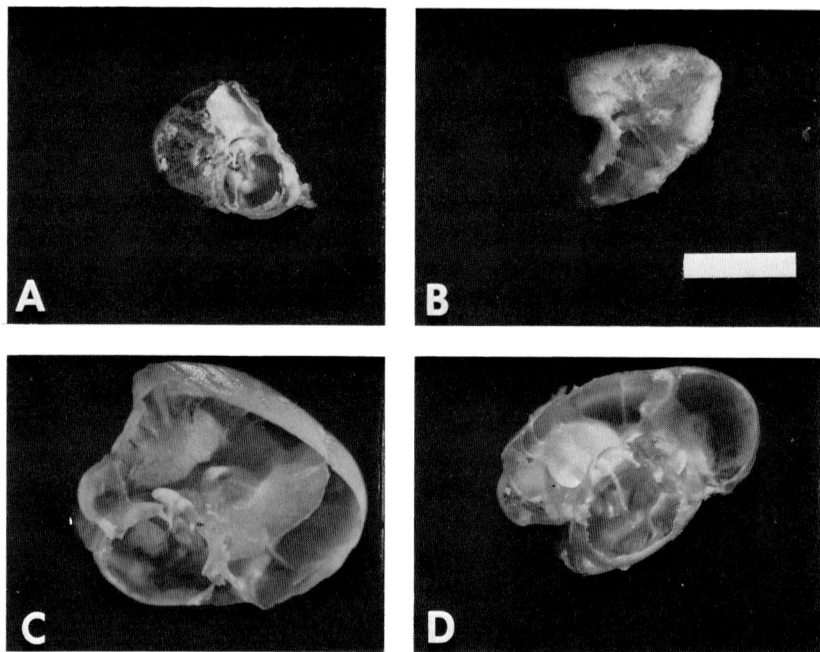

FIG. 16. Ventrolateral views of dissected temporal bones of *Liomys* (A), *Perognathus* (B), *Dipodomys* (C), and *Microdipodops* (D), demonstrating the differences in size and trabeculation. Bar equals 5.0 mm.

much smaller than that of kangaroo rats) (Webster and Webster, 1975a). The antrum and the epitympanum are enlarged, and the hypotympanum is somewhat expanded, but all three portions of the middle ear cavity contain thick bone. The outer wall is of hard compact bone; the inner walls are of trabeculated bone containing numerous tiny interconnecting air cells communicating with and thus part of the middle ear cavity (Fig. 16). Like the spiny pocket mice, *Perognathus* has very small ossicles; the stapes is about the same size as in spiny pocket mice, the manubrium of the malleus is longer, while the long process of the incus is shorter. The tympanic membrane is slightly larger. Like spiny pocket mice, *Perognathus* lacks a stapedius muscle; unlike them, it has a large stapedial artery. Its stapedial annular ligament is even finer than that of spiny pocket mice, with connective tissue fibers only on the middle ear side of the oval window. These morphological features suggest that the middle ear of *Perognathus* will transmit low frequencies somewhat better than that of spiny pocket mice, but not as well as that of kangaroo rats (Webster and Webster, 1975a).

Relative to body size, the largest heteromyid middle ear (Fig. 17) is found in kangaroo mice (*Microdipodops*) (Webster and Webster, 1975a). All three portions of the cavity (hypotympanum, epitympanum, and antrum) are maximally inflated and bounded by paper-thin bony walls (Fig. 16). Relative to body size, the tympanic membrane and auditory ossicles are also larger than in any other heteromyid, although in absolute size they are slightly smaller than those of kangaroo rats. As in kangaroo rats, the auditory ossicles are delicately suspended and the stapedial footplate is convex and bullate shaped, with a fine annular ligament. These morphological features should favor good low-frequency transmission but, due to the somewhat smaller absolute size, it should not be quite as good as in kangaroo rats. Like kangaroo rats, kangaroo mice also have a stapedius muscle and a large stapedial artery (Webster and Webster, 1975a).

In order to obtain functional data on the efficiency of sound transmission in the Heteromyidae, CMs were recorded from 93 animals representing all 5 genera

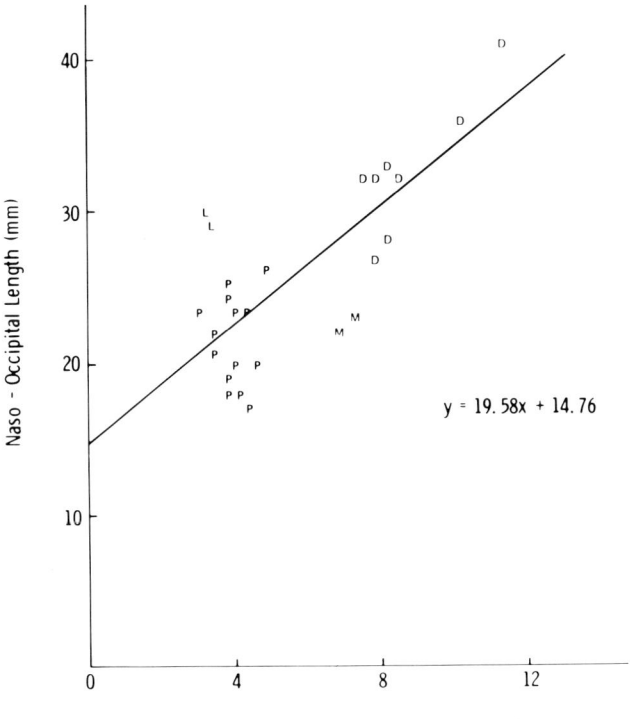

FIG. 17. Relation of middle ear volume to skull length among Heteromyidae. L, *Liomys;* P, *Perognathus;* M, *Microdipodops;* D, *Dipodomys.* Each letter indicates a separate species. (From Webster and Webster, 1975a, with permission.)

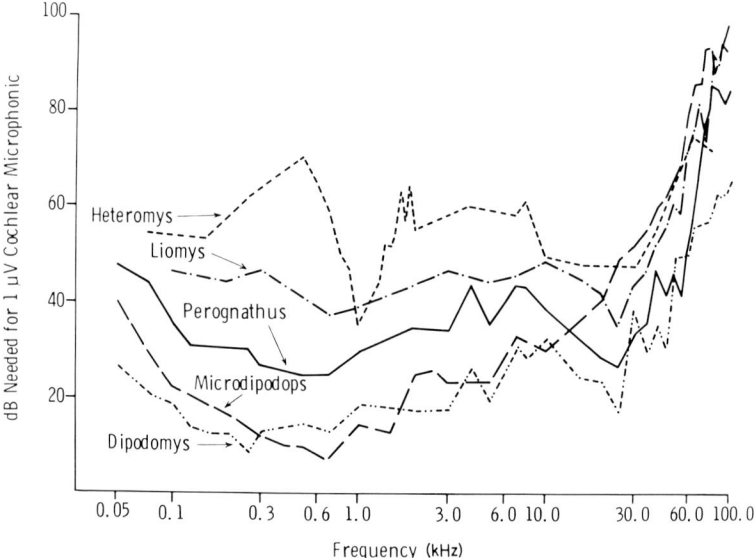

Fig. 18. Average cochlear microphonics (1-μV thresholds) for each of the five genera of heteromyid rodents. (From Webster and Webster, 1980, with permission.)

(Fig. 18). The intensity of sound necessary to produce a 1-μV CM was determined in the frequency range from 0.05 to 100.0 kHz (Webster and Strother, 1972; Webster and Webster, 1980; Peterson, unpublished data); the results are pleasingly consistent with what would be predicted from the morphological data. The low-frequency sensitivity of both *Dipodomys* and *Microdipodops* is remarkable for such small rodents, particularly below 1 kHz. In addition, although the high-frequency sensitivity of *Microdipodops* falls off rapidly above 10 kHz, *Dipodomys* retains the good high frequency sensitivity that is characteristic of most small rodents. *Perognathus* has very good low-frequency sensitivity but is still about 15 dB less sensitive than *Dipodomys* and *Microdipodops*. *Liomys* and *Heteromys* have relatively poor sensitivity throughout their hearing spectrum. Although we would not expect these two genera to be unusually sensitive at low frequencies, their insensitivity at high frequencies is surprising, for their middle ear morphology, with small mass and much stiffness, would suggest good high-frequency transmission. However, *Heteromys* has best hearing at 1 kHz, where it is 34 dB more sensitive than at 0.5 kHz and 20 dB more sensitive than at 2 kHz. Nothing that we have found in their middle ear morphology predicts or explains this sensitivity peak at 1 kHz (Webster and Webster, 1975b).

III. THE COCHLEA

A. Must the Cochlea Match the Middle Ear?

Humans, guinea pigs, and chinchillas all have good low-frequency sensitivity but no obvious cochlear specializations; should we not have expected the same situation in the kangaroo rat? No, and size and impedance explain why not.

The basis for impedance matching within the cochlea is the increase in width of the basilar membrane from base to apex, which makes it progressively wider and less stiff, and impedance matched to lower frequencies. However, there is a physical limit to how wide the basilar membrane of a very small mammal can become. If it is to respond to the physical stimulation of low-frequency, long wavelength sounds transmitted from a specialized middle ear, it must have some specializations to render it far less stiff and/or more massive than is usual in small mammals. As we know, kangaroo rats are much smaller than other low-frequency-sensitive species, and therefore cochlear specializations are to be expected.

B. Structure of the Kangaroo Rat Cochlea

These specializations are found principally in the basilar membrane and the border cells of Hensen and Claudius (Fig. 19). The cochlear partition of *D. merriami* is 9.8 mm long, with four and a quarter turns (Webster, 1961). Basilar membrane width increases along the partition, as in all mammals, but not linearly; it more than doubles in the basal turn, increases only slightly to a maximum width of over 250 μm near the apex, and finally becomes slightly narrower at the extreme apex. The zona pectinata of the basilar membrane is greatly hypertrophied, containing an amorphous hyaline mass between two layers of radial fibers. Ultrastructural examination reveals that this mass is actually a proliferation of the same cottony ground substance found in other mammalian species (Webster, 1977). This basilar membrane hyaline mass is smallest basally; it gradually increases to a thickness of more than 40 μm in the upper third turn, and then gradually and slightly decreases (Webster and Webster, 1977).

The border cells of Hensen and Claudius are even more unusual. The extraordinary Hensen's cells rest upon the innermost row of Claudius' cells, which extend from the outer sulcus cells inward to the Deiters' cells. Each Hensen's cell has a flask-shaped main portion, or "body," with a centrally placed nucleus (Webster, 1961). A single cytoplasmic process extends from the body toward the scala media and then expands as an umbrella-shaped canopy (Fig. 20), the edges of which make tight junctions with the canopy of adjacent Hensen's cells, or,

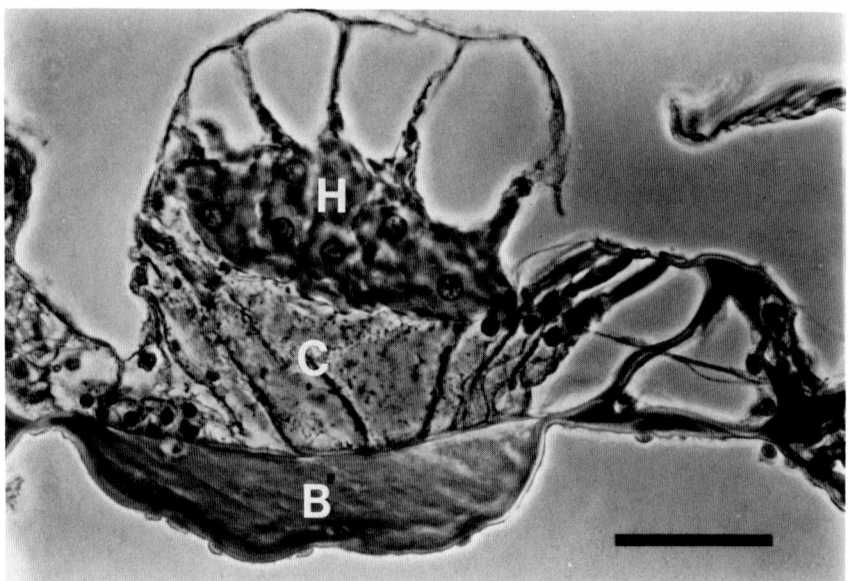

FIG. 19. Phase-contrast photomicrograph of a radial section of the organ of Corti of *Dipodomys merriami*. Note the specialized cells of Hensen (H) and Claudius (C) and the thickening of the zona pectinata of the basilar membrane (B). Bar equals 40 μm.

internally, with the phalangeal expansions of Deiters' cells (Webster, 1977). Moreover, unlike the Hensen's cells of most mammals, kangaroo rat Hensen's cells have a high protein content, including very high concentrations of nonspecific, noncholinergic esterases (Webster and Stack, 1968). Ultrastructurally, the Hensen's cells contain a rich, smooth endoplasmic reticulum, scattered large mitochondria, free ribosomes, and microfilaments. The microfilaments are randomly oriented in the "body" of the cells but become organized in parallel groups in the apical processes and canopy, where they apparently act as a cytoskeleton for these tenuous portions of the cell. Nevertheless, where it is unsupported by the apical processes the canopy is fragile and easily develops tears and holes in the fixed preparation (Webster, 1977).

The size of these unusual Hensen's cells varies along the basilar membrane (Fig. 21). They are quite small basally, but increase in size to more than 100 μm in height in the upper third turn; then they decrease slightly in the apical one and a quarter turns (Webster, 1961).

These morphological specializations adapt this small cochlea for low-frequency stimulation. The doubling in width of the basilar membrane in the basal turn causes stiffness to decrease very rapidly; thus more of the basilar membrane is available for low-frequency stimulation. The enlargement of both zona pectinata

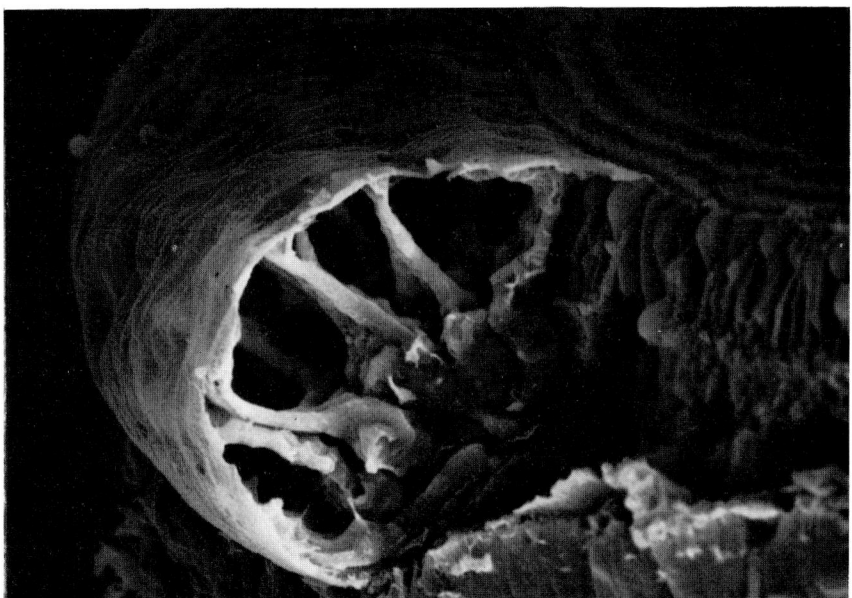

Fig. 20. Scanning electron micrograph showing the specialized Hensen cells of the kangaroo rat, with their apical processes extending up to form the canopy.

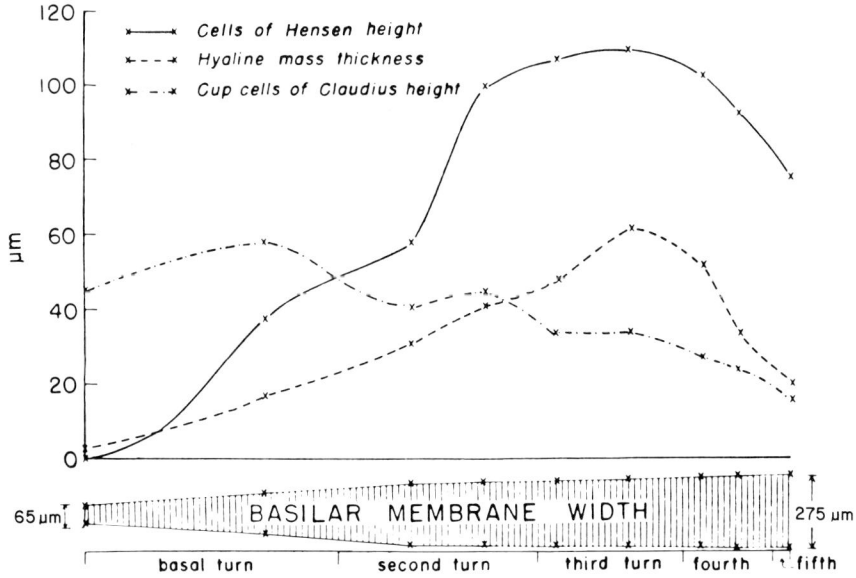

Fig. 21. Graph showing the sizes of organ of Corti components along the basilar membrane of *Dipodomys merriami*. (From Webster, 1961, with permission.)

and Hensen's cells in the wide apical portion must mass load the system. The combination of decreased stiffness and increased mass, found throughout the apical half of the kangaroo rat cochlea, causes the cochlea to be impedance matched to low frequencies.

Other structures in the kangaroo rat cochlea are "normal," such as the stria vascularis, tectorial membrane, hair cells, pillar cells, and supporting cells (Webster, 1961), but these structures are more involved with the transducer mechanism than with transferring energy from stapes to cochlear partition. Because the modifications described allow low-frequency stimulation to affect the cochlear partition, no unusual modifications of the transducer mechanism would be expected.

C. Development of the Kangaroo Rat Cochlea

As is true of all altricial rodents, the cochlea in the newborn kangaroo rat is immature and generalized, being at this early stage almost identical to those of laboratory mice and rats of similar ages (Fig. 22). Hair cells, supporting cells, pillar cells, border cells, etc., are discernible but do not yet have the distinct

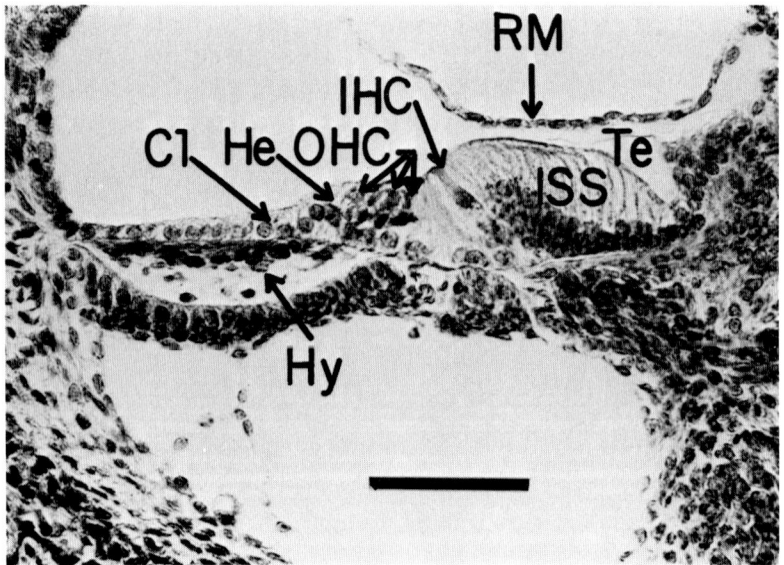

FIG. 22. Radial section of the organ of Corti of a 3-day-old *Dipodomys merriami*. Cl, Cells of Claudius; He, cells of Hensen; Hy, hyaline mass of basilar membrane; IHC, inner hair cell; ISS, inner spiral sulcus; OHC, outer hair cells; RM, Reissner's membrane; Te, tectorial membrane. Bar equals 100 μm. (From Webster, 1975, with permission.)

characteristics of the mature kangaroo rat. Only the zona pectinata of the basilar membrane gives any hint of its adult specializations; at birth it shows some thickening, caused by a small hyaline mass with fibroblasts interspersed within the cottony ground substance (Webster, 1975).

Neither the process nor the timetable of cochlear differentiation in the first 2 weeks after birth is unusual. In the organ of Corti, the large, immature inner spiral sulcus cells regress in size to become the small, nondescript cuboidal cells of the adult. The supporting cells, hair cells, and pillar cells mature while the extracellular spaces of the tunnel of Corti and spaces of Nuel develop. The border cells differentiate, the cells of Claudius migrate internally under the Hensen's cells to abut against the Deiters' cells, and the Hensen's cells themselves enlarge and send up apical processes, finally forming the canopy. The hyaline mass of the zona pectinata hypertrophies and the fibroblasts within it gradually disappear. By 14 days after birth, the immature cochlear partition has developed its distinctive kangaroo rat characteristics (Webster, 1975).

Because of this developmental pattern we can be confident that, in spite of their unusual nature, what we are calling the border cells of Claudius and Hensen are homologous to those of other mammals. The relatively late differentiation of both zona pectinata and border cells indicates that they are more recently evolved structures, which, during ontogeny, appear almost "added on" to a typical and earlier evolved mammalian cochlear partition.

D. Cochleae of Other Heteromyid Rodents

We have seen that we can predict a relationship between specialized middle ears and good low-frequency sensitivity in heteromyids; these two features are also correlated with specialized cochleae. We would expect that kangaroo rats (*Dipodomys*) and kangaroo mice (*Microdipodops*) would have the most specialized cochleae; that the pocket mice (*Perognathus*) would have some cochlear specializations but that they would be less extreme; and that the spiny pocket mice (*Liomys* and *Heteromys*) would have the least cochlear specializations.

The cochlear partition is 8–10 mm long in *Dipodomys, Microdipodops, Liomys*, and *Heteromys*, and only 6.5 mm long in *Perognathus* (Webster and Webster, 1977). Because many species of *Perognathus* are extremely small (8–10 g adult weight), their shorter cochlear partition is not surprising; what is remarkable is that the cochlear partition of *Microdipodops*, which is as small as many species of *Perognathus*, is 9 mm long. Basilar membrane width is most extreme in *Dipodomys* and *Microdipodops*, in which it more than doubles in the first turn to become, and remain, wider than 200 μm for the rest of its length. The basilar membrane widens much more slowly in the other three genera and in no case even reaches 150 μm. A hyaline mass is present in the zona pectinata of the basilar membrane in all five genera, and, in all five, becomes larger from the base through the third turn, and then somewhat smaller. However, both absolutely and relative to body size, this hyaline mass is greatest in *Dipodomys, Microdipodops,* and *Perognathus* and significantly smaller in *Liomys* and *Heteromys* (Webster and Webster, 1977).

The modified border cells of Hensen and Claudius described here for *Dipodomys* are also found in all species of *Microdipodops* and *Perognathus;* relative to body size, they are largest in *Microdipodops* and only slightly smaller in *Dipodomys* and *Perognathus.* They are always smallest at the cochlear base, reach their maximum size in the upper third turn, and then diminish slightly at the extreme apex. The border cells are unmodified in *Liomys* and *Heteromys,* and resemble those of such diverse animals as laboratory mice, cats, and humans (Webster and Webster, 1977; Webster, 1975).

One can take organ of Corti height plus basilar membrane thickness as a measure of mass; this value is greatest in *Dipodomys* and *Microdipodops,* intermediate in *Perognathus,* and least in *Liomys* and *Heteromys.* Relative to body size (using naso-occipital length as a conservative measure) it is greatest in *Microdipodops,* intermediate in *Dipodomys* and *Perognathus,* and least in *Liomys* and *Heteromys* (Webster and Webster, 1977) (Fig. 23).

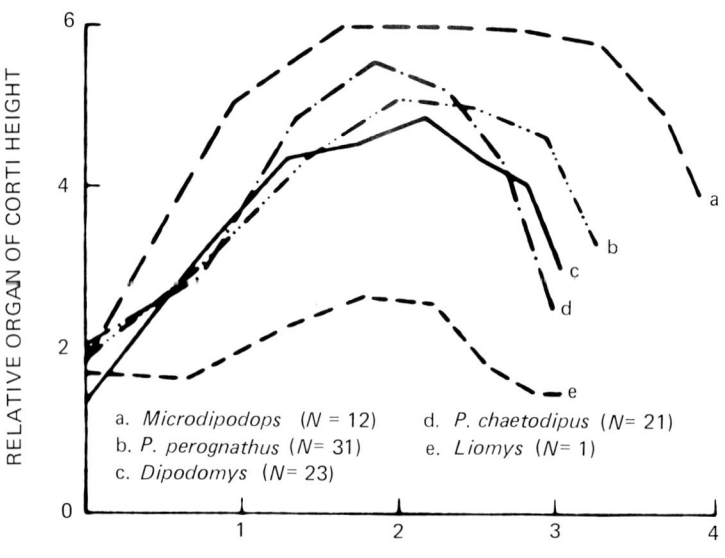

FIG. 23. Mean relative organ of Corti height among groups of heteromyids. (From Webster and Webster, 1977, with permission.)

IV. THE CENTRAL AUDITORY SYSTEM

A. Theoretical

Because the transduction of mechanical to neural energy occurs in the organ of Corti, one would not necessarily expect to find qualitative modifications of the central auditory system accompanying those of the peripheral system; however, we know that there are *quantitative* central modifications in many mammals. For instance, the large spherical cell area of the cochlear nuclei is large in mammals with good low-frequency sensitivity, such as cats (Osen, 1969) and guinea pigs (Pirsig, 1968), but very small in mammals with poor low-frequency sensitivity, such as mice (Ollo and Schwartz, 1979). Furthermore, the medial superior olivary nucleus of the superior olivary complex is considerably larger in mammals with good low-frequency hearing than in those without (Irving and Harrison, 1967; Masterton *et al.*, 1975). And, of course, physiological recordings show a preponderance of units with low best frequencies throughout the central auditory pathways of predominantly low-frequency-sensitive mammals (e.g., Moushegian and Rupert, 1970b; Caspary, 1972). It is also true that animals such as bats and owls, whose survival is dependent upon audition, have large, prominent central auditory pathways (Zook and Casseday, 1982; Knudsen and Konishi, 1978). One would expect the same to be true of kangaroo rats.

B. Kangaroo Rat Central Auditory Pathway

There are no real surprises in the morphology of the central auditory system of the kangaroo rat. All the central auditory nuclei and tracts are large and prominent (Fig. 24), as would be expected (Webster *et al.*, 1968). The afferent projections to and efferent projections from the cochlear nuclei are essentially what have been demonstrated in other mammals (Webster, 1971; Browner and Webster, 1975). The neuronal types present in the cochlear nuclei, and their distribution, are comparable to those of other mammals (Webster, 1971; Webster *et al.*, 1968). As expected, the large spherical cell area of the anterior ventral cochlear nucleus is much more prominent in kangaroo rats than in mammals such as the mouse, which has poor low-frequency sensitivity (Webster, 1971).

In the superior olivary complex, the lateral superior olivary nuclei, medial superior olivary nuclei, and medial nucleus of the trapezoid body are all prominent, which reflects both the low- and high-frequency sensitivity of these rodents (Webster *et al.*, 1968). The afferent and efferent projections from the superior olivary nuclei are also "conventionally" mammalian in their distributions (Browner and Webster, 1975). Similarly, the nuclei of the lateral lemniscus, inferior colliculus, and medial geniculate bodies contain no apparent specializa-

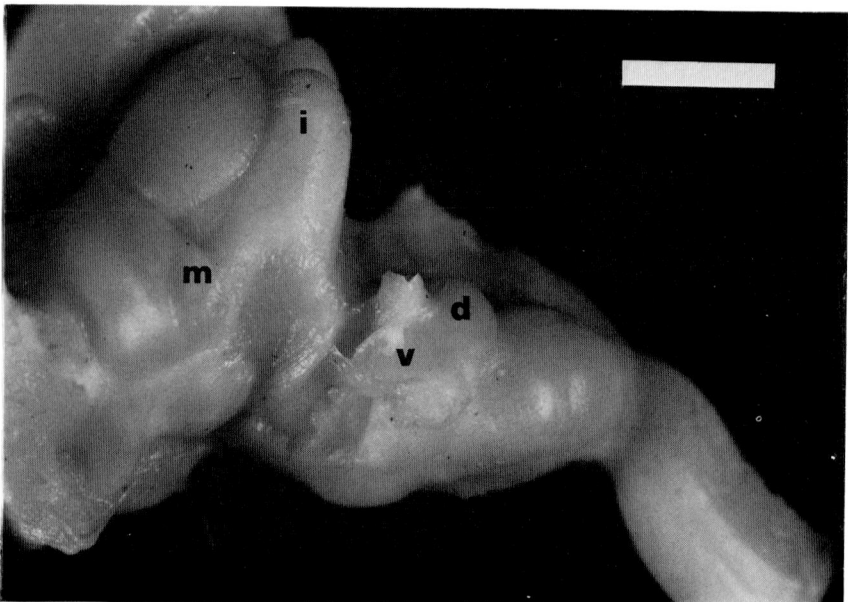

FIG. 24. Brainstem of *Dipodomys merriami*. d, Dorsal cochlear nucleus; i, inferior colliculus; m, medial geniculate body; v, ventral cochlear nucleus. Bar equals 2.0 mm.

tions except that they are all very prominent (Carey and Webster, 1971). The kangaroo rat auditory cortex has not been described.

There have been many electrophysiological studies on the kangaroo rat central auditory pathway (Moushegian and Rupert, 1970a,b, 1974; Moushegian *et al.*, 1975; Rupert *et al.*, 1977; Caspary *et al.*, 1977; Caspary, 1972; Bledsoe *et al.*, 1982; Crow *et al.*, 1978; Bledsoe and Moushegian, 1980). The principal finding of interest to the present discussion is that the great majority of single units have best frequencies below 1 kHz—which is, of course, in accord with the available middle ear, cochlear, and behavioral data. In fact, the major reason for using kangaroo rats in these studies (in addition to their freedom from otitis media) is that they are one of the few inexpensive mammals with low-frequency reception comparable to that of humans. Except for this, response characteristics of single units in the auditory brainstem are essentially similar to those of other species.

C. Central Auditory System of Other Heteromyids

No central physiological studies have been reported on other heteromyids and morphological data are scant; we have studied the cochlear nuclei to a limited extent (Webster, 1970) and the superior olivary nuclei in greater detail (Webster,

1969; Trune *et al.*, 1976). The cochlear nuclei have been studied only qualitatively and estimates have been made about quantitative aspects.

The normal cochlear nuclear cytoarchitectonic regions seen in other rodents are present in all heteromyids. However, there apparently are distinct quantitative differences: in the tropical genera, *Liomys* and *Heteromys,* the octopus cell area and small spherical cell area are particularly prominent. In the most arid genera, *Dipodomys* and *Microdipodops,* the large spherical cell and multipolar cell areas are most prominent. The relative sizes of cytoarchitectonic areas in the semiarid genus, *Perognathus,* fit neatly between those of the tropical and arid forms.

In the superior olivary complex, detailed cell counts were made for the lateral superior olivary nucleus (LSO), the medial superior olivary nucleus (MSO), and the medial nucleus of the trapezoid body (MNTB) (Trune *et al.,* 1976). Work on other mammals has shown that the MSO has a predominance of low-frequency units whereas the LSO and the MNTB have both high- and low-frequency units. Comparative studies have also shown that in most mammals there is a positive correlation between the sizes of the LSO and the MNTB, and that these nuclei

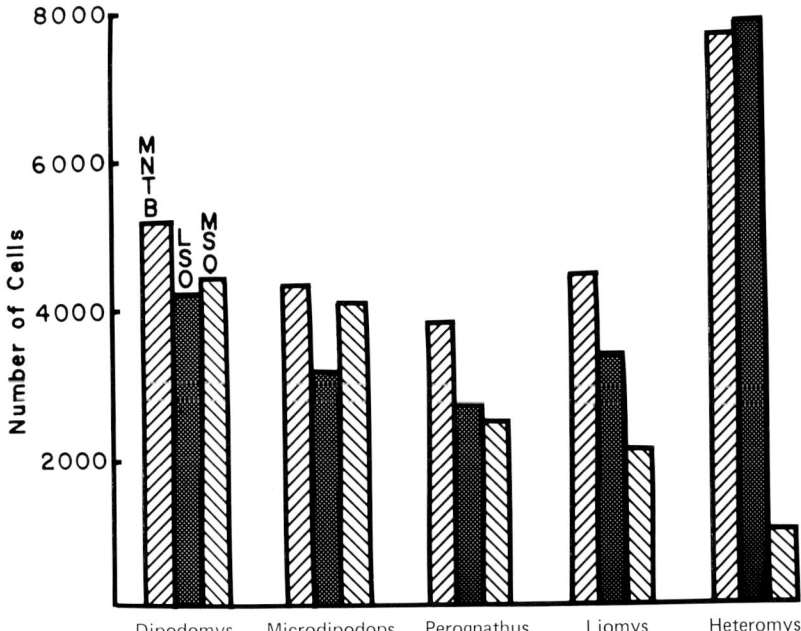

FIG. 25. Number of neurons in the medial nucleus of the trapezoid body (MNTB), lateral superior olivary nucleus (LSO), and medial superior olivary nucleus (MSO) in each of the five genera of Heteromyidae.

are particularly large in most nonprimate mammals. The MSO is particularly large in species with good low-frequency hearing. Our comparative data on the five heteromyid genera demonstrate a highly positive correlation between the numbers of cells in the LSO and the MNTB; these two nuclei have the greatest number of neurons in *Heteromys,* and the next largest number in *Dipodomys.* In the other three genera they have about the same number of neurons, which is decidedly less than in *Heteromys* and *Dipodomys.* Most interestingly, the low-frequency nucleus, the MSO, is largest in *Dipodomys* and *Microdipodops,* intermediate in *Perognathus,* and by far the smallest in *Liomys* and *Heteromys* (Fig. 25). Therefore, there is a very strong positive correlation between the size of the MSO and acute low-frequency hearing.

V. SUMMARY

Kangaroo rats are small, nocturnal rodents living in some of the most arid regions of the southwestern United States and northern Mexico. Their middle ear cavities are so hypertrophied that the combined volume of the right and left middle ears is greater than their brain volume. The combination of their enlarged middle ears, delicately balanced tympano-ossicular system, and cochlear modifications adapt these small rodents for better low-frequency hearing than almost any other very small mammal.

The primary predators of kangaroo rats are rattlesnakes and owls, both of which can hunt in total darkness and both of which produce some low-intensity, low-frequency noise while attacking their prey. Normal kangaroo rats can avoid these predatory strikes. Kangaroo rats with experimentally reduced middle ear volumes cannot do so in the dark, but can avoid the strikes of rattlesnakes if there is sufficient light; those who were also blinded could not. Kangaroo rats whose olfactory bulbs were removed showed no caution when near rattlesnakes, and were thus more susceptible to predation. In a natural selection experiment, more kangaroo rats with reduced middle ear volumes disappeared from a natural habitat than either normal or sham-operated kangaroo rats, and most of those that disappeared did so during the dark phase of the moon. It is concluded that the specializations of the middle ear and cochlea of the kangaroo rat facilitate low-frequency sensitivity, which is highly adaptive in predator avoidance.

The central auditory pathways and the portions of the cochlea involved in transduction are prominent in kangaroo rats, but not specialized. This is understood to be because there are enough other modifications to allow cochlear partition deflections in response to low-frequency stimulation; once that occurs, a normal transducer mechanism and central auditory system are evidently sufficient for central processing of low-frequency information.

Studying the five genera of Heteromyidae has aided in understanding the

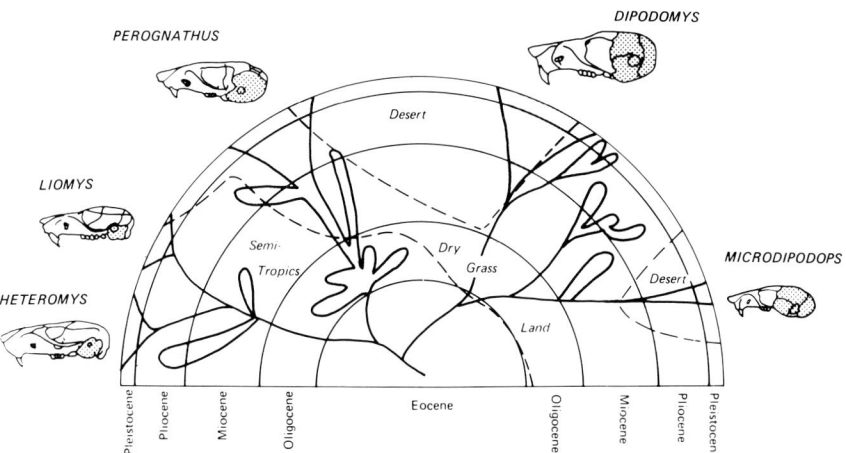

FIG. 26. Phylogeny of Heteromyidae based on both the fossil record and auditory specializations. Temporal bones of the skulls are stippled. (From Webster and Webster, 1975a, with permission.)

evolution of this specialized auditory system (Fig. 26). The semitropical to tropical genera, *Liomys* and *Heteromys,* have the least modified middle and inner ears and basically a "high-frequency" central auditory system; they have very poor low-frequency auditory sensitivity. The semiarid genus, *Perognathus,* has some but not all of the middle ear and cochlear modifications found in kangaroo rats (*Dipodomys*) and its central auditory structures, such as the medial superior olivary nucleus, are fairly well formed; *Perognathus* is more sensitive to low frequencies than *Heteromys* or *Liomys* but less so than *Dipodomys.* The two most arid genera, *Dipodomys* and *Microdipodops,* have the greatest middle ear and cochlear modifications and a "low-frequency" central auditory system. They have the best low-frequency sensitivity within the family Heteromyidae.

One can imagine a scenario of increasing aridity in the western United States during the Cenozoic, causing hot weather and sparse, discontinuous vegetation. Heteromyids adapting to this climate were forced to forage farther, with less natural cover, and at night, for sparser food supplies. This put extreme selective pressure on modifications such as low-frequency sensitivity that would enable the animals to detect and evade predators, which presumably, then as now, produced some low-frequency noise during strikes.

ACKNOWLEDGMENTS

The work reported on in this article was carried out over about a 20-year period. During this time a large number of students, colleagues, technicians, and friends have made substantial contributions to the work. We particularly wish to acknowledge and thank our former students, including Robert Ackerman, Peter Brown, Robert Browner, Charlotte Carey, Donald Caspary, Carol Stack, and Dennis Trune. Dr. Ernest A. Peterson graciously allowed us access to his unpublished data on heteromyid cochlear microphonics. Many of our own cochlear microphonics data were obtained with the assistance of Dr. William Strother. Some of the field studies were carried out when we were guests of the Southwest Research Station of the American Museum of Natural History and the Deep Canyon Desert Research Station of the University of California at Riverside. We also gratefully acknowledge the help of many ranchers in the southwestern United States who allowed us to use parts of their properties for our studies.

The research has been supported by a grant from the National Science Foundation and Grants NB-04365, NS-05800, and NS-11459 from the National Institutes of Health.

REFERENCES

Bledsoe, S. C., Jr., and Moushegian, G. (1980). The 500Hz frequency-following potential in kangaroo rat: An evaluation with noise masking. *Electroencephalogr. Clin. Neurophysiol.* **48,** 654–663.

Bledsoe, S. C., Jr., Rupert, A. L., and Moushegian, G. (1982). Response characteristics of cochlear nucleus neurons to 500-Hz tones and noise: Findings relating to frequency-following potentials. *J. Neurophysiol.* **47,** 113–127.

Browner, R. H., and Webster, D. B. (1975). Projections of the trapezoid body and the superior olivary complex of the kangaroo rat (*Dipodomys merriami*). *Brain Behav. Evol.* **11,** 322–354.

Bullock, T. H., and Diecke, F. P. J. (1956). Properties of an infrared receptor. *J. Physiol. (London)* **134,** 47–87.

Carey, C. L., and Webster, D. B. (1971). Ascending and descending projections of the inferior colliculus in the kangaroo rat (*Dipodomys merriami*). *Brain Behav. Evol.* **4,** 401–412.

Caspary, D. (1972). Classification of subpopulations of neurons in the cochlear nuclei of the kangaroo rat. *Exp. Neurol.* **37,** 131–151.

Caspary, D. B., Rupert, A. L., and Moushegian, G. (1977). Neuronal coding of vowel sounds in the cochlear nuclei. *Exp. Neurol.* **54,** 414–431.

Crow, G., Rupert, A. L., and Moushegian, G. (1978). Phase locking in monaural and binaural medullary neurons: Implications for binaural phenomena. *J. Acoust. Soc. Am.* **64,** 493–501.

Dalland, J. I. (1965). Hearing sensitivity in bats. *Science* **150,** 1185–1186.

Dallos, P. (1973). "The Auditory Periphery: Biophysics and Physiology." Academic Press, New York.

Heffner, H., and Masterton, B. (1980). Hearing in Glires: Domestic rabbit, cotton rat, feral house mouse, and kangaroo rat. *J. Acoust. Soc. Am.* **68,** 1584–1599.

Heffner, R. S., and Heffner, H. E. (1982). Hearing in the elephant (*Elaphas maximus*): Absolute sensitivity, frequency discrimination, and sound localization. *J. Comp. Psychol.* **96,** 926–944.

Hodos, W., and Campbell, C. B. G. (1969). *Scala Naturae:* Why there is no theory in comparative psychology. *Psychol. Rev.* **76,** 337–350.

Howell, A. B. (1932). The saltatorial rodent *Dipodomys:* The functional and comparative anatomy of its muscular and osseous systems. *Proc. Am. Acad. Arts Sci.* **67,** 377–536.

Irving, R., and Harrison, J. M. (1967). The superior olivary complex and audition: A comparative study. *J. Comp. Neurol.* **130,** 77–86.

Knudsen, E. I., and Konishi, M. (1978). Space and frequency are represented separately in auditory midbrain of the owl. *J. Neurophysiol.* **41,** 870–884.

Konishi, M. (1973). How the owl tracks its prey. *Am. Sci.* **61,** 414–424.
Lay, D. M. (1972). The anatomy, physiology, functional significance, and evolution of specialized hearing organs of gerbilline rodents. *J. Morphol.* **138,** 41–120.
Legouix, J. P., and Wisner, A. (1955). Rôle functionnel des bulles tympaniques géantes de certains rongeurs (Meriones). *Acoustica* **5,** 209–216.
Legouix, J. P., Petter, F., and Wisner, A. (1954). Étude de l'audition chez des mammifères à bulles tympaniques hypertrophées. *Mammalia* **18,** 262–271.
Masterton, B., Thompson, G. C., Bechtold, J. K., and RoBards, M. J. (1975). Neuroanatomical basis of binaural phase-difference analysis for sound localization: A comparative study. *J. Comp. Physiol. Psychol.* **89,** 379–386.
Møller, A. R. (1972). The middle ear. *In* "Foundations of Modern Auditory Theory" (J. V. Tobias, Ed.), Vol. 2, pp. 133–194. Academic Press, New York.
Moushegian, G., and Rupert, A. L. (1970a). Neuronal response correlates of cochlear nucleus: Evidence for restrictive and multiple parameter information transfer. *Exp. Neurol.* **29,** 349–365.
Moushegian, G., and Rupert, A. L. (1970b). Response diversity of neurons in ventral cochlear nucleus of kangaroo rat to low-frequency tones. *J. Neurophysiol.* **33,** 351–364.
Moushegian, G., and Rupert, A. L. (1974). Relations between the psychophysics and the neurophysiology of sound localization. *Fed. Proc. Fed. Am. Soc. Exp. Biol.* **33,** 1924–1927.
Moushegian, G., Rupert, A. L., and Gidda, J. S. (1975). Functional characteristics of superior olivary neurons to binaural stimuli. *J. Neurophysiol.* **38,** 1037–1048.
Noble, G. K., and Schmidt, A. (1937). The structure and function of the facial and labial pits of snakes. *Proc. Am. Philos. Soc.* **77,** 263–288.
Oaks, E. C. (1967). Structure and function of inflated middle ears of rodents. Doctoral dissertation, Yale University.
Ollo, C., and Schwartz, I. R. (1979). The superior olivary complex in C57BL/6 mice. *Am. J. Anat.* **155,** 349–374.
Osen, K. K. (1969). Cytoarchitecture of the cochlear nuclei in the cat. *J. Comp. Neurol.* **136,** 453–483.
Payne, R. S., and Drury, W. H. (1958). *Tyto alba* II. Marksmen of the darkness. *Nat. Hist.* **67,** 316–323.
Pirsig, W. (1968). Regionen, Zelltypen und Synapsen im ventralen Nucleus cochlearis des Meerschweinchens. *Arch. Klin. Exp. Ohren Nasen Kehlkopfheilk.* **192,** 333–350.
Reeder, W. G. (1957). A review of tertiary rodents of the family Heteromyidae. Doctoral dissertation, University of Michigan.
Rupert, A. L., Caspary, D. M., and Moushegian, G. (1977). Response characteristics of cochlear nucleus neurons to vowel sounds. *Ann. Otol. Rhinol. Laryngol.* **86,** 37–49.
Schmidt-Nielsen, B., and Schmidt-Nielsen, K. (1951). A complete account of the water metabolism in kangaroo rats and an experimental verification. *J. Cell. Comp. Physiol.* **38,** 165–181.
Shotwell, J. A. (1967). Late tertiary geomyoid rodents of Oregon. *Bull. Mus. Natl. Hist. Univ. Ore.*, No. 9, pp. 1–51.
Trune, D., Webster, D. B., and Webster, M. (1976). Quantitative studies of the superior olivary complex in Heteromyidae. *Am. Zool.* **16,** 208.
Webster, D. B. (1961). The ear apparatus of the kangaroo rat, *Dipodomys. Am. J. Anat.* **108,** 123–148.
Webster, D. B. (1962). A function of the enlarged middle-ear cavities of the kangaroo rat, *Dipodomys. Physiol. Zool.* **35,** 248–255.
Webster, D. B. (1969). Comparative morphology of the superior olivary complex in Heteromyidae. *Am. Zool.* **9,** 1148–1149.
Webster, D. B. (1970). The cochlear nuclei of Heteromyidae. *Am. Zool.* **10,** 554–555.

Webster, D. B. (1971). Projection of the cochlea to cochlear nuclei in Merriam's kangaroo rat. *J. Comp. Neurol.* **143,** 323–340.

Webster, D. B. (1973). Audition, vision, and olfaction in kangaroo rat predator avoidance. *Am. Zool.* **13,** 1346.

Webster, D. B. (1975). Auditory systems of Heteromyidae: Postnatal development of the ear of *Dipodomys merriami*. *J. Morphol.* **146,** 377–393.

Webster, M. (1977). Kangaroo rat cochlea: Qualitatively and quantitatively unique features. *Trans. Am. Acad. Ophthalmol. Otolaryngol.* **84,** ORL-223–ORL-232.

Webster, D. B., and Stack, C. R. (1968). Comparative histochemical investigation of the organ of Corti in the kangaroo rat, gerbil, and guinea pig. *J. Morphol.* **126,** 413–434.

Webster, D. B., and Strother, W. F. (1972). Middle ear morphology and auditory sensitivity of heteromyid rodents. *Am. Zool.* **12,** 727.

Webster, D. B., and Webster, M. (1971). Adaptive value of hearing and vision in kangaroo rat predator avoidance. *Brain Behav. Evol.* **4,** 310–322.

Webster, D. B., and Webster, M. (1972). Kangaroo rat auditory thresholds before and after middle ear reduction. *Brain Behav. Evol.* **5,** 41–53.

Webster, D. B., and Webster, M. (1975a). Auditory systems of Heteromyidae: Functional morphology and evolution of the middle ear. *J. Morphol.* **146,** 343–376.

Webster, D. B., and Webster, M. (1975b). Ear structure and sensitivity compared in tropical and desert-dwelling heteromyid rodents. *J. Acoust. Soc. Am.* **58**(Suppl. 1), S124.

Webster, M., and Webster, D. B. (1975c). Maze running in kangaroo rats with sensory deprivations. *Physiol. Psychol.* **3,** 195–200.

Webster, D. B., and Webster, M. (1977). Auditory systems of Heteromyidae: Cochlear diversity. *J. Morphol.* **152,** 153–170.

Webster, D. B., and Webster, M. (1980). Morphological adaptations of the ear in the rodent family Heteromyidae. *Am. Zool.* **20,** 247–254.

Webster, D. B., Ackerman, R. F., and Longa, G. C. (1968). Central auditory system of the kangaroo rat, *Dipodomys merriami*. *J. Comp. Neurol.* **133,** 477–494.

Wood, A. E. (1935). Evolution and relationships of the heteromyid rodents. *Ann. Carn. Mus.* **24,** 73–262.

Zook, J. M., and Casseday, J. H. (1982). Cytoarchitecture of auditory system in lower brainstem of the mustache bat, *Pteronotus parnellii*. *J. Comp. Neurol.* **207,** 1–13.

Zwislocki, J. (1965). Analysis of some auditory characteristics. *In* "Handbook of Mathematical Psychology" (R. Luce, R. Bush, and E. Galanter, eds.), Vol. III, pp. 1–97. Wiley, New York.

Index

A

Axons
  classical approaches to identifying populations of, 100–119
  organization in cat medial superior olivary nucleus, 99–129
Amino acid labeling
  differential studies on, in medial superior olivary nucleus, 119–126
  limitations, 126
  SOC compared to, 121–124
Auditory information, medial superior olivary nucleus and new possibilities for processing of, 119
Auditory system, 2-deoxyglucose studies on stimulus coding in, 79–97
Auditory system of kangaroo rats, 161–195
  auditory ossicles and intraneural muscles, 168–169
  central auditory system, 189–190
  cochlea, 183–188
    development, 186–187
    structure, 183–186
  low-frequency hearing and, 172–177
  middle ears, 165–182
    anatomy, 165–167
    evolution, 177–182
    function, 169–170
  tympanic membrane, 167–168
Auditory temporal integration, 131–159
  current research on, 151–156
    integration and resolution, 151–154
  empirical findings on, 132–140
    graphic presentations, 133–137
    review of, 137–140
  recent models of, 154–156
  theories of, 140–151
    exponential models of integration, 145–149
    hyperbolic models of integration, 143–145
    nonsummation interpretations, 143
    short time constants vs long time constants, 149–151

statistical probability formulations, 141–142

B

Brainstem, 2-deoxyglucose role in stimulus coding of auditory system of, 79–97

C

Cat
  2-deoxyglucose studies on brainstem auditory system of, 79–97
  medial superior olivary nucleus axons in, 99–129
Central auditory system of kangaroo rats, 189–190
Cerebellum, connections of with superior colliculus, 29–30
Cochlea
  of kangaroo rat, 183–188
  of other heteromyid rodents, 187–188

D

2-Deoxyglucose (2-DG)
  autoradiographs of, interpretation, 81–85
  in stimulus coding of brainstem auditory system, 79–97
  sound variation effects on, 85–89

F

Frequency of sound, 2-deoxyglucose studies on, 89–93

H

Heteromyid rodents
  central auditory system of, 190–191
  cochlea of, 187–188
  phylogeny of, 193

I

Intensity of sound, 2-deoxyglucose studies on, 93–95

K

Kangaroo rats, auditory system of, 161–195

L

Lateral geniculate nucleus (LGN)
  layer definition in, 43–44
  layer development in, 41–77
    afferent projection patterns, 56–62
    cytoarchitectural and cytological features, 50–56
    early stages, 49–50
    enucleation effects on, 69–71
    model of, 71–73
  retinogeniculate fiber role in, 62–71
    enucleation effects on, 63–69

M

Medial superior olivary (MSO) nucleus
  amino acid-labeling studies on, 119–126
    anatomical and chemical correlations, 124–125
    transmitter identification, 125–126
  axonal organization in, 99–129
    arborization patterns, 116
    Golgi studies on axons of, 107–113
      intrinsic axons, 113
      periolivary inputs, 107–109
      presumed extrinsic inputs, 109–113
    input segregation within, 116–117
    periolivary inputs into, 117–118
    principal axonal input into, 102–106
Middle ears of kangaroo rats, 165

N

Neurotransmitters, identification by amino acid labeling, 125–126

O

Occipital lobe, effects superior colliculus, 17–19

R

Retina, effects on superior colliculus layers, 13–15
Retinogeniculate fibers, role in lateral geniculate nucleus lamination, 62–71

S

Sensorimotor transformations in superior colliculus, 1–40
Sound
  2-deoxyglucose studies on, 85–95
    frequency variations, 89–93
    intensity variations, 93–95
    sound onset, 85–89
Superior colliculus
  behavioral studies of tectal organization of, 5–7
  cerebellar connections with, 29–30
  cortical input into deep tectum of, 27–29
  cytoarchitecture of, 3
  efferent connections of, 3–5
  laminar organization in, 3–12
  occipital lobe influences on, 17–19
  optic tectum and basal ganglia relationships in, 22–26
  organization models for, 13–20
  physiological distinctions between layers of, 7–12
  retinal influences on deep tectal layers of, 13–15
  sensorimotor transformations in, 1–40
  tectoreticular cell distribution in, 21–22
  ventral lateral geniculate nucleus projections to, 19

T

Tectoreticular cells
  distribution in superior colliculus, 21–22
Tree shrew
  lateral geniculate nucleus studies on, 41–77
  laminar organization, 44–49
Tympanic membrane of kangaroo rat, 167–168

V

Ventral lateral geniculate nucleus, projections to superior colliculus, 19
Visual pathways to superior colliculus deep layers, 21–30

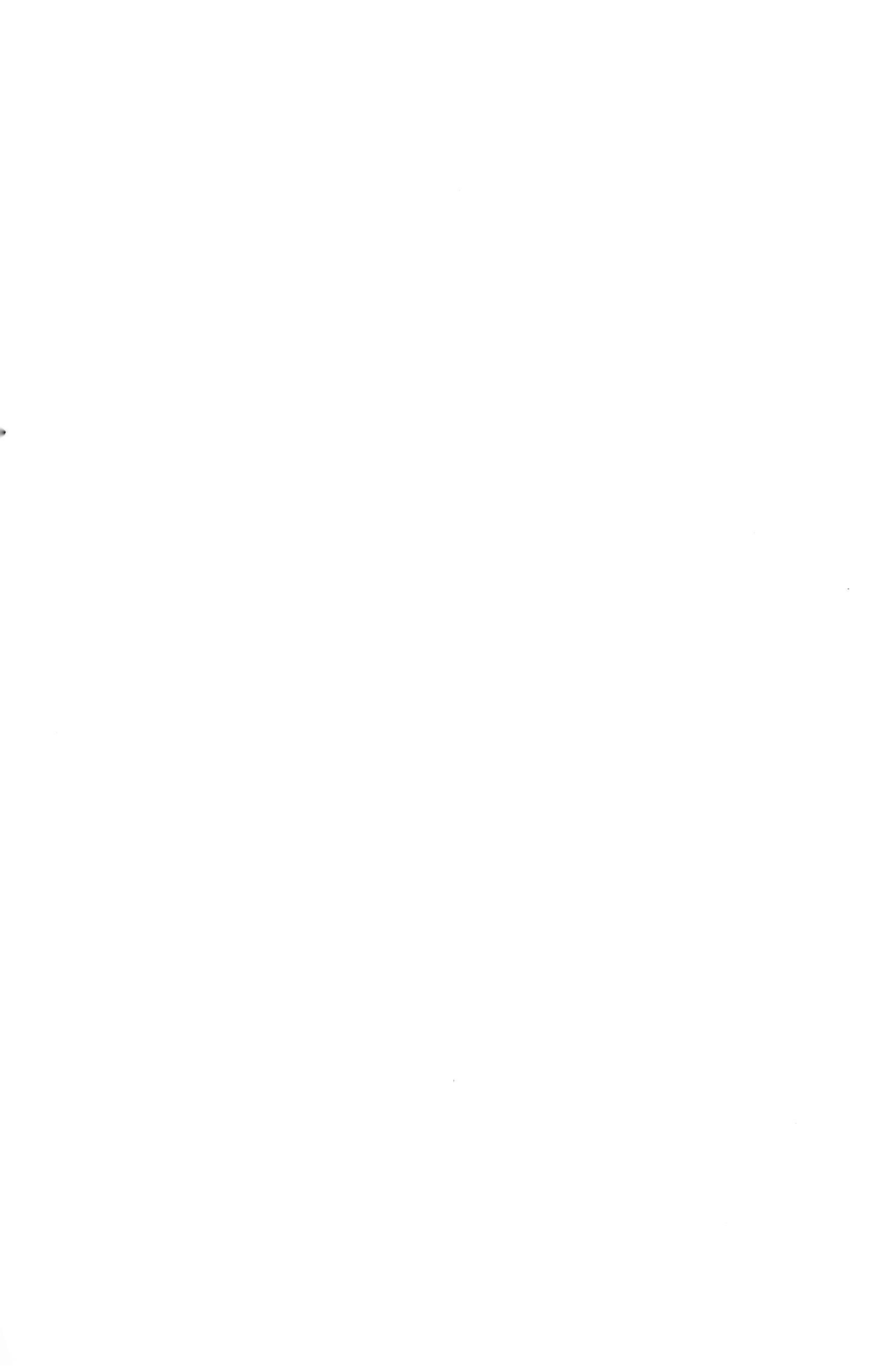